Practice Guidelines for

Pediatric
Nurse
Practitioners

Practice Guidelines
for
Pediatric
Nurse
Practitioners

BETH RICHARDSON, DNS, RN, CPNP
Associate Professor and Assistant Dean for Student Affairs
Indiana University School of Nursing
Indianapolis, Indiana

ELSEVIER
MOSBY

ELSEVIER
MOSBY

11830 Westline Industrial Drive
St. Louis, Missouri 63146

PRACTICE GUIDELINES FOR PEDIATRIC NURSE PRACTITIONERS
Copyright © 2006 by Elsevier, Inc.

Notice

Knowledge and best practice in this field are constantly changing. As new research and experience broaden our knowledge, changes in practice, treatment and drug therapy may become necessary or appropriate. Readers are advised to check the most current information provided (i) on procedures featured or (ii) by the manufacturer of each product to be administered, to verify the recommended dose or formula, the method and duration of administration, and contraindications. It is the responsibility of the practitioner, relying on their own experience and knowledge of the patient, to make diagnoses, to determine dosages and the best treatment for each individual patient, and to take all appropriate safety precautions. To the fullest extent of the law, neither the Publisher nor the Author assumes any liability for any injury and/or damage to persons or property arising out or related to any use of the material contained in this book.

The Publisher

ISBN-13: 978-0-323-02977-3
ISBN-10: 0-323-02977-9

Executive Publisher: Barbara Nelson Cullen
Editor: Sandra Clark Brown
Senior Developmental Editor: Sophia Oh Gray
Publishing Services Manager: John Rogers
Senior Project Manager: Cheryl A. Abbott
Senior Designer: Teresa McBryan

Working together to grow
libraries in developing countries

www.elsevier.com | www.bookaid.org | www.sabre.org

ELSEVIER   BOOK AID
International   Sabre Foundation

Printed in the United States of America

Last digit is the print number: 9   8   7   6   5   4

Acknowledgments

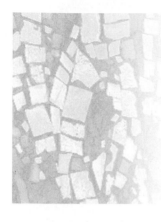

I would like to thank my late husband Wally; my children Jason, Sarah, and Joanie; my grandchildren Caroline and Darren; and my friends for all their love and support.

To students and colleagues, thank you for all you do in caring for children and their families.

Beth

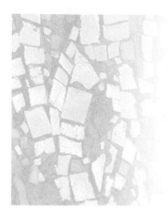

Contributors

MARY J. ALVARADO, MSN, RN, CPNP
Clinical Instructor, Department of Family Health
Indiana University School of Nursing
Indianapolis, Indiana
18. 11- to 13-Year Visit (Preadolescent)

PATRICIA CLINTON, RN, MA, PhD, CPNP
Director, Master's Programs
Director, Pediatric Nurse Practitioner Program
University of Iowa College of Nursing
Iowa City, Iowa
9. 4-Month Visit
10. 6-Month Visit
11. 9-Month Visit
12. 12-Month Visit

KAREN M. CORLETT, MSN, RN, CPNP
Pediatric Nurse Practitioner, Cardiac Intensive Care Unit
Children's Medical Center
Dallas, Texas
25. Cardiovascular Disorders

MARY JO EOFF, MSN, RN, CPNP
Clinical Associate Professor
Indiana University School of Nursing
Indianapolis, Indiana;
Staff Nurse, Hematology/Oncology
Riley Children's Hospital
Indianapolis, Indiana
3. Performing a Physical Examination

AMY L. FELDMAN, MSN, RN, CPNP, IBCLC, CIMI
Nurse Consultant, Shapiro Center for Infant Development
ARC of Essex County
East Orange, New Jersey;
Formerly Coordinator Lactation Service
St. Peters University Hospital
New Brunswick, New Jersey
5. Guidelines for Breastfeeding

JANE A. FOX, EdD, APRN, CS, PNP
Founder and President
Fox Educational Systems, Inc.
Southampton, New York
22. Ear Disorders

LINDA S. GILMAN, EdD, RN, CPNP
Associate Professor Emeritus
Indiana University School of Nursing
Indianapolis, Indiana
29. Endocrine Disorders

DONNA HALLAS, PhD, APRN, BC, CPNP
Associate Professor and Chair, Department of Undergraduate Studies
Pace University Lienhard School of Nursing
Pleasantville, New York;
Pediatric Nurse Practitioner, Pediatric Primary Health Care
St. Vincent's Medical Center
Jamaica, New York
2. Obtaining an Interval History
33. Behavioral Disorders

BETSY ATKINSON JOYCE, EdD, MSN, CPNP
Associate Professor Emeritus
Indiana University School of Nursing
Indianapolis, Indiana
15. 3-Year Visit (Preschool)
32. Hematologic Disorders

SHELLY J. KING, MSN, RN, CPNP
Pediatric Urology Nurse Practitioner
Riley Children's Hospital
Indianapolis, Indiana
27. Genitourinary Disorders

MARTI MICHEL, MSN, RN, CNS, CPNP
Adjunct Faculty
Indiana University School of Nursing
Indianapolis, Indiana;
Certified Nurse Specialist, Pediatric Nurse Practitioner
Clarian Health Partners, Methodist Campus
Indianapolis, Indiana
24. Respiratory Disorders

PAMELA MEADOR NICKELL, MSN, RN, CPNP
Pediatric Nurse Practitioner
Riley Hospital for Children
Indianapolis, Indiana;
Program Coordinator, Department of Developmental Pediatrics Intrathecal
  Baclofen Pump Program
Indiana University School of Medicine
Indianapolis, Indiana
16. 6-Year Visit (School Readiness)

MIKI M. PATTERSON, PhD(c), APRN, NP, ONC
President-Elect, National Association of Orthopedic Nurses
Doctoral Student, University of Massachusetts School of Nursing
Amherst, Massachusetts;
Orthopedic Nurse Practitioner, Harvard Vanguard Medical Association
Cambridge, Massachusetts
30. Musculoskeletal Disorders

FRANCES K. PORCHER, EdD, RN, CPNP
Director of Graduate Programs and Associate Professor
Medical University of South Carolina College of Nursing
Charleston, South Carolina
14. 2-Year Visit
21. Eye Disorders

SUSAN G. RAINS, BSN, MA, CPNP
Pediatric Nurse Practitioner
CHS Pediatrics
Muncie, Indiana
13. 15- to 18-Month Visit
23. Sinus, Mouth, Throat, and Neck Disorders

BETH RICHARDSON, DNS, RN, CPNP
Associate Professor and Assistant Dean for Student Affairs
Indiana University School of Nursing
Indianapolis, Indiana
1. Obtaining an Initial History

MARY LOU C. ROSENBLATT, MS, RN, CPNP
Senior Pediatric Nurse Practitioner
Harriet Lane Primary Care Center for Children and Adolescents
Johns Hopkins Hospital
Baltimore, Maryland
19. 14- to 18-Year Visit (Adolescent)
28. Gynecologic Disorders

SUSAN M. ROWLEY, MS, CPNP, ARNP
Nurse Practitioner, School-Based Health Centers and Child Neurology
Blank Children's Hospital
Des Moines, Iowa
31. Neurologic Disorders

ROBIN SHANNON, MS, RN, CPNP
Clinical Instructor
Medical University of South Carolina College of Nursing
Charleston, South Carolina;
Pediatric Nurse Practitioner, Pediatric GI
Medical University of South Carolina
Charleston, South Carolina
26. Gastrointestinal Disorders

ELIZABETH GODFREY TERRY, MSN, RN, CPNP
Health Writer/Research Editor
Children's Better Health Institute
Indianapolis, Indiana
17. 7- to 10-Year Visit (School Age)

PEGGY VERNON, RN, MA, CPNP
Associate Faculty
Regis University, Department of Nursing
Denver, Colorado
20. Dermatologic Disorders

KIM WALTON, MSN, CNS
Director of Youth Services
Community Health Network
Indianapolis, Indiana
34. Mental Health Disorders

CANDACE F. ZICKLER, MSN, RN, CPNP
Adjunct Faculty, Adolescent Clinic
Wright State University College of Nursing and Health
Dayton, Ohio;
Team Clinics, Pediatric Nurse Practitioner
Children's Memorial Center
Dayton, Ohio
4. Making Newborn Rounds
6. 2-Week Visit
7. 1-Month Visit
8. 2-Month Visit

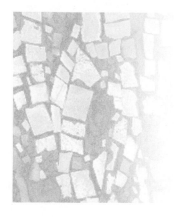

Reviewers

STEPHANIE BONNEY, MS, RN, CPNP
Pediatric Nurse Practitioner
St. Mary's Hospital for Children
Bayside, New York

SHARON M. COYER, PhD, CPNP, APRN
Assistant Professor
Northern Illinois University School of Nursing
DeKalb, Illinois

AMY SUZANNE QUIRKE, RNC, BSN, CPNP
Captain
United States Air Force, Nurse Corp
Dayton, Ohio

CAROL ANN SHERMAN, RN, BSN, MSN, CPNP
Pediatric Nurse Practitioner
McGill University School of Nursing
Montreal, Quebec
Canada

ELIZABETH ANN O'ROURKE SWEET, MSN, CPNP
Pediatric Nurse Practitioner
Alfred I. DuPont Hospital for Children
Wilmington, Delaware

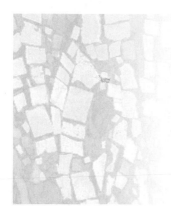

Preface

Practice Guidelines for Pediatric Nurse Practitioners was developed as a reference for nurse practitioners, as well as a guide for student education. This book is to be used as a quick guide when caring for children and families.

Practice Guidelines for Pediatric Nurse Practitioners can be used as a source of information including treatment strategies and is divided into three sections. The first section includes history taking with a family seen for the first time, taking an interval history, newborn rounding, and breastfeeding. Well-child visits are included and information about nutrition, elimination, sleep patterns, growth and development, and injury prevention are provided. The second section is organized by body system and is written in outline format, making it easy to read and find information quickly. Common medical conditions are presented with information about etiology, occurrence, clinical manifestations, physical findings, diagnostic tests, differential diagnosis, treatment, follow-up, complications, and patient/family education. The third section includes common medications used in pediatrics, and information is provided about common uses, availability, adverse effects, and nursing implications.

The Appendixes have several charts, including growth charts, BMI, asthma guidelines, and fluoride dosing. The charts are to be used to locate needed information quickly.

Beth Richardson

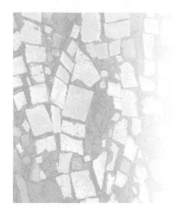

Contents

Section **TWO**

COMMON CHILDHOOD DISORDERS

Section **THREE**

APPENDIXES

Child Health Care

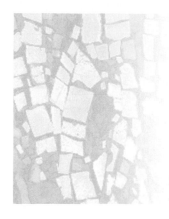

CHAPTER I

Obtaining an Initial History

BETH RICHARDSON

I. Introduction

A. The complete health history taken at the first visit is an opportunity for the practitioner to establish a relationship with the child and family, gain insight into family relationships, and obtain pertinent health information.

II. Initial information

A. Parent(s).
   1. Name(s).
   2. Age(s).
   3. Health status.
B. Sibling(s).
   1. Age(s).
   2. Health status.

III. Reason for current visit

A. Current problem or illness.
   1. Background information.
      a. When did it start?
      b. What are the symptoms?
      c. Others in family ill with similar symptoms?
      d. What has been done to treat symptoms?

IV. Past history

A. Prenatal history and care if child <5 years.
   1. Was pregnancy planned?
   2. Did the mother smoke? Drink alcohol? Take any medications or drugs?
   3. Any problems such as:
      a. Vaginal infection?
      b. Kidney infection?
      c. High blood pressure?

      d. Diabetes?

      e. Edema?

      f. Bleeding?

      g. Any accidents during pregnancy?

B. Natal history and care.

  1. Labor and delivery.

      a. Where was infant born?

      b. Type of delivery?

      c. Length of labor?

      d. Anesthesia used during labor?

      e. Any problems with mother or infant after birth?

      f. Infant's birth weight? Length? Head circumference? Gestational age?

      g. Did infant go home with the mother?

  2. Feeding.

      a. Baby fed by bottle or breast?

      b. Type of formula used?

      c. Frequency of feedings?

      d. Pattern of weight gain?

  3. Childhood illness.

      a. Rheumatic fever, chickenpox, number of ear infections, strep throat, respiratory syncytial virus (RSV), whooping cough, mononucleosis, sexually transmitted infections (STIs).

  4. Hospitalizations.

      a. Dates, names of hospitals, diagnoses.

  5. Surgeries.

      a. Dates, names of hospitals, diagnoses, complications.

  6. Immunizations (see Appendix A).

      a. Dates, reactions.

  7. Screening tests.

      a. Vision, hearing, speech, hemoglobin, urine, tuberculosis skin test, x-rays, other laboratory tests.

  8. Allergies.

      a. Medications, environment, foods.

  9. Transfusions.

      a. Dates, number of units transfused, reactions.

  10. Medications.

      a. Prescription; over the counter; herbal; current/recent medications including dosage, length of time taking medication, adverse/side effects.

V. Review of systems

  A. History.

    1. Head, eyes, ears, nose, throat.

      a. Head: headaches or head injuries?

      b. Eyes: tearing, strabismus? Has child had vision test? Does child wear glasses/contacts?

      c. Ears: Ear infections? Drainage? Has child had hearing test?

    d. Nose: Allergies? Frequency of colds? Does child snore, have nosebleeds or postnasal drip?

    e. Throat: sore throat, dental hygiene, lymph glands, hoarseness.

2. Cardiovascular.
   a. Heart murmur.
   b. Congenital heart disease.
   c. Cyanosis.
   d. Edema.
   e. Activity tolerance, shortness of breath, syncope.

3. Respiratory.
   a. Pneumonia, bronchitis.
   b. Asthma.
   c. Cystic fibrosis.
   d. Croup, cough.

4. Gastrointestinal.
   a. Diarrhea, constipation.
   b. Vomiting, reflux, upset stomach, abdominal pain.
   c. Bloody stools, rectal bleeding.
   d. Fissures, ulcer.
   e. Jaundice.

5. Genitourinary.
   a. When did child achieve night dryness?
   b. Frequency of urination, urinary tract infections, dysuria, polyuria.
   c. Hematuria.
   d. Menstrual history (pain, flow), vaginal drainage.
   e. Penis or testes abnormalities, STIs, sexual activity.

6. Musculoskeletal.
   a. Painful joints, swelling, strains, sprains, fractures.
   b. Deformities.
   c. Activity tolerance.

7. Neurologic.
   a. Headaches.
   b. Seizures, epilepsy.
   c. Fainting, dizziness, tremors.
   d. Clumsy, uncoordinated.
   e. ADD/ADHD, learning disabilities, developmental delay.

8. Endocrine.
   a. Sexual maturation.
   b. Diabetes.
   c. Thyroid or adrenal diseases.

9. Skin.
   a. rashes, birth marks.

VI. Family history

A. History of any of following in family members:

1. High blood pressure.

2. Heart disease, stroke.
3. Diabetes.
4. Cataracts, glaucoma.
5. Anemia.
6. High cholesterol levels.
7. Asthma, allergies.
8. Kidney infections
9. Colitis, ulcers.
10. Cancer.
11. Thyroid problems.
12. Epilepsy.
13. Dysplasia of hip.
14. Mental retardation.
15. Alcoholism or substance abuse.

VII. Disease history

1. Disease/problem.
   a. When was patient diagnosed?
   b. How was patient treated? Response to treatment?
   c. How have symptoms changed? How is patient doing now?
   d. Is patient taking medications to treat problem?

VIII. Social history

A. Parent/guardian's employment site(s) and hours worked.
B. Child care.
   1. Day care or sitter?
   2. Preschool or after-school programs?
C. Family relationships: How do family members get along?
D. Home life.
   1. Does home have a yard where child can play?
   2. Stairs in house?
   3. City, well, or bottled water?
   4. Is home in safe neighborhood?
E. School life.
   1. How is child's progress.
      a. What are child's grades?
      b. What are child's strengths and weaknesses in learning? Does child need extra help in learning?
      c. What type of classroom (advanced, regular, learning disability)?
   2. Does this child bully others or is child a victim of bullying? What is child's behavior in learning situations? History of absenteeism or truancy?
   3. Classmates/friends.
      a. How does child relate to and play with those in classroom, day care, or preschool? Does child have a best friend?
      b. What does child like to play?

IX. Development

A. For child <2 years ask when first:
1. Smiled.
2. Rolled.
3. Sat alone.
4. Crawled.
5. Walked alone.
6. Said 2 words.
7. Fed self.
8. Said 10 words.

B. Behavior.
1. Temper tantrums, whining.
2. Thumb sucking.
3. Sleep patterns.
4. Temperament.

BIBLIOGRAPHY

Fox J: *Primary health care of infants, children, & adolescents,* ed 2, St Louis, 2002, Mosby.
Jarvis C: *Physical examination and health assessment,* ed 4, Philadelphia, 2004, Lippincott.

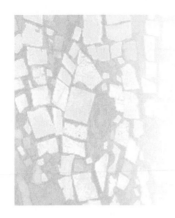

CHAPTER 2

Obtaining an Interval History

DONNA HALLAS

I. The interval history

A. Definition.

1. *Interval history:* data collection that occurs at subsequent visits to one in which comprehensive history and physical examination were completed.

2. Amount of information reviewed and collected for interval history depends on child's age and length of time since either comprehensive history was obtained and/or prior appointments in which interval history was updated.

3. General guideline for obtaining interval history: review and update data every 6 months for infants, toddlers, preschool-age children and every year for school-age children, adolescents.

B. Significance of interval history.

1. Although comprehensive history is used to establish initial health promotion plan, analysis of data collected during interval history is often used in one of three ways:

   a. To continue established health promotion plan.

   b. To make changes to health promotion plan.

   c. To establish new health promotion plan.

C. Preparation for obtaining interval history.

1. Prior to beginning data collection for interval history, review comprehensive history and any prior interval histories available on medical record.

   a. Helps nurse practitioner focus questions that will elicit data needed to complete interval history.

   b. Sample data contained in comprehensive history that may need further exploration during interval history are listed in Table 2-1.

D. Elements of an interval history.

1. Elements included in interval history should be related to the age of the child.

TABLE 2-1 • Focusing the interval history from details in the comprehensive history

Comprehensive history	Interval history
Past medical history	Any data in past medical history that is significant and requires further clarification?
	Consider previous acute illnesses including hospitalizations; injuries, accidents, surgeries, chronic illnesses.
	Review problem list.
	If all prior problems are listed as resolved, then no further data should be elicited at this visit.
	If problems still exist, then ask questions specific to identified problem.
Allergies	Always obtain update on allergies to foods, medications, environmental pollutants.
Developmental history	Review results of prior DDST.
	Note achievement of developmental milestones at each interval visit.
	If delays are noted, question status of intervention services (early intervention for children <5 years old; OT; PT; speech; special education services for all children).
Social history	Exercise and activity.
	Wellness behaviors.
	Behavior issues.
	Review family structure and family support systems.
	If data contained in comprehensive history suggest dysfunctional family, ask about present family structure and function.
Family history	Review genogram.
	Review significant family history prior to interview.
	Pay particular attention to strong family history of conditions in which family lifestyle modifications can have significant impact (i.e., cardiovascular conditions, hypertension, diabetes, obesity). Implementing lifestyle modifications in early childhood years may significantly affect health throughout lifetime.
Medication history	Prescription.
	Over the counter.
	Homeopathic remedies.
Nutritional history	Timing and frequency of meals.
	Ethnic and cultural considerations in food choices.
Immunization history	Immunization records should be reviewed at each visit.

2. Major focus for interval history for each age child and adolescent should include questions concerning eating, sleeping, bladder, and bowel patterns. Additional questions are then age related.
3. Infant, toddler, and preschool-age children
   a. Ask questions related to achievement of developmental milestones.
   b. Denver Developmental Screening Test (DDST) may be used as guide for questioning patterns concerning achievement of developmental milestones.

       c. Toddlers and preschoolers: assess information regarding speech and language development and development of social skills.

    4. School-age children.

        a. Should also include questions related to sociobehavioral development with peers and progress in school.

        b. If female school-age child has secondary sex characteristics, then ask about menstrual cycle: age of onset, frequency, length of cycle, any discomfort prior to or during menstruations.

        c. Children >10 years of age should be asked:

- Alcohol and drugs: have they or their friends tried?
- Home life okay?
- What is their diet?
- Happy with appearance/weight?
- Thought about harming themselves or others?
- Sexually active?

    5. Adolescents.

        a. Adolescent female: ask questions related to menstrual cycle.

        b. At each visit: ask about hobbies, education, alcohol, drugs, diet, suicide.

        c. Ask about high-risk social behaviors (smoking, alcohol/drug use, sexual activity, including diagnosis and treatment of sexually transmitted infections [STIs]) and other high-risk social behaviors (driving motor vehicle in reckless manner, use of guns, etc.).

  E. Review of systems (ROS).

    1. Age-appropriate ROS: conduct in head-to-toe manner as identified in comprehensive physical examination (Table 2-2).

II. Interval history for athletic child and adolescent

  A. Pre-participation sports history and physical have well-established guidelines; follow explicitly.

  B. Interval history is integral part of assessment.

    1. Question parent and child about significant family history changes (i.e., sudden death from cardiovascular condition of relative who was <50 years old). Include questions that elicit information about significant episodes (red flags) of chest pain, dyspnea, syncope, palpitations, loss of consciousness (Table 2-3).

III. Focused history

  A. Focused history: used to collect data about specific problem, usually chief complaint identified by parent/child (Table 2-4).

  B. Focus all questions on eliciting data about chief complaint.

  C. Focused history usually limited to one or two systems.

IV. Applying data obtained in interval history to clinical practice

  A. After completing interval history and physical examination, compare findings in comprehensive history to data obtained in interval history.

    1. If no significant changes found in interval history: advise parent, infant/child to continue to follow established health promotion plan.

TABLE 2-2 • Review of system (ROS) in an interval history

System	ROS—gathering the interval history*
On a regular basis, do you have problems with:	
Head and neck	Headaches
	Blurred vision or any vision problems
	Earaches
	Nose bleeds
	Sore throats
	Any lumps in head or neck area
Chest and lungs	Chest pain
	Heart beating fast in chest (palpitations)
	Shortness of breath
	Fainting
	Cough
Abdomen	Nausea
	Vomiting
	Diarrhea
	Urinating or bowels
	Menstruation
	Testicular pain
Musculoskeletal	Leg pain or cramps
	Stiffness, swelling, bone deformities
Skin, hair, and nails	Rashes
	Moles
	Darkened or discolored areas
	Abnormal hair growth
	Clubbing of nails
	Bruising easily
Endocrine	Excess thirst, urination, hunger
	Unexplained weight changes
	Intolerance to heat and/or cold
Neurologic	Syncope, seizures, weakness, paralysis
Psychiatric	Depression, mood changes, difficulty concentrating, nervousness, anxiety

*This information is gathered in addition to the details related to eating, sleeping, bladder, and bowel patterns.

2. If significant changes are found in interval history: revise health promotion plan.
   a. Example: if interval family history reveals family members have diabetes mellitus, evaluate and modify family/child exercise and dietary patterns.
3. If significant changes are found in interval history in relation to child's health: establish new health promotion plan with input from parent and child/adolescent.
   a. Example: if interval history reveals significant change in frequency of coughing and upper respiratory symptoms, complete a detailed focused history and establish a new health promotion plan.

TABLE 2-3 • Red flags: the interval history for the athletic child or adolescent

Interval history questions that may elicit red flag data	System	Red flag data
Any relatives <50 years of age die as result of sudden unexpected cardiac death?	Cardiovascular	Change in family history Sudden death of relative <50 years of age

Child report chest pain or palpitations during or after exercise?		Chief complaint from child:
		  Chest pain
		  Palpitations

Child report any breathing problems during or after exercise?	Respiratory	Chief complaint from child:
		  Dyspnea
		  Wheezing

Child had any episodes of dizziness, syncope, loss of consciousness during or after exercise?	Neurologic	Chief complaint from child:
		  Syncope
		  Loss of consciousness

TABLE 2-4 • Sample focused history

Subjective data	Questions to focus the history
"My child has a chronic cough." "My child begins coughing each night. I cannot remember the last time he didn't cough at night."	What do you mean by a chronic cough? Does child cough during day or just at night? What time of night does child begin coughing? Describe the cough. Is cough productive or nonproductive? Does cough affect child's sleeping pattern? Any products currently being used in household that weren't being used before child began having this "chronic" cough? Pets in your household? Did you change pillow your child uses? Use any over-the-counter or prescription medications to treat this cough? Has child been evaluated for asthma or allergies? Anything make cough better or worse?

BIBLIOGRAPHY

Bickley LS, Hoekelman RA: *Bates' guide to physical assessment,* ed 8, Philadelphia, 2002, Lippincott.

Coylar MR: *Well-child assessment for primary care providers,* Philadelphia, 2003, FA Davis.

Engel J: *Pocket guide to pediatric assessment,* ed 3, St Louis, 1997, Mosby.

Siberry GK, Iannone R, editors: *The Harriet Lane handbook: a manual for pediatric house officers,* ed 16, St Louis, 2003, Mosby.

CHAPTER 3

Performing a Physical Examination

MARY JO EOFF

I. Introduction

A. Pediatric physical assessment is continual process that includes interviews, inspection, observation of children.

B. Physical growth, motor skills, cognitive, and social development change as the child matures.

C. The assessment of the pediatric patient must include what is considered to be normal within the child's age limits.

D. Children will differ among themselves at various stages of development.

E. The following is an outline that can be used as a guide in doing a comprehensive physical assessment.

II. Pediatric physical examination

A. Growth measurements.
  1. Length/height.
    a. Recumbent (<2 years).
    b. Standing height.
  2. Weight.
  3. Head circumference (occipital frontal circumference [OFC]).
  4. Chest circumference (up to 1 year).
  5. Skinfold thickness.

B. Vital signs.
  1. Temperature, heart rate, respirations, blood pressure.

C. General appearance.
  1. Cleanliness, posture, hygiene.
  2. Nutrition.
  3. Behavior, ability to cooperate.
  4. Development.
  5. Alertness.

D. Skin.
  1. Color: pallor, cyanosis, erythema, ecchymosis, petechiae, jaundice.

    2. Texture.

    3. Temperature.

    4. Turgor.

    5. Describe size, shape, and location of rashes, eruptions, and lesions.

    6. Sweating.

E. Hair: color, texture, quantity, distribution, infestations (nits).

F. Nails.

    1. Inspect color, texture, quality, distribution, hygiene.

    2. Observe for nail-biting.

G. Hands and feet.

    1. Observe flexion crease on palm.

    2. Assess for foot and ankle deformities.

H. Lymph nodes.

    1. Palpate for nodes in following areas:

        a. Submaxillary.

        b. Cervical.

        c. Axillary.

        d. Inguinal.

    2. Note size, mobility, or tenderness of any enlarged node.

I. Head.

    1. Assess shape and symmetry.

    2. Assess head control; should be well established by 6 months of age.

    3. Palpate skull.

        a. Fontanels (<2 years of age).

        b. Suture ridges and grooves (up to 6 months of age).

        c. Nodes.

        d. Any swelling.

    4. Examine scalp for hygiene, lesions, signs of trauma, loss of hair, or discoloration.

    5. Percuss frontal sinuses (children >7 years of age).

J. Neck.

    1. Palpate trachea for deviation.

    2. Palpate thyroid, noting size, shape, symmetry, tenderness, or nodules.

    3. Palpate carotid arteries.

    4. Palpate neck structure.

        a. Pain or tenderness.

        b. Enlargement of parotid gland.

        c. Web-like tissue.

K. Eyes.

    1. Check peripheral vision.

    2. Check visual acuity.

        a. Snellen E chart.

        b. Allen test.

    3. Note whether eyelashes curl away from eye.

    4. Note whether eyebrows are above eye and do not meet in midline.

   5. Test for any strabismus.
      a. Hirschberg test.
      b. Cover–uncover test.
   6. Observe for nystagmus or ptosis.
   7. Inspect conjunctiva for drainage, redness, swelling, pain.
   8. Inspect sclera, cornea, iris.
   9. Check: pupils equal, round, react to light.
  10. Examine with ophthalmoscope.
      a. Optic disk, macula, arteriole/vein, fovea centralis, red reflex.
  11. Inspect lachrymal ducts: tears, drainage.
  12. Inspect placement, alignment of outer eye: palpebral slant, epicanthus, lids.
L. Ears.
   1. Inspect placement and alignment of pinna.
   2. Inspect auditory canal: color, cerumen, patency.
   3. Observe for skin tags and hygiene.
   4. Examine middle ear with otoscope.
      a. Color of tympanic membrane, light reflex, bony landmarks.
   5. Check hearing.
      a. Rinne test.
      b. Weber test.
M. Nose.
   1. Observe mucosal lining for color, discharge, patency.
   2. Observe color of the turbinates and meatus.
   3. Note if septum is midline.
N. Mouth and throat.
   1. Observe internal structures.
      a. Hard and soft palate, palatoglossal arch, palatine tonsil, tongue, oropharynx, palatopharyngeal arch, uvula.
   2. Palpate ethmoid, frontal, and maxillary sinuses.
   3. Observe lip edges.
   4. Observe eruption of teeth.
      a. Number appropriate for age.
      b. Color and hygiene.
      c. Occlusion of upper and lower jaw.
   5. Check salivation.
   6. Check drooling.
   7. Check swallowing reflex.
   8. Note color, texture, or any lesions of the lips.
   9. Observe gingiva and mucous membranes for color, texture, moistness.
O. Tongue.
   1. Observe for smoothness, fissuring, coating, or redness.
   2. Tongue able to extend forward to lips?
   3. Tongue interfere with speech?
P. Chest.
   1. Observe shape of thorax.

2. Check costal angles; should be between 45 and 50 degrees.
3. Check points of attachments between ribs and costal cartilage smooth.
4. Check movement.
    a. Inspiration: chest expands, costal angle increases, diaphragm descends.
    b. Expiration: reverse occurs.
Q. Lungs.
    1. Evaluate respiratory movement: rate, rhythm, depth, quality, character.
    2. Auscultate breath sounds.
        a. Vesicular breath sounds.
        b. Bronchovesicular breath sounds.
        c. Bronchial breath sounds.
    3. Note adventitious breath sounds.
        a. Crackles, wheezes, stridor, pleural friction rub.
    4. Check for cough.
        a. Productive/nonproductive.
        b. Color of secretions.
    5. Check retractions.
    6. Check abdominal breathing.
    7. Check thoracic expansion.
    8. Palpate tactile fremitus.
R. Heart.
    1. Auscultate heart sounds.
        a. Aortic area, pulmonic area, Erb's point, tricuspid area, mitral or apical area.
    2. Check S1–S2.
    3. Palpate for thrill.
    4. Record murmurs.
        a. Area best heard.
        b. Timing within S1–S2 cycle.
        c. Change with position.
        d. Loudness and quality.
        e. Grade intensity of murmur.
S. Vascular.
    1. Assess capillary refill; should occur in 1–2 seconds.
    2. Assess circulation.
        a. Color and texture of skin.
        b. Nail and hair distribution.
    3. Assess perfusion.
        a. Edema.
        b. Pulses (4+-0).
    4. Assess collateral circulation.
T. Abdomen.
    1. Inspect contour and size of abdomen.
    2. Note condition of skin.
    3. Inspect umbilicus for hernias, fistula, discharge.

      4. Auscultate bowel sounds.

      5. Auscultate for any aortic pulsations.

      6. Percuss abdomen.

      7. Palpate outer edge of liver.

      8. Palpate spleen.

      9. Elicit abdominal reflux.

      10. Palpate femoral pulses.

U. Neurologic.

      1. Observe behavior, mood, affect, interaction with environment, level of activity, positioning, level of consciousness, orientation to surroundings.

      2. Check reflexes of the infant.

          a. Rooting (present birth to 6 months of age).

          b. Sucking (present birth to 10 months of age).

          c. Palmer grasp (present birth to 4 months of age).

          d. Tonic neck (present at 6–8 weeks of age and lasts until 6 months).

          e. Stepping (present birth to 3 months of age).

          f. Plantar grasp (present birth to 8 months of age).

          g. Moro (present birth to 4–6 months of age).

          h. Babinski (child <15–18 months of age normally fans toes outward and dorsiflexes greater toe).

          i. Gallant (present birth to 1–2 months of age).

          j. Placing (lack of response is abnormal).

          k. Landau (present 3 months to 2 years of age).

      3. Test cranial nerves.

          a. I: Olfactory.

          b. II: Optic.

          c. III: Oculomotor.

          d. IV: Trochlear.

          e. V: Trigeminal.

          f. VI: Abducens.

          g. VII: Facial.

          h. VIII: Acoustic.

          i. IX: Glossopharyngeal.

          j. X: Vagus.

          k. XI: Spinal accessory.

          l. XII: Hypoglossal.

      4. Test cerebellar functioning: finger-to-nose test, heel-to-shin test, Romberg.

      5. Test deep tendon reflexes (grading 4+-0): biceps, triceps, brachioradialis, patellar, Achilles.

      6. Check sensory functioning: pain, temperature, touch.

V. Musculoskeletal.

      1. Inspect curvature and symmetry of spine.

      2. Test for scoliosis.

      3. Inspect all joints for size, temperature, color, tenderness, mobility.

      4. Test for developmental dysplasia of the hips (DDH).

      a. Ortolani maneuver (evaluate up to 12 months of age).

      b. Barlow's maneuver.

      c. Trendelenburg's test (used after child walking).

  5. Examine tibiofemoral bones: knock knee, bow legs.

  6. Inspect gait: waddling gait (DDH), scissor (cerebral palsy [CP]), toeing-in.

  7. Note flexibility and range of motion of joints.

  8. Elicit planter reflex.

  9. Test motor strength of arms, legs, hands, feet (grading 4+-0).

W. Breast.

  1. Pigmentation.

  2. Location.

  3. Tanner stages (sexual maturity rating).

X. Genitalia.

  1. Male.

      a. Inspect size of penis.

      b. Inspect glands and shaft for swelling, skin lesions, inflammation.

      c. Inspect uncircumcised male: prepuce.

      d. Inspect location of urethral meatus, note any discharge.

      e. Inspect scrotum for size, location, skin and hair distribution.

      f. Palpate each scrotal sac for testes.

      g. Tanner stages (sexual maturing rating)

  2. Female.

      a. Palpate genitalia for any masses, cysts.

      b. Observe for any venereal warts.

      c. Inspect for location of urethral meatus, Skene glands, mons pubis, Bartholin gland, clitoris, labia majora, labia minora.

      d. Note any discharge: color and odor.

      e. Tanner stages (sexual maturity rating).

Y. Anus.

  1. Inspect anal area for firmness and condition of skin.

  2. Elicit anal reflex.

BIBLIOGRAPHY

Jarvis C: *Physical examination and health assessment,* ed 4, Philadelphia, 2004, WB Saunders.

Weber J, Kelley J: *Health assessment in nursing,* ed 2, Philadelphia, 2003, Lippincott.

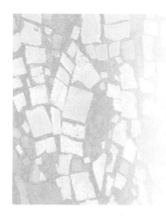

CHAPTER 4

Making Newborn Rounds

CANDACE F. ZICKLER

Asthma, **493.9**	Jaundice, **774.6**
Breathing difficulties, **786.09**	Meconium stools, **777.1**
Café au lait spots, **709.09**	Nares patent (choanal atresia), **748.0**
Coarctation of aorta, **747.10**	Neck short/masses (cystic hygroma), **228.1**
Cyanosis, **770.83**	No urine in 12 hours, **788.20**
Cytomegalovirus (CMV), **078.5**	Pallor, **782.61**
Decreased bowel movements, **564.00**	Petechiae, **772.6**
Epispadius, **752.62**	Poor feeding, **779.3**
Gestational diabetes (GD), **648.8**	Port wine stain, **757.32**
Gonorrhea, **098.0**	Pregnancy-induced hypertension
Group B streptococcus, **041.02**	(PIH), **642.9**
Heart rate with murmur, **785.2**	Rash or pustules, **782.1**
Hemangioma, **228.01**	Rubella, **056.9**
Hematoma/caput succedaneum, **767.19**	Seizures, **779.0**
Herpes simplex virus (HSV) **054.9**	Sickle cell disease, **282.60**
Human immunodeficiency virus (HIV), **042.**	Spontaneous abortions, **634.9**
Hypoglossia/macroglossia, **529.8**	Stillbirths/perinatal deaths, **779.9**
Hypospadias, **752.6**	Supernumerary nipples, **757.6**
Infant galactosemia, **271.1**	Toxoplasmosis, **130.9**
Infertility, **628.9**	Umbilicus with hernia, **553.1**
Irritability, **799.2**	Vomiting, **787.03**

I. **Making newborn rounds**
   A. Determine number of newborns in last 24 hours.
   B. Prioritize assessments by birth time and concerns of nurses in nursery.
   C. Evaluate each infant within 12–24 hours of age.
II. **Review of the individual records**
   A. Mother.
      1. Past obstetric history: infertility, spontaneous abortions, stillbirths/
         perinatal deaths, parity, gravity, duration of pregnancy, congenital

anomalies, isoimmune disease (Rh, ABO), pregnancy-induced hypertension (PIH), cesarean births, vaginal birth after cesarean, gestational diabetes. Current pregnancy history: maternal age, overall health (asthma, sickle cell disease), estimated date of confinement, prenatal care, number of previous pregnancies, multiple fetuses or single fetus, presentation/position of fetus, amount of amniotic fluid, fetal growth/size (small, appropriate, or large for gestational age).
2. Results of prenatal lab work: blood type, rubella IgG level, hepatitis B immunization status, serologic tests, HIV status (elective), gonorrhea and chlamydia cultures, maternal alpha fetal protein, urinalysis (bacteria, blood, protein), glucose screen, exposure to drugs, alcohol, tobacco, or teratogenic medications (valproate, tetracycline), exposure to viruses (TORCH: toxoplasmosis, rubella, cytomegalovirus, herpes simplex virus), sexually transmitted infections, Group B streptococcus status.
B. Newborn
1. Prenatal history: vaginal or cesarean delivery, length of labor and delivery, tocolytics, narcotics, anesthesia, or analgesics mother received, presentation, placental abnormalities (three-vessel cord), amniotic fluid color/volume, Apgar scores (heart rate, respirations, muscle tone, reflex irritability, color) with 5-minute Apgar >7.
2. Since birth: delivery weight/length/occipital frontal circumference (OFC), temperature, blood pressure, pulse, respirations, nursing with bottle or breast, voiding, passage of meconium, contact with mother/parents.

III. Physical assessment of the newborn
A. General appearance.
B. Current weight, length, OFC, color, heart rate, respirations, response to stimuli, posture, gestational age (38–42 weeks = term gestation).

IV. Abnormal physical findings
Consult with staff physician and/or refer for evaluation, as indicated.
A. Dysmorphic facies.
1. Skin and scalp with plethora, pallor, jaundice, cyanosis, bruising, abrasions, petechiae, hemangioma, port wine stain, café au lait spots.
2. Shape of skull.
3. Bruising, hematoma/caput succedaneum.
4. Size and tone of anterior and posterior fontanelles.
B. Pupils without red reflex and unequal pupillary sizes, nares patent (choanal atresia), mouth with teeth, hypoglossia/macroglossia, palate high arched or missing. External ears with tags or pinhole openings. Neck short/masses (cystic hygroma) or webbing.
C. More/less than five fingers/toes on each hand/foot.
D. Check clavicles for fractures. Chest shape with pectus excavatum/carinatum, and supernumerary nipples. Breath sounds that are moist and grunting/retractions after 4 hours of age, apnea/respirations <30 or >60 bpm.

    E. Heart rate with murmur (soft III/IV systolic murmur normal for first 12–24 hours since patent ductus may not be closed), or an irregular rate/rhythm <100 or >180 bpm, a cuff blood pressure <65 or >95 mm Hg of systolic pressure, and diastolic <30 or >60 mm Hg. Absent or decreased femoral pulses (coarctation of aorta), slow capillary refill is indicative of poor perfusion.

    F. Temperature instability <97.7°F (36.5°C) after 4 hours of age.

    G. Abdominal skin thin or missing, asymmetrical, distended, umbilicus with hernia, discharge, redness, odor. Missing or overactive bowel sounds. Lower liver edge 3 cm below costal margin (heart disease), infection, hemolysis, palpable spleen (infection or hemopoiesis), enlarged bladder (1–4 cm above symphysis).

    H. Female

        1. Masses in labia (hernia, enlarged Bartholin gland), vesicles.

    I. Male

        1. Meatal opening on penis placed abnormally (hypospadias or epispadius), absence of testes in either inguinal canals or scrotal sac, hydrocele, bifid scrotum, discoloration or bruising.

    J. Anus absent or not patent.

    K. Absent or missing extremities, bands, masses, inequality from side to side. Abnormal Ortolani or Barlow sign. Bowing of extremities, abnormal foot positions, flaccid upper extremity. Lesions or dimpling of lower spine.

    L. Abnormal posturing, floppy or very jittery, abnormal cry. Exaggerated tonic neck, Moro reflex, poor sucking, or poor rooting.

V. Laboratory assessment of newborn

    A. Glucose screening (normal 40–90 mg/dL), venous hematocrit (normal 45–65%), cord blood (ABO, Rh). If baby is Rh−, maternal RhoGAM status should be Rh+.

    B. Bilirubin (total, direct, indirect) (under 24 hours of age, bilirubin 1 mg/dL is normal; <15 mg/dL in term infant is considered normal). Anything above considered pathologic.

VI. Meeting with the parent

    A. Introduce self and sit by bedside. Describe your role.

    B. Praise parents, compliment baby.

    C. Call baby by name.

    D. Determine mother's health/wellness/contact with infant so far.

    E. Review your findings, briefly.

    F. If male, determine if baby is to be circumcised. Discuss pros and cons.

    G. Ask about method of feeding, car seat, help when home, concerns.

VII. Nutrition

    A. Breastfeeding is encouraged for all newborns (see Chapter 5).

        1. No breastfeeding if HIV infected, active herpes of breast, untreated tuberculosis, maternal debilitating disease (cancer), illicit drug use by mother, infant galactosemia.

    B. If bottle feeding, reassure that baby will grow and thrive on formula.

      1. Only commercially prepared, iron-fortified formulas should be used: powder, concentrate, ready-to-feed. Do not dilute ready-to-feed; do not reuse if >4 hours since opened.

      2. Mix formulas with bottled water for first month, continue if on well or unsure of water quality. Store in refrigerator if open no longer than 24 hours.

      3. Specialized formulas have similar preparation directions. Goat's milk, whole cow's milk, rice milk have inadequate amounts of vitamins and minerals.

      4. Serve formula at room temperature. Do not microwave to heat. Do not let formula sit out at room temperature to warm for more than 15–20 minutes.

  C. Clean technique is sufficient for mixing formulas. Clean off cans with soap and water before opening. Use hot soapy water and bottlebrush to clean nipples and bottles or clean in dishwasher.

  D. Hold during feedings; burp every 1–2 ounces.

  E. Hold in upright, semireclined position for feedings. No bottle propping.

  F. Newborn will suckle 0.5–1 ounce of formula/feeding every 2–3 hours for first 24 hours (60–100 mL/kg/day). Volume increases to 12–24 ounces/day and interval between feedings >3–4 hours in first month. May be days when baby takes more or less, depending on sleep pattern. Baby should take in 90% of feeding in first 20 minutes.

VIII. Elimination

  A. Meconium stools in first 48 hours, transition stools green-brown, change to yellow pasty after 2–3 days of oral feeding.

  B. Infant should have 1–6 yellow pasty stools/24 hours.

  C. Breastfed baby may have upper range of frequency, bottle-fed may have less.

  D. Void every 1–3 hours or with each feeding and diaper change.

IX. Sleep

  A. Awake for feedings; feed every 2–4 hours. Should be alert for feedings, nurse vigorously for 15–20 minutes, then fall back to sleep. Respirations may be slightly irregular.

  B. Babies should sleep on back or on side in cribs to decrease incidence of sudden infant death syndrome (SIDS). No pillows/toys that baby could get face against and smother.

  C. Babies should sleep in own cribs, not with parents, to decrease potential injury.

X. Growth and development

  A. Newborn can lose up to 10% of body weight in first 10 days of life. Should regain birth weight by 2 weeks of age.

  B. Infant grows 1 inch, on average, per month for first 6 months.

  C. Head circumference increases 9 cm in first year.

  D. Has minimal head control.

  E. Looks at person during feeding.

  F. Tracks 45 degrees.

XI. Social development
- A. Babies have different cries, will fuss/cry 1 to 2 hours per day.
    1. Similar time/pattern daily.
    2. Provide for infant's needs and crying should cease.
    3. Cry gradually decreases by 3 months of age.
- B. Refer all high-risk infants/mothers to social worker before release. High-risk situations include:
    1. Adolescent pregnancy.
    2. No prenatal care.
    3. Consideration about giving up the baby for adoption.
    4. Unwanted pregnancy.
    5. Insufficient support when home.
    6. Physical limitations of parent.
    7. Inadequate housing/finances.
    8. Domestic violence.
    9. Positive toxicology.
    10. Incarcerated parent.
    11. Emotional disorders.
    12. Parent with mental retardation.
    13. Multiple small children in home.

XII. Immunizations (see Appendix A)
- A. Only monovalent hepatitis B can be used for birth dose. Monovalent or combination vaccine can be used to complete series. Four doses of hepatitis B may be given if newborn dose is received.
- B. Newborns with mothers who are HBsAg + or whose hepatitis B status is unknown, also get 0.5 mL of hepatitis B immune globulin IM within first 12 hours of life, given in site other than at site of hepatitis B immunization.

XIII. Safety/anticipatory guidance
- A. Sleep position "back to sleep."
- B. Not safe for baby to sleep in adult bed; must discuss with parents.
- C. Use federal motor vehicle safety tested and approved car seat; install properly in backseat, facing backward in automobile. Contact local hospital, fire department, or March of Dimes chapter for car seat rental program.
- D. No smoking around infant.
- E. One-piece pacifiers only.
- F. No corn syrup (Karo) for constipation.
- G. No solids, only breast or formula fed to infant.
- H. When to call health care provider.
    1. Breathing difficulties, seizures, irritability, poor feeding, vomiting, no urine in 12 hours, black or decreased bowel movements, reddened, draining umbilical site, jaundice, rash or pustules not present on discharge, concerns.
- I. Give office phone number, explain how to use system.

XIV. Discharge to home

    A. Review all records/progress.

    B. Repeat complete physical examination.

    C. Identify abnormal findings that require ongoing monitoring.

    D. Review hearing screen.

    E. Collect newborn blood screen.

    F. Administer hepatitis B immunization.

    G. Complete all consults.

    H. Staff nurses will have covered discharge instructions of bathing, cord care, bulb syringe, diapering, dressing, fingernail care, holding, feeding.

    I. Review recommendations/follow-up appointments with parents. Make them aware that they can call with any concerns.

BIBLIOGRAPHY

2004 Immunization for Infants and Children, retrieved from *www.cdc.gov/nip/acip/hepatitis.*

Carroll JL, Siska E: SIDS: counseling parents to reduce the risk (sudden infant death syndrome), retrieved from *www.findarticles.com/cf_dls/m3225.*

Finn-Davis K, Parker KP, Montgomery GL: Sleep in infants and young children: part one: normal sleep, *J Pediatr Health Care* 18 (2):65-71, March-April 2004.

Newborn visit. In Green M, Palfrey J, editors: *Bright futures: guidelines for health supervision of infants, children, and adolescents,* ed 2 rev, Arlington, VA, 2002, National Center for Education in Maternal and Child Health.

Schrag SJ et al: Prenatal screening for infectious diseases and opportunities for prevention, *J Obstetr Gynecol* 102 (4), October 2003, retrieved from *www.acog.org/from_home/publications/green_journal.*

Shelov SP, Hanneman RE: *Caring for your baby and young child: birth to 5 years of age,* ed rev, Chicago, IL, 2004, American Academy of Pediatrics.

Sudden infant death in infants, retrieved from *www.sidscenter.org/SIDSWEB.HTM.*

TIPP Safety sheet, birth to 6 months, January 2004, retrieved from *www.aap.org/tippsafetysheets.*

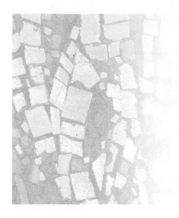

Guidelines for Breastfeeding

AMY L. FELDMAN

I. Introduction

A. Breastfeeding provides optimal nutrition for newborns and infants, protecting against many diseases and infections and improving maternal health.

II. Physiology of lactation

A. Mammary glands are endocrine organs that respond to complex combination of hormones and stimulation to produce milk. After expulsion of placenta following delivery, significant change in maternal hormones and suckling infant readies body for milk production (Figure 5-1).

B. Predominant hormones of lactation are prolactin and oxytocin.

C. Quantity of milk production depends on several factors including release of lactation hormones, effective milk removal, breast stimulation.

D. Full lactation can be produced by breasts from 16 weeks of pregnancy forward.

E. Imperative to understand balance of supply and demand to optimize lactation.

F. Baby needs to frequently and effectively remove milk to maximize production.

III. Human milk

A. Human milk is exceptional in its ability to sustain appropriate growth and development for infants.

B. "Liquid gold," as human milk is often referred to, is living tissue, which encompasses fats, proteins, carbohydrates, antibodies, hundreds of components.

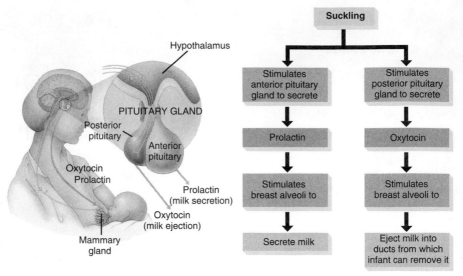

FIGURE 5-1 • Physiology of lactation. (From Thibodeau GA, Patton KT: *Anatomy and physiology,* ed 5, St Louis, 2003, Mosby.)

    C. Composition of human milk changes to provide optimal nutrition as infant grows.
        1. Colostrum is first milk, produced during pregnancy, considered infant's first immunization, providing protection to newborn from viruses and bacteria.
        2. Transitional milk is produced after colostrum, then mature milk as lactogenesis stage II (production of large quantities of milk) begins (Box 5-1).

IV. Contraindications for breastfeeding

    A. Occasionally there are circumstances that preclude mothers from breastfeeding.
        1. Maternal contraindications include:
            a. HIV+ mother (in the United States).
            b. Maternal drug abuse.
            c. Maternal chemotherapy.
            d. Herpetic lesions on mother's nipple, areola (breast lesions must be covered).
            e. Untreated, active tuberculosis.
            f. Certain radioactive compounds may require temporary cessation of breastfeeding (list available in resources).
        2. Infant contraindications include:
            a. Galactosemia in infant.

V. Maternal assessment

    A. Breastfeeding goals and family support.
    B. Previous breastfeeding experience.

> **BOX 5-1** • Description of Secretions from the Breast during Lactogenesis and Lactation
>
> *Colostrum*, the first "milk," is a thick substance that appears yellow because of its high carotene content. Colostrum is contained in the ducts during the later part of pregnancy and is secreted the first few days postpartum. Colostrum is especially important for the newborn; it is rich in immunoglobulins and has a laxative effect on the gut, aiding with the passage of newborn meconium. Compared with mature milk, colostrum is higher in protein, lower in fat, and lower in carbohydrate. Colostrum is lower in energy than mature milk, containing about 67 kcal/100 mL (about 20 calories per ounce), whereas mature milk has about 75 kcal/100 mL (about 22.5 calories per ounce).
>
> *Transitional* milk is produced in the very early postpartum period as the colostrum diminishes and mature milk develops.
>
> *Mature* milk is produced after lactogenesis stage II. The energy content is different from colostrum, as is the proportion of many nutrients.
>
> *Foremilk* is produced and stored between feeding and released at the beginning of the next feeding. It has an appearance similar to skimmed milk, with a characteristic blue tinge. *Hindmilk* is produced during and released at the end of the feeding. It looks much like heavy cream.
>
> From Lawrence RA, Lawrence RM: *Breastfeeding: a guide for the medical profession,* ed 5, St Louis, 1999, Mosby.

    C. General health and nutritional status.
    D. Breast, nipple, or thoracic surgery.
    E. Medications, both prescription and OTC.
    F. Pregnancy, labor, birth history.
    G. Inverted or flat nipples.
VI. Infant assessment
    A. General health, including gestational age.
    B. Congenital circumstances.
    C. Birth history.
    D. Medications received and procedures experienced.
    E. Initial feeding attempts.
    F. Oral facial assessment.
VII. Breastfeeding in the early days
    A. If mother and baby are discharged <48 hours after delivery, visit within 2–4 days to observe breastfeeding and ascertain that breastfeeding is successful.
    B. Initial feedings.
        1. Encourage breastfeeding within first hour after birth during quiet alert phase. Do not restrict length or frequency of feedings.
        2. Facilitate skin-to-skin contact during this initial period and as often as possible.
        3. Promote rooming in 24 hours a day.
        4. Encourage exclusive breastfeeding; this helps to establish sufficient milk supply.

5. Instruct parents in correct latch-on techniques (see below).
6. Educate parents regarding initial feedings of colostrum: quantity is very small, but sufficient nutrition as baby is learning to breastfeed.
7. Discourage use of any supplements unless medically indicated.
8. Avoid use of bottles and pacifiers until breastfeeding is well established.
9. Teach parents to breastfeed in response to infant feeding cues (rooting, increased alertness, fists in mouth), at least 8–12 times/day. Crying is late sign of hunger.
10. Baby should finish feeding on one breast, then be offered second if he/she will take more. Fat content of milk is higher at end of feeding than at beginning. Forcing baby to switch breasts too soon may decrease amount of higher calorie milk consumed.
11. Babies who sleep for long periods of time without eating or feed only for few minutes should be stimulated (i.e., unwrap, tickle feet), encouraged to nurse.

C. Positioning and latch.
1. Mother and infant should be comfortable with infant on his/her side at nipple height supported by pillows or blankets.
2. Support infant's head so can easily reach areola without turning neck.
3. Infant's ear, shoulder, hips should be in alignment.
4. Mother quickly brings infant to breast only when infant's mouth is open widely.
5. Infant's lips should be flanged outward with chin touching breast (Figure 5-2).
6. Infant's tongue will protrude over gum ridge and "cup" breast.
7. Repeat latch-on attempts until baby is on correctly.
8. Common breastfeeding positions are cradle position (Figure 5-3), cross cradle (Figure 5-4), football hold (Figure 5-5), and side-lying position (Figure 5-6).

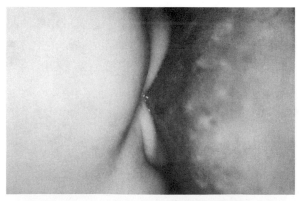

FIGURE 5-2 • UNICEF positioning slide. (From UNICEF/WHO 1993, C-107#7.)

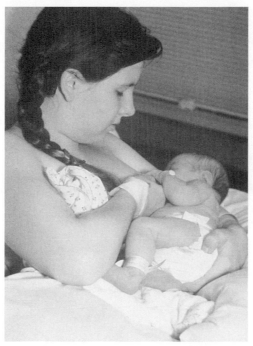

FIGURE 5-3 • Cradle position.(From Biancuzzo M: *Breastfeeding the newborn,* ed 2, St Louis, 2003, Mosby.)

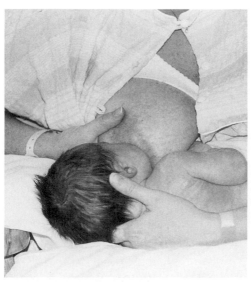

FIGURE 5-4 • Cross cradle position. (From Biancuzzo M: *Breastfeeding the newborn,* ed 2, St Louis, 2003, Mosby.)

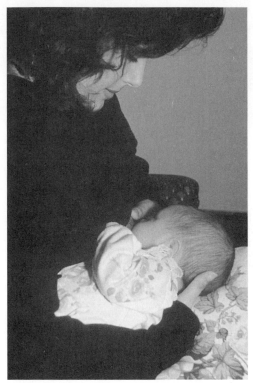

FIGURE 5-5 ● Football hold position. (From Biancuzzo M: *Breastfeeding the newborn,* ed 2, St Louis, 2003, Mosby.)

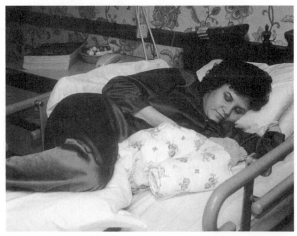

FIGURE 5-6 ● Side-lying position. (From Biancuzzo M: *Breastfeeding the newborn,* ed 2, St Louis, 2003, Mosby.)

9. Have Mom insert small finger between baby's gums to release latch.
10. Practitioner should observe a latch-on and feeding.
D. Signs of milk transfer in infant.
   1. Observe sustained, rhythmic suck/swallow pattern with intermittent pauses.
   2. Listen for audible swallowing.
   3. Baby's arms and hands should be relaxed.
   4. Baby's oral mucous membranes should be moist after feedings.
   5. Baby appears satisfied after feedings.
E. Signs of milk transfer in mother.
   1. Mother feels strong tugging sensation when baby is sucking that is not painful.
   2. Mother feels uterine contractions or increased lochia flow during initial days postpartum.
   3. Milk may leak from opposite breast during feedings.
   4. Mother may feel relaxed or drowsy during feedings.
   5. Breast softens after feeding (after milk supply is established).
   6. Nipples are elongated, but not pinched or bruised after release of latch.
   7. Assessing infant weight gain.
      a. Parents should be aware of baby's birth and discharge weight.
      b. Encourage parents to keep daily journal of first week to track feedings, output.
      c. Healthy, breastfeeding infants may lose 3–7% of birth weight in initial days.
      d. After Mom's milk is in, infant should gain 0.5–1 ounce/day (4–7 ounces/week).
      e. Babies often regain birth weight by 2 weeks of age, double it by 6 months, triple it by a year.
      f. Exclusively breastfed infants tend to be leaner than bottle-fed infants in second 6 months of life.
F. Assessing infant output.
   1. Colostrum acts as laxative, encouraging expulsion of meconium in first days.
   2. Effective and regular breastfeeding helps to prevent jaundice in early days.
   3. Infants showing signs of jaundice should be assessed carefully for ineffective breastfeeding.
   4. Bowel movements become lighter in color, then turn to a mustard color/seedy consistency by day 4 or 5.
   5. Babies who are breastfeeding well should have 2–3 large mustard color, seedy stools/day.
   6. Inadequate stools are red flag for ineffective breastfeeding.
   7. Stool output may decrease to one stool every few days after first few weeks.
   8. Urine output is less helpful than stool output in assessing adequate milk intake.

9. Exclusively breastfed baby should produce one wet diaper on day 1, two on day 2, three on day 3, etc., for first week.
10. By end of first week, baby should have six soaking wet, pale yellow diapers/day.

VIII. Separation of mother and infant
  A. Pumping.
   1. If small number of feedings must be missed, teach mother hand expression or use of hand/battery-operated pump to express milk from both breasts every few hours.
   2. Lengthy separation warrants use of hospital-grade, piston-style pump with double hookup system to efficiently remove breast milk 6–8 times per 24 hours for 15 minutes each session.
   3. Even the smallest quantity of expressed colostrum or milk should be fed to infant via eyedropper, syringe, cup, or feeding tube taped to breast.
  B. Milk collection and storage.
   1. Recommendations for collection and storage of mother's milk for hospitalized infant differ from that of the following instructions for well child at home.
   2. Mothers should wash hands thoroughly prior to pumping.
   3. Follow manufacturer's instructions for cleaning of pump parts.
   4. Plastic bags made specifically for storing breast milk; plastic bottles or glass containers can be used.
   5. Encourage milk let down by looking at picture of baby, smelling piece of baby's clothing.
   6. Warm, wet washcloths on breast combined with breast massage may be helpful in starting milk flow.
   7. Breastfeeding on one breast, while pumping from other breast is an option.
   8. All pumps are different. Encourage mother to find one that creates comfortable seal, which provides appropriate suction. Pumping should not be painful.
   9. Expressed milk can be kept at room temperature for about 10 hours, refrigerated for about 5 days, or frozen for 6 months or longer. It will keep in freezer compartment of a refrigerator for 2–4 months.

IX. Supporting breastfeeding past the early days
  A. Maternal diet.
   1. Encourage mother to eat wide variety of healthy foods, eating when hungry, drinking to quench her thirst.
     a. Forcing large quantities of fluids will not increase her milk production.
     b. No specific foods must be avoided by breastfeeding mothers.
     c. Most foods do not bother most babies.
     d. If particular food seems to bother baby, decrease/eliminate for week to 10 days.
     e. Maternal diet does not significantly affect quantity of vitamin D in breast milk.
   2. It is recommended that all breastfed babies be supplemented with vitamin D 200 IU starting within first 2 months of life.

3. Families with significant allergies should receive knowledgeable dietary counseling regarding possible need to eliminate certain foods while breastfeeding.
B. Growth spurts.
   1. Regardless of culture, women frequently worry about ability to provide enough milk for baby.
   2. Teach parents that growth spurts (periods when babies want to nurse more frequently to meet rapid growth) usually occur around 2–3 weeks, 6 weeks, 3 months.
   3. Feed as often as baby wants to nurse to maintain adequate milk supply.
   4. Reinforce concept of supply and demand.
   5. Supplementing with formula is strongly discouraged; mother's milk supply will not increase without adequate stimulation to meet baby's growing demand for more milk.
C. Medications and breastfeeding.
   1. It is imperative that nurse practitioners make recommendations to mothers who breastfeed on the safety of medications based on appropriate, current research. An excellent reference guide such as Hale (2002) should be available in every clinical setting that deals with breastfeeding mothers.
   2. Nearly all medications likely to be prescribed to breastfeeding mother should not affect maternal milk supply or infant's safety.
   3. Dose of medication transferred through breast milk is almost always too low to be clinically significant or it is poorly bioavailable to infant.
   4. Extensive benefits of breastfeeding far outweigh any potential risks in majority of cases.
      a. Medications should be safe for infants to consume.
      b. Choose drugs with breastfeeding information whenever possible.
      c. Choose shortest acting form of medication.
      d. Encourage feeding when maternal drug level is lowest.
      e. Educate parents as to potential side effects to observe in infant.
      f. Be extra cautious with preterm, low-birth-weight or sick infants.
      g. Certain herbal substances may be harmful to infants.
D. Maternal employment.
   1. Women who return to work must be well supported in effort to continue providing breast milk for infant.
   2. Women need private, clean place to pump every few hours while separated from infant.
   3. Expressed milk can be kept at room temperature for short periods, in insulated bag with cooler pack, or, if available, in refrigerator. Encourage mothers to rent or purchase pump that is comfortable and is efficient for their particular needs.
   4. Provide information on how to introduce bottle to the infant, as well as suggestions for caregiver that will promote extended breastfeeding (i.e., not bottle feeding immediately before mother will pick up infant, proper handling, storage of breast milk).

5. Returning to workplace while continuing to provide breast milk for her baby may initially seem overwhelming to some mothers. Strong encouragement, praise, support can make difference between mother being successful and giving up.

X. Common problems

A. Mothers can complain about pain even when damage cannot be visualized. Determine that baby is positioned properly at breast height with adequate support and is latching on correctly. Mother's often describe sensation of baby feeding as strong tugging sensation. Breastfeeding should not be painful. Nipples do not "toughen up" as breastfeeding proceeds. Assess for other causes of sore nipples such as trauma, improper latch release, thrush, milk plugs on nipple, incorrect use of breastfeeding devices.

B. Sore nipples management includes:
   1. Correct positioning and latch-on.
   2. Teach mothers to express colostrum/hindmilk to rub into nipples after each feeding.
   3. Allow nipples to dry before putting bra back on.
   4. Offer use of breast shells to prevent fabric from rubbing against nipple.
   5. Breastfeed from least sore side first.
   6. Change positions at each feeding to decrease pressure on sore area.
   7. Suggest moist wound healing methods (i.e., modified lanolin or hydrogel dressings).
   8. Analgesics as needed.

C. Flat or inverted nipples.
   1. Can initially make breastfeeding more of a challenge, may be difficult for baby to latch on, suck well.
   2. "Pinch test": determines if nipple is flat or inverted (Figure 5-7). With thumb behind nipple and first two fingers underneath, grasp about 1 inch back from base of nipple and compress skin.
      a. Normal nipple will evert.
      b. Flat nipple remains flat with compression.

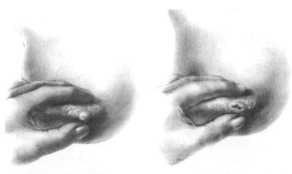

FIGURE 5-7 • Pinch test. (From Lawrence RA, Lawrence RM: *Breastfeeding: a guide for the medical profession,* ed 5, St Louis, 1999, Mosby.)

    c. Inverted nipple looks sunken in.

    d. Nipples can look flat or inverted, but evert on compression.

  3. Flat or inverted management includes:

    a. Encouraging deepest possible latch onto breast.

    b. Making sure infant is at breast height and well supported to prevent sliding to base of nipple.

    c. Release latch and repeat attempts until proper latch is obtained. Allowing baby to suck at base of nipple prevents stimulating milk supply, will cause sore nipples.

    d. Encourage offering flat/inverted breast first when baby is hungriest and sucking is strongest.

    e. Teach mother to evert nipple with gentle pulling/rolling immediately prior to latch.

    f. Hand express few drops of colostrum to entice baby to latch on.

    g. Use hand/electric pump for few minutes immediately prior to latch.

    h. If supplement is medically indicated, use expressed milk first using an eyedropper, syringe, cup, or feeding tube at the breast.

    i. Avoid pacifiers and bottle nipples until breastfeeding is well established.

D. Severe engorgement.

  1. Milk stasis caused by inefficient, infrequent removal of milk, results in extremely full, swollen, lumpy, painful breasts.

  2. Result is different from transient breast fullness associated with milk "coming in" 2–4 days after birth.

  3. Breastfeeding emergency: milk stasis can cause damage to tissue, decrease milk supply, difficult to impossible for infant to compress areola and remove milk.

  4. Severe engorgement management includes:

    a. Analgesics as necessary.

    b. Warm, wet compresses to breast prior to feedings to help increase milk flow.

    c. Soften areola using hand expression so baby can latch properly.

    d. Use breast compression during feedings to improve milk flow. Using her thumb on top of breast, her fingers underneath, the mother brings her fingers together, which compresses breast.

    e. Use of cold compresses may help to decrease engorgement after feeding. Some mothers like to use this prior to feeding as well.

    f. Use of chilled green cabbage leaves left on breast for short period several times/day has been helpful to some mothers. Stop using this as soon as engorgement decreases.

    g. Express milk after feeding as needed for comfort. Any expressed milk can be fed to baby using alternative feeding methods.

E. Mastitis.

  1. Infection of breast, usually caused by *Staphylococcus aureus*.

TABLE 5-1 • Comparison of findings of engorgement, plugged duct, and mastitis

Characteristics	Engorgement, 611.79	Plugged duct	Mastitis, 611.0
Onset	Gradual, immediately postpartum	Gradual, after feedings	Sudden, after 10 days
Site	Bilateral	Unilateral	Usually unilateral
Swelling and heat	Generalized	May shift a little or no heat	Localized, red, hot, and swollen
Pain	Generalized	Mild but localized	Intense but localized
Body temperature	<38.4°C	<38.4°C	<38.4°C
Systemic symptoms	Feels well	Feels well	Flu-like symptoms

From Lawrence RA, Lawrence RM: *Breastfeeding: a guide for the medical profession,* ed 5, St Louis, 1999, Mosby.

    2. Frequently occurs in upper outer quadrant of breast at 2–3 weeks postpartum.

    3. Symptoms commonly include hard, swollen, reddened area on breast accompanied by flu-like symptoms.

    4. Difficult to differentiate between engorgement, plugged duct, mastitis (Table 5-1).

    5. Mastitis management includes:

        a. Rest (decrease stress and fatigue by enlisting support from friends, family).

        b. Antibiotics, analgesics as needed.

        c. Increase maternal fluid intake.

        d. Frequent effective emptying of breasts (important to continue breastfeeding, milk is not infected, fine for baby).

        e. Abrupt weaning can predispose to an abscess.

        f. Analgesics as needed.

        g. Correct latch to prevent further nipple trauma (cracked, bleeding nipples allow bacteria to enter milk ducts).

        h. Mother's preference of warm or cool packs for comfort.

  F. Jaundice.

    1. Rarely requires cessation of breastfeeding.

    2. Galactosemia, uncommon metabolic disorder: stop breastfeeding.

    3. Pathologic jaundice, with onset in first 24 hours of life, warrants medical evaluation in addition to lactation support.

    4. Encourage early initiation of breastfeeding, then frequent, effective, unrestricted feedings to minimize jaundice.

    5. Colostrum acts as laxative, eliminating bilirubin through meconium expulsion.

    6. Physiologic jaundice, which begins 48–72 hours after birth and peaks on day 3–5, is seen in thriving infants with normal weight gain and output.

7. Observe for effective breastfeeding and continue assessment for normal weight gain and output. Onset and peak of breastfeeding associated with jaundice is similar to physiologic jaundice, but infant is fussy/sleepy with poor feeding, inadequate weight gain, output.
8. Assist with frequent, unrestricted effective breastfeeding.
9. Teach parents to watch for signs of milk transfer during feedings. If necessary, express milk in addition to feedings, use alternate feeding methods to give baby milk.

G. Thrush.
   1. Described as burning, itching, stinging lasting throughout feeding and beyond, radiating from nipple and breast to shoulder and back.
   2. Nipple or areolar skin is often red and shiny.
   3. May have period of pain-free nursing, then have sudden onset of pain.
   4. Pain from poor latch is often described as feeling like a knife or being stabbed, dissipates as feeding progresses, frequently limited to nipple and areola.
   5. Regardless of nipple pain, poor latch must be corrected immediately.
   6. Broken skin is perfect environment for organisms to invade.
   7. Signs in infant may range from nothing to white patches on buccal mucosa, tongue, and palate, which may bleed when scraped with tongue blade. Fiery red diaper rash with shiny red patches and pustules may also be present.
   8. Both mother and baby should be treated simultaneously to prevent reinfection from one to the other.
   9. All objects coming in contact with baby's mouth should be boiled/bleached daily.
   10. Mothers can be treated with gentian violet (0.5% solution painted on nipple/areola immediately prior to feedings once a day for 4–7 days.)
   11. All-purpose nipple cream, Mupirocin 2% (15 grams), Nystatin ointment (1,000,000 units/mL: 15 grams), Clotrimazole (vaginal cream: 15 grams), Betamethasone 0.1% ointment (15 grams) can be mixed by pharmacist, applied to nipples after all feedings except one when gentian violet is used. Preparation does not need to be washed off prior to feedings. Mixture is not adequate to treat infant's mouth alone, whereas gentian violet is. Oral Fluconazole can be prescribed to mother for at least 2 weeks if above treatments are not bringing relief.
   12. Mothers should be encouraged to continue breastfeeding while treating infection.
   13. Because *Candida albicans* thrives in warm, moist, dark areas, nipples can be rinsed with clear water or vinegar solution of 1 Tbsp vinegar in cup of water after each feeding, exposed to air after each feeding.
   14. Bed linens, sheets, bras can be rinsed in vinegar solution after hot wash cycle. Breast pads should be disposable and changed as soon as wet.
   15. Sexual contact between mother and partner can spread infection. Partner should be treated appropriately.

H. Weight gain concerns.
1. Breastfed infants gaining less than appropriate amount for age should be carefully evaluated. Often, correcting latch and positioning is enough to facilitate efficient breastfeeding and improve weight gain.
2. Do not recommend formula supplementation without evaluating breastfeeding. If extra calories are needed, have mother hand express or pump in addition to breastfeeding and use alternative feeding methods to give baby milk.
3. Allowing baby to finish feeding on one breast before feeding on second allows sufficient amounts of higher calorie breast milk.
4. Review with parents appropriate signs of infant hunger, encourage frequent (8–12 or more/24 hours) unrestricted feedings.
5. Keeping written log of feedings and output is also helpful. Imperative that infant have adequate caloric intake.
6. If after evaluation and management with skilled breastfeeding consultant, breastfeeding is not going well, formula supplementation is appropriate. Plan for maintaining/increasing mother's milk supply must be implemented.
7. Return office visit within 24–48 hours to monitor situation should be scheduled. Frequent phone follow-up, support are necessary.
8. Standard growth charts are not necessarily reflective of breastfed infants.
   a. Breastfed infants grow more quickly in first 2 months, then slow down compared to present NCHS growth charts.
   b. Breastfed infants gain weight more quickly in second year than charts mirror; in general, by end of second year, charts accurately reflect breastfed infant's weight.
   c. Educate parents that breastfed infants are leaner than formula-fed babies; if plotted on NCHS growth charts, growth may appear to be deficient compared with formula-fed counterparts.

XI. Helpful breastfeeding resources

A. Board-certified lactation consultants (Table 5-2).
B. Books
Biancuzzo M: *Breastfeeding the newborn: clinical strategies for nurses,* ed 2, St Louis, 2003, Mosby.
Hale TW: *Medications and mother's milk,* ed 10, Amarillo, TX, 2002, Pharmasoft Medical Publishers.

TABLE 5-2 • Locating a board-certified lactation consultant

International Lactation Consultant Association	919-861-5577	*www.ilca.org*
International Board of Lactation Consultant Examiners	703-560-7330	*www.iblce.org*
Medela	800-453-8316 or 815-363-1166	*www.Medela.com*

Newman J: *The ultimate breastfeeding book of answers,* Rocklin, CA, 2000,
Prima Publishing.

Riordan J, Auerbach K: *Breastfeeding and human lactation,* ed 2, Sudbury,
MA, 1999, Jones & Bartlett.

Walker M: *ILCA core curriculum for lactation consultant practice,* Sudbury,
MA, 2002, Jones & Bartlett.

C. Breastfeeding information.

Academy of Breastfeeding Medicine

877-836-9947, ext. 25 or 609-799-6327; *www.bfmed.org*

American Academy of Pediatrics

847-434-4000; *www.aap.org*

Hotline for health care professionals for drug information, unusual
breastfeeding circumstances: 716-275-0088

Human Milk Banking Association of North America

919-861-4530; *www.hmbana.com*

International Lactation Consultant Association

919-861-5577; *www.ilca.org*

Lactation Study Center, Department of Pediatrics, University of Rochester
Medical Center

La Leche League International

847-519-7730; *www.lalecheleague.org*

Rocky Mountain Drug Consultation Center (information on medications)
800-332-3073

United States Breastfeeding Committee

202-367-1132; *www.usbreastfeeding.org*

BIBLIOGRAPHY

American Academy of Breastfeeding Work Group on Breastfeeding: Breastfeeding and the use
of human milk, *Pediatrics* 100 (6):1035-1039, 1997.

American Academy of Family Physicians: Breastfeeding position paper 2002, retrieved
February 11, 2004, from *www.uufp.org/x6633.xml.*

American Academy of Pediatrics Committee on Drugs. The transfer of drugs and other
chemicals into human milk, *Pediatrics* 108(3):776-789, September 2001.

Ball T, Wright A: Health care costs of formula-feeding in the first year of life, *Pediatrics*
103(4):870-876, 1999.

Hale TW: *Medications and mother's milk,* ed 10, Amarillo, TX, 2002, Pharmasoft Medical
Publishing.

Human Milk Banking Association of North America: *Recommendations for collection, storage
and handling of a mother's milk for her own infant in the hospital setting,* Raleigh, NC, 1999.

International Lactation Consultant Association: *Evidence based guidelines for breastfeeding
management during the first fourteen days,* Raleigh, NC, April 1999.

Lu MC, et al: Provider encouragement of breast-feeding: Evidence from a national survey,
Obstet Gynecol 97(2):290-295, February 2001.

Marks JM, Spatz DL: Medications and lactation: What PNPs need to know, *J Pediatr Health
Care* 17(6):311-319, November-December 2003.

NAPNAP breastfeeding position statement, *J Pediatr Health Care* 15(5):22A, 2001.

Newman J, Pitman T: *The ultimate breastfeeding book of answers,* Rocklin, CA, 2000, Prima Publishing.

US Breastfeeding Committee: Breastfeeding in the United States: a national agenda. Rockville, MD, 2001, US Department of Health and Human Services, Health Resources and Services Administration, Maternal and Child Health Bureau.

US Department of Health and Human Services. HHS blueprint for action on breastfeeding. Washington, DC, 2000, US Department of Health and Human Services, Office on Women's Health.

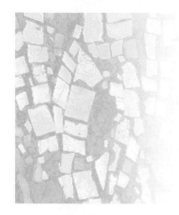

CHAPTER **6**

2-Week Visit

CANDACE F. ZICKLER

Breathing difficulties, 786.09	Poor feeding, 783.3
Decreased bowel movements, 564.00	Rash, 782.1
Irritability, 799.2	Reddened, draining umbilical site, 789.9
Jaundice, 782.4	Seizures, 780.39
Jaundice, newborn, 774.6	Vomiting, 787.03
No urine in 12 hours, 788.20	

I. General impression

A. Parents are settling in with 2-week-old; each getting acquainted with other.

B. Infant's cord should have fallen off or be about ready to fall off.

C. Jaundice should be resolved except in some breastfed infants.

D. Newborn screen results should be negative and hearing test should be passed.

E. Reflexes present are for rooting, Galant's (trunk incurvation), placing and stepping, Landau (infant lifts head when suspended in prone position), asymmetric tonic neck reflexes are present.

II. Nutrition

A. Breastfeeding is encouraged for all newborns. If breastfeeding, review all medications that mother may be taking (see Chapter 5).

1. Commercially prepared-iron fortified formulas come in powder, concentrate, ready-to-feed. Do not dilute ready-to-feed. Follow directions for mixing concentrate and powder.

2. Do not reuse bottle if over 4 hours since opened.

3. Mix formulas with bottled water for first month, continue to use bottled water if house is on well/unsure of water quality. Store mixed and open formula in refrigerator; refrigerate no longer than 24–36 hours. Specialized formulas have similar preparation directions; read labels. Goat's milk, whole cow's milk, rice milk have inadequate amounts of vitamins and minerals.

4. Serve formula at room temperature. Do not microwave to heat. Do not let formula sit out to warm for more than 15–20 minutes.
5. Clean technique is sufficient for mixing formulas. Clean off cans with soap and water before opening. Use hot soapy water and bottlebrush to clean nipples bottles or clean in dishwasher.
6. Hold infant in upright, semireclined position; burp every 1–2 ounces. No bottle propping.
7. No smoking or drinking hot beverages while holding baby.
8. Baby should take in 90% of feeding in first 20 minutes. 2-week old infant takes 3–5 ounces per feeding, 5–6 feedings per 24 hours (90–120 cal/kg/day).

III. Elimination
A. Bowel movements should be formed or soft with no green color. Infant should have 1–6 yellow pasty stools/24 hours. Breastfed infant may have upper range of frequency with less formed texture. Void every 1–3 hours or with each feeding and diaper change.

IV. Sleep
A. Awake and alert for feedings, every 2–4 hours. Should nurse vigorously for 15–20 minutes, then fall back to sleep.
B. Babies should sleep in own cribs, not with parents, to decrease smothering or injury. Babies should sleep on back or side in cribs to decrease incidence of sudden infant death syndrome (SIDS).

V. Growth and development
A. Growth.
   1. Should regain birth weight by 2 weeks. Should gain 0.5–1 ounce per day or approximately 2 pounds per month for next 5 months.
   2. Infant grows 1 inch, on average, per month for first 6 months.
   3. Head circumference increases 0.5 cm per month in first year.
B. Development.
   1. Moves all 4 extremities, keep hands fisted, and has flexed posture.
   2. Has startle response to noises.
   3. May have a smile. May begin to look for "who is talking."
   4. May have "fussy" time of 1–2 hours per day, oftentimes in evening.
   5. Should have some supervised, "tummy" play time.
   6. Do not mention colic unless parents indicate that crying is a problem/ worry for them.

VI. Social development
A. Babies have different cries, will fuss/cry 1–2 hours per day. Providing for infant's needs should stop the crying. Crying gradually decreases by 3 months of age.
B. Infant needs holding, touching, feeding, dry clean diaper, warm yet comfortable environment.
C. Discourage taking baby to public places or visiting relatives because no immunizations as yet. Ill adults should stay away from infant.
D. Encourage mother to rest when baby rests/sleeps.

VII. Immunizations (see Appendix A).
   A. If mother is HBsAg–, infant may not have received hepatitis B #1 in newborn nursery and will need to get it today or before 2 months of age. If infant received hepatitis B immunization in the nursery, he/she will need to get 4 immunizations.
   B. Infant should not have fever or fussiness from the immunization.

VIII. Safety/anticipatory guidance
   A. Sleep position "back to sleep."
      1. Not safe for baby to sleep in adult bed.
      2. Discuss room temperature (comfortable), amount of clothing to put on baby (not to overdress infant).
      3. No pillows/toys that baby could get face against and smother.
      4. Federal motor vehicle safety tested and approved car seat: installed properly in backseat, facing backward in automobile. Contact local hospital, fire department, or March of Dimes chapter for car seat rental programs.
   B. No smoking around infant.
   C. Reassure parents they cannot spoil infant at this age.
   D. Discuss sibling jealousy and possible regression of toddler.
   E. Discuss pet safety: do not leave infant unattended near pet.
   F. Discuss toys.
   G. Discuss what to look for when choosing babysitter or day care (e.g., handwashing, number of children, sick policy, feeding techniques).
   H. One-piece pacifiers only, discuss appropriate use of pacifiers, wean from pacifier when can sit up and spoon feed.
   I. No corn syrup (Karo) for constipation.
   J. No solids or extra water.
   K. Remind parents of when and how to call health care provider. Review call-in phone policy and explain hours that are best to call office.
      a. Breathing difficulties.
      b. Seizures.
      c. Irritability.
      d. Poor feeding, vomiting.
      e. No urine in 12 hours, black or decreased bowel movements.
      f. Reddened, draining umbilical site.
      g. Jaundice.
      h. Rash or pustules not present on discharge.
      i. Concerns.

BIBLIOGRAPHY

Crying in babies, retrieved from *www.AskDrSears.com* (click on "fussybabies").
FDA/CFSAN Infant Formula: Frequently asked questions, retrieved from *www.keepkidshealthy.com/nutrition/infant_formula_basics.html*.
Finn-Davis K, Parker KP, Montgomery GL: Sleep in infants and young children: part 1: normal sleep, *J Pediatr Health Care* 18 (2):65-71, March-April, 2004.

Hepatitis B immunization, retrieved from *www.cdc.gov/nip/acip.*

Newborn screening, retrieved from *www.modimes.org.*

Oral health care for infants, retrieved from *www.childhealthalert.com/Jan1999/pacifiers.*

Recommendations for car seat use, retrieved from *www.aap.org/family/carseatguide.htm.*

Scheers NJ, Rutherford GW, Kemp JS: Where should infants sleep? A comparison of risk for suffocation of infants sleeping in cribs, adult beds, and other sleeping locations: *Pediatrics* 112:883-889, October 2003.

Sudden infant death syndrome, retrieved from *www.sidscenter.org/SIDSWEB.HTM.*

Szilagyi PG: Assessing children: infancy through adolescence. In Bickley LS, Szilagyi PG, editors: *Bates' guide to physical examination and history taking,* ed 8, Philadelphia, 2003, Lippincott Williams & Wilkins.

Tien-Lan C, Kleinman RE: Standard and specialized enteral formulas. In Walker WA, Watkins JB, Duggan C: *Nutrition in pediatrics: basic science and clinical applications,* ed 3, Hamilton, Ontario, 2003, BC Decker.

Ziegler EE, Foman SJ, Carlson SJ: The term infant. In Walker WA, Watkins JB, Duggan C: *Nutrition in pediatrics: basic science and clinical applications,* ed 3, Hamilton, Ontario, 2003, BC Decker.

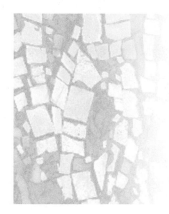

CHAPTER 7

1-Month Visit

CANDACE F. ZICKLER

Breathing difficulties, **786.09**	Poor feeding, **783.3**
Decreased bowel movements, **564.00**	Seizures, **780.39**
Irritability, **799.2**	Vomiting, **787.03**
No urine in 12 hours, **788.20**	

I. General impression

    A. Parents and infant should be settled into routine and more comfortable with each other.

II. Nutrition

    A. Mix formula with bottled water for first month, continue to use bottled water if house is on well/unsure of water quality. Have well water tested at local health department for small fee.

        1. Store ready-to-feed and open formula bottles in refrigerator. Refrigerate no longer than 24–36 hours.

        2. Specialized formulas have similar preparation directions; read labels. Goat's milk, whole cow's milk, rice milk have inadequate amounts of vitamins and minerals.

        3. Serve formula at room temperature. Do not microwave to heat. Do not let formula sit out to warm for more than 15–20 minutes.

    B. Clean technique is sufficient for mixing formulas.

        1. Clean off cans with soap and water before opening.

        2. Use hot soapy water and bottlebrush to clean nipples and bottles or clean in dishwasher.

    C. Hold infant in upright, semireclined position; burp every 1–2 ounces.

        1. No bottle propping.

        2. No smoking or drinking hot beverages while holding baby.

    D. 1-Month old infant will take 4–6 ounces per feeding and 5–6 feedings per 24 hours (90–120 cal/kg/day).

III. Elimination
A. Should have 1–6 yellow pasty stools/24 hours.
B. With each feeding, breastfed infant may have softer, formed/seedy stools.
C. Void every 1–3 hours or with each feeding.

IV. Sleep
A. Awake and alert for feedings, every 2–4 hours. Baby will suck vigorously for 15–20 minutes, then fall back to sleep.
B. Babies should sleep in own cribs, not with parents, to decrease risk of smothering or injury.
C. Babies should sleep on back or side in cribs to decrease risk of sudden infant death syndrome (SIDS).
D. No pillows/toys that baby could get face against and smother.

V. Growth and development
A. Growth.
   1. Should gain 0.5–1 ounce per day or approximately 2 pounds per month for next 4 months.
   2. Infant grows 1 inch, on average, per month for first 6 months.
   3. Head circumference increases 0.5 cm per month in first year.
B. Development.
   1. May be able to lift head off bed if on tummy.
   2. May have a smile.
   3. Responds to sounds of voices. May begin to look for "who is talking."
   4. Looks at faces when awake.
   5. Moves all 4 extremities, usually simultaneously.
   6. May cry but parents are learning what each cry means; crying ceases with needs being met. Cry gradually decreases by 3 months of age.
   7. May have "fussy" time of 1–2 hours per day, often in evening. Use "fussy" time as interaction time, not extra feeding.
   8. Should have some supervised, "tummy" play time each day.
   9. Baby may have symptoms of "colic" start around 2–3 weeks of age. Infant cries for prolonged periods, no specific cause or pathology identified. Infant requires additional comfort measures to quiet and settle.

VI. Social development
A. Parent should be assessed for sadness, depression, fatigue. Parent should show attentive, animated behavior toward baby. Listen carefully for frustration, potential for abuse/neglect.
B. Discourage taking baby to public places or visiting relatives because no immunizations as yet.
C. Encourage mother to rest when baby rests/sleeps.
D. Baby is learning to "trust" parent and caretakers.

VII. Immunizations (see Appendix A)
A. If mother is HBsAg⁻, infant may not have received hepatitis B #1 in newborn nursery or at 2-week visit. Will need to get it today.
B. Infants should not have fever or fussiness from immunization.

VIII. Safety/anticipatory guidance
    A. Sleep position "back to sleep."
        1. Not safe for baby to sleep in adult bed.
        2. Temperature of room comfortable.
        3. Amount of clothing needed to dress infant is discussed.
    B. Federal motor vehicle safety tested and approved car seat should be installed properly in backseat, facing backwards in automobile. Contact local hospital, fire department, or March of Dimes chapter for car seat rental program.
    C. No smoking around infant.
    D. One-piece pacifiers only.
    E. No corn syrup (Karo) for constipation.
    F. No solids or extra water.
    G. Remind parents of when and how to call the health care provider.
        a. Breathing difficulties.
        b. Seizures.
        c. Irritability.
        d. Poor feeding, vomiting.
        e. No urine in 12 hours, black or decreased bowel movements.

BIBLIOGRAPHY

Asch-Goodkin J: The 2004 immunization schedule: Small change and shorter shelf life. *Contemp Pediatr* 21(2):89-90, 93, 2004.

Dixon SD, Stein MT: *Encounters with children: pediatric behavior and development*, ed 3, St Louis, 2000, Mosby.

One month visit. In Green M, Palfrey J, editors: *Bright futures: guidelines for health supervision of infants, children, and adolescents*, ed 2 rev, Arlington, VA, 2002, National Center for Education in Maternal and Child Health.

www.aap.org/tippsafetysheets
www.AAPpolicy.org/infantsleepposition
www.cdc.gov/nip/acip/hepatitis
www.childhealthalert.com/April2002/infantbotulism
www.childhealthalert.com/Jan1999/pacifiers

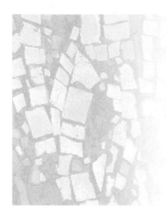

CHAPTER 8

2-Month Visit

CANDACE F. ZICKLER

Breathing difficulties, **786.09**	No urine output in 12 hours, **788.20**
Colic, **789.0**	Poor feeding, **783.3**
Decreased bowel movements, **564.00**	Seizures, **780.39**
Fever, **780.6**	Vomiting, **787.03**
Irritability, **799.2**	

I. General impression

   A. Parents should be enjoying their infant and taking joy from accomplishments.

   B. Infant is more responsive with smiling and cooing.

II. Nutrition

   A. 2-Month old infant will take 6–8 ounces per feeding, 4–6 feedings per 24 hours (94–130 cal/kg/day).

   B. Baby should take in 90% of feeding in first 20 minutes.

   C. Hold infant in semireclined position; burp every 1–2 ounces.

   D. Specialized formulas have similar preparation directions; read labels. Goat's milk, whole cow's milk, rice milk have inadequate amounts of vitamins and minerals.

   E. Serve formula at room temperature. Do not microwave to heat. Do not let formula sit out to warm for more than 15–20 minutes.

   F. Clean technique is sufficient for mixing formulas.

      1. Clean off cans with soap and water before opening.

      2. Use hot soapy water and bottlebrush to clean nipples and bottles or clean in dishwasher.

   G. No bottle propping.

   H. No smoking or drinking hot beverages while holding baby.

III. Elimination

   A. Should have 1–5 yellow pasty, but formed stools/24 hours.

   B. Breastfed babies may have more stools than bottle-fed babies.

   C. Void every 1–3 hours or with each feeding and diaper change.

IV. Sleep
  A. Babies sleep 16–18 hours per 24 hours. Infant is developing sleep pattern. May sleep through night. May have longer awake periods during day.
  B. Sleep cycles have both active and quiet sleep periods in equal proportions. Each sleep cycle lasts 50–60 minutes. Infants are less efficient with sleep and easily interrupted with noise. Should be alert for feedings, nurse vigorously for 15–20 minutes, then fall back to sleep/stay awake for short periods.
  C. Babies should sleep in own cribs, not with parents, to decrease smothering injury to infant.
    1. Babies should sleep on back or on side in cribs to decrease incidence of sudden infant death syndrome (SIDS).
    2. No pillows/toys that baby could get face against and smother.

V. Growth and development
  A. Growth.
    1. Babies should gain 0.5–0.75 ounce per day or approximately 2 pounds per month for next 5 months.
    2. Infant grows 1 inch, on average, per month for first 6 months.
    3. Head circumference increases 0.5 cm per month in first year.
  B. Development.
    1. Holds head upright for short periods. Follows people and looks for voice.
    2. Responds to smiling with return smile.
    3. Babbles and makes sounds with prompt of verbal cue.
    4. Shows interest in what is happening in room.
    5. Moves all 4 extremities, usually simultaneously.
    6. May cry but parents are learning what each cry means. Crying ceases when needs are met.

VI. Social development
  A. Baby learning to "trust" parent and caretakers to meet needs.
  B. Parent shows attentive and animated behavior toward baby. Family is settling in to routines with infant.
  C. Listen carefully for frustration, potential for abuse/neglect. Discuss child's unique temperament characteristics, relate to parents' feelings.
  D. Parent should be assessed for sadness, depression, fatigue.
    1. Encourage mother to rest when baby rests/sleeps.
    2. Encourage mother to take breaks away from baby to do self-nurturing (needs designated sitter).
  E. Take baby on selective, limited outings because infant is not fully immunized; will only receive first set today.
  F. Ask about plans for returning to work. Discuss guidelines for selecting sitter/day care.
  G. May have "fussy" time of 1–2 hours per day, often in evening. Use "fussy" time as interaction time, not extra feeding. Cry gradually decreases by 3 months of age.
  H. Baby may have symptoms of "colic" (starts 2–3 weeks of age, ceases by 12 weeks). Infant cries for prolonged periods, no specific cause or

pathology identified. Infant continues to grow well. Infant requires additional comfort measures to quiet and settle.

I. Should have some supervised, "tummy" play time while awake.

J. Encourage parent to actively talk, play with infant. Select age-appropriate toys.

VII. Immunizations (see Appendix A)

A. Infant will receive first set of immunizations today. Combinations are available that decrease number of injections. Need to discuss risks and benefits of immunizations and have parent sign consent. Required:
   1. Hepatitis B #1 or #2 (hepatitis B) depending if had #1 in nursery.
   2. DTaP #1 (diphtheria-tetanus-acellular pertussis).
   3. IPV #1 (inactivated poliovirus).
   4. Hib #1 (*Haemophilus influenzae* type b).
   5. PnC #1 (pneumococcal conjugate).

B. Infants should not have fever or constitutional symptoms from immunizations.

C. May give weight/age-appropriate dose of acetaminophen before immunizations and for 24 hours after administration.

VIII. Safety/anticipatory guidance

A. Needs safe sleep position "back to sleep."
   1. Not safe for baby to sleep in adult bed.
   2. Discuss temperature of room, temperature of water, bathing safety guidelines.
   3. Discuss appropriate amount of clothing to keep baby comfortable in varied environments.

B. Never leave baby unattended near pet or sibling.

C. Keep hand on baby when on changing tables, sofas, when risk of falling.

D. Review need for car seat that is federal motor vehicle safety tested and approved, installed properly in backseat, facing backward in automobile. Contact local hospital, fire department, or March of Dimes chapter for car seat rental program.

E. No smoking around infant.

F. Use only one-piece pacifiers and mention that weaning from pacifier begins when infant can sit up and begins finger feeding.

G. To treat constipation, advise giving extra water or dilute apple juice. No corn syrup (Karo) or honey.

H. No solids should be offered.

I. Make sure smoke detectors are installed and functioning in home. Home should have fire plan.

J. Limit sun exposure, use sunscreen with SPF rating of 15+ if out for even 30 minutes of direct sun exposure.

K. Baby will be seen for regular appointment again at 4 months. By then infant will be babbling more; will get second set of immunizations, similar to what baby had at this visit.

L. Remind parents of when and how to call the health care provider.
   a. Breathing difficulties.

    b. Seizures.

    c. Irritability.

    d. Poor feeding, vomiting.

    e. No urine output in 12 hours, black/decreased bowel movements.

    f. Any fever.

BIBLIOGRAPHY

Asch-Goodkin J: The 2004 immunization schedule: Small change and shorter shelf life. *Contemp Pediatr* 21 (2):89-90, 93, 2004.

Botulism in infants under one year of age, retrieved from *www.childhealthalert.com/ April,2002/infantbotulism.*

Dixon SD, Stein MT: *Encounters with children: pediatric behavior and development,* ed 3, St Louis, 2000, Mosby.

Finn-Davis K, Parker KP, Montgomery GL: Sleep in infants and young children: Part one: Normal sleep, *J Pediatr Health Care* 18 (2):65-71, March-April 2004.

Humiston SG, Judelsohn RG: A practical guide to using the new combination vaccines, *Contemp Pediatr* 20 (2):36-38, 43-46, 48, 50, 52, 2003.

National Fire Protection Association fact sheets, retrieved from *www.nfpa.org/Research/ NFPAFactsheets/Alarms.*

Shelov SP, Hanneman RE: *Caring for your baby and young child: birth to 5 years of age,* ed rev, Chicago, IL, 2004, American Academy of Pediatrics.

Two month visit. In Green M, Palfrey J, editors: *Bright futures: guidelines for health supervision of infants, children, and adolescents,* ed 2 rev, Arlington, VA, 2002, National Center for Education in Maternal and Child Health.

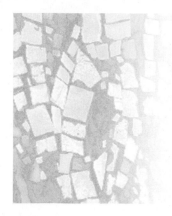

4-Month Visit

PATRICIA CLINTON

| Dehydration, 276.5 | Fever, 780.6 |
| Diarrhea, 787.91 | Vomiting, 787.03 |

I. General impression

A. 4-Month-old infant is generally well integrated into family unit, interacts with family members, is beginning to actively explore environment by making more purposeful movements.

B. Patterns of sleeping, eating, elimination are fairly well established.

II. Nutrition

A. Caloric needs: 98–108 kcal/kg/day.

B. Breastfeeding.
1. Recommended as sole source of nutrition.
2. Infant easily distractible.
3. Support mother in continuing to nurse.

C. Formula feeding.
1. Iron-fortified only.
2. No cow's milk of any kind.

D. Introduction of solids.
1. May begin after 4-month visit.
2. Introduce solids when tongue thrust diminishes, infant has good head control.
3. Introduce solids with spoon; do not put cereal in bottle.
4. Begin with iron-fortified rice cereal; prepare with either breast milk or formula.
5. Add new foods one at a time and start with 1–2 teaspoons.
6. Limit to cereal, vegetables, fruit initially.
7. Goal is to accustom infant to new textures and tastes.

III. Elimination

A. Voiding pattern.
1. Average 6–8 wet diapers/day.

　　　2. Illness (fever, vomiting, diarrhea) associated with decreased voiding and concerns of dehydration.

　B. Stooling pattern.

　　　1. Breastfed infants generally have 1 stool per day to 1 stool every 7–10 days.

　　　2. Consistency more important than frequency.

　　　3. Stools should be soft, semiformed, odor not offensive.

　　　4. Formula-fed infants generally have 1 or more stools per day, color varies by formula, may be more odiferous.

IV. Sleep

　A. Requirements.

　　　1. Nighttime 9–12 hours; may still waken for nighttime feedings.

　　　2. Naps 2–4 per day; 30 minutes to 2 hours.

　B. Environment.

　　　1. Begin to establish consistent bedtime routine.

　　　2. Put to bed drowsy but awake.

　　　3. Temperature should be temperate and not excessively warm.

　　　4. Transitional object such as blanket may be comforting.

　　　5. Room dim, may use night-light.

　　　6. Cosleeping is family/culturally determined; encourage discussion, avoid being judgmental; safety should be focus.

　　　7. Avoid bottles in bed.

　C. Safety.

　　　1. Put to bed on back. Once rolls over, infant determines position during sleep.

　　　2. Sleeping surface should be firm; avoid pillows, comforters. Slats $<2\frac{3}{8}$ inches apart; corner posts $<\frac{1}{16}$ inch high.

　　　3. Smoke-free environment.

　　　4. Remove mobiles, Venetian blind cords, other hanging toys before infant learns to pull up in crib.

V. Growth and development

　A. Growth.

　　　1. Infants should gain 0.5–1 ounce per day or about 2 pounds per month.

　　　2. Infants grow 1 inch, on average, per month.

　　　3. Head circumference increases 0.5 cm per month.

　B. Development.

　　　1. Grasps objects.

　　　2. Brings hands together.

　　　3. Follows objects with eyes to 180 degrees.

　　　4. Good head control. Lifts head and chest when prone.

　　　6. Bears weight on legs.

　　　7. Rolls from front to back.

　　　8. Rooting and palmar grasp disappear.

　　　9. Moro and tonic neck no longer as prominent, may disappear by 4 months.

10. Begins to link event with action such as quieting when put in nursing position.
11. Ability to wait begins to develop as infant learns to anticipate response from caregiver.
12. Cooing, laughing, squealing. Vocalizes in variety of ways to sustain interaction.
14. Beginning to listen when others speak.

VI. Social development
A. Relationships.
  1. Recognizes primary caregiver.
  2. Enjoys being cuddled.
B. Environment: conditions that foster trust, positive psychosocial feelings, development.
  1. Learning to trust caretakers.
  2. Smiles are purposeful.

VII. Immunizations (see Appendix A)
A. Review immunization schedule: DTaP #2, Hib #2, IPV #2, PCV #2, HepB #2 or 3.
B. Review immunization reactions.

VIII. Safety/anticipatory guidance
A. Always check bath water temperature.
B. Never leave infant alone in tub or on changing table.
C. Use sunscreen of SPF 15+ and avoid prolonged sun exposure.
D. Use car seat consistently. Never leave infant alone in car.
E. Avoid use of walkers.
F. Begin "baby proofing": outlet covers, door and drawer latches, safety gates. Remove cords, wires, string, plastic bags from baby's environment.
G. Maintain smoke-free environment.
H. If mother is returning to work, plan strategies for breastfeeding.
I. No honey or corn syrup (Karo). Use of cool mist vaporizers only.
J. Do not prop bottles. Do not put cereal in bottles.
K. Allow infant to self-regulate amount eaten: watch for cues, i.e., turning head away.
L. Secure infant in highchair. Never leave infant alone in highchair.
M. Encourage floor "tummy" time so infant can begin to explore surroundings.
N. Talk, read, sing to infant.
O. Use variety of toys/other household objects to stimulate infant. Introduce infant to different textures in toys, objects.
P. Discuss infant's temperament and how it relates to sleep/wake activities.
Q. Begin exploring parental ideas about discipline.
R. Cleanse gums with soft cloth after feeding.
S. Increased drooling indicates functional salivary glands, not teething.
T. Stress hand washing by all caregivers.
U. Review guidelines for calling health care provider, illness signs (i.e., fever, vomiting, diarrhea).

BIBLIOGRAPHY

Behrman RE, Kliegman RM: *Nelson essentials of pediatrics,* ed 4, Philadelphia, 2002, WB Saunders.

Burns CE et al: *Pediatric primary care: a handbook for nurse practitioners,* ed 3, Philadelphia, 2004, WB Saunders.

Colyar MR: *Well-child assessment for primary care providers,* Philadelphia, 2003, FA Davis.

Dixon SD, Stein MT: *Encounters with children: pediatric behavior and development,* St Louis, 2000, Mosby.

Fox J, editor: *Primary health care of infants, children, and adolescents,* ed 2, St Louis, 2002, Mosby.

Green M, Palfrey J, editors: *Bright futures: guidelines for health supervision of infants, children, and adolescents,* ed 2 rev, Arlington, VA, 2002, National Center for Education in Maternal and Child Health.

Mindell JA, Owens JA: *A clinical guide to pediatric sleep: diagnosis and management of sleep problems,* Philadelphia, 2003, Lippincott Williams & Wilkins.

Recommended childhood immunization schedule, United States, January-December 2004, *MMWR* 53:01, 2004.

Samour PQ, Helm KK, Lang CE: *Handbook of pediatric nutrition,* ed 2, Gaithersburg, MD, 2004, Aspen.

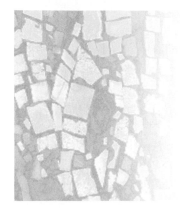

CHAPTER 10

6-Month Visit

PATRICIA CLINTON

Breathing difficulties, 786.09   Rash, 782.1
Irritability, 799.2   Seizures, 780.39
No urine output in 12 hours, 788.20

I. General impression
   A. 6-Month old infant is active, social person in family and with others although new people may be cause for some anxiety.
   B. Parents are comfortable in their role, look forward to infant's new achievements.

II. Nutrition
   A. Caloric and nutrient needs.
      1. 95–105 kcal/kg/day.
      2. Iron stores may not meet needs; encourage iron-fortified cereals and formulas.
      3. Nutrient needs cannot be generally met from breast milk or formula alone.
   B. Breastfeeding.
      1. Continue to encourage breastfeeding through first year.
   C. Formula feeding.
      1. Continue with iron-fortified formula.
      2. No cow's milk until after first birthday.
   D. Solid foods.
      1. Should be offering solid foods by 6 months.
      2. Progress from iron-fortified cereals to fruits and vegetables.
      3. Meat not added until later in first year.

III. Elimination
   A. Continues to have 6+ wet diapers per day.
   B. Stool consistency and color change with intake of solid foods.

IV. Sleep

    A. Should be sleeping through night; 9–12 hours.

    B. Naps in morning and afternoon from 30 minutes to 2 hours.

    C. Regular patterns are established although there may be occasional lapses. Continue to put to bed drowsy but awake. Encourage consistent bedtime rituals.

    D. Transitional objects continue to be important.

V. Growth and development

    A. Doubles birth weight between 5 and 6 months. Length increases ½ inch per month. Growth may occur in spurts; always plot.

    B. Anterior fontanel still open, no overriding sutures palpated.

    C. Grasps objects with hands. Rakes objects. Transfers objects between hands.

    D. "Plays" with objects: drops, shakes, bangs.

    E. Sits alone or with minimal support and no head lag.

    F. Rolls over both directions.

    G. Bears weight on legs.

    H. Moro and tonic neck reflex have disappeared.

    I. Responds to name.

    J. Babbles.

VI. Social development

    A. Enjoys interacting with parents.

    B. Expects that needs will be met and expresses frustration when they are not.

    C. May begin to show wariness of strangers.

    D. Begins to differentiate angry or friendly tone of others and respond accordingly.

VII. Immunizations (see Appendix A)

    A. DTaP #3.

    B. Hib (depending on which vaccine used).

    C. IPV #3.

    D. PCV #3.

VIII. Safety/anticipatory guidance

    A. Always check bath water temperature. Never leave infant alone in tub or on changing table.

    B. Use sunscreen of SPF 15+ and avoid prolonged sun exposure.

    C. Use car seat consistently. Never leave infant alone in car.

    D. Avoid use of walkers.

    E. Baby proof environment with outlet covers, door and drawer latches, safety gates. Remove cords, wires, string, or plastic bags from baby's environment. Avoid tablecloths; remove heavy/hot objects from tables that have tablecloths.

    F. Maintain smoke-free environment, ensure smoke alarms in baby's home.

    G. Do not leave alone in room with pets or siblings.

    H. Monitor for small objects or toys especially if other young children present.

I. Keep bathroom door closed, toilet lid down, remove buckets with water.
J. Use protective enclosures around swimming pools, hot tubs, other water sites (ponds, fountains).
K. Provide poison control number to be placed by telephone; syrup of ipecac no longer recommended.
L. Eating is social time; include infant in family meals. Introduce cup. As infant's pincer grasp develops, may offer finger foods.
M. Avoid allergenic foods until end of first year (strawberries, eggs).
N. Play games such as "peek-a-boo." Encourage reading activities with picture books, infant board books.
O. Treat teething discomfort with oral massage, frozen wet washcloths, other cold hard objects for chewing; acetaminophen or ibuprofen. Discourage use of numbing gels because of likelihood of numbing entire oral cavity, suppressing gag reflex.
P. Assess fluoride source, supplement as necessary (see Appendix B).
Q. Review illness symptoms and interventions.
R. Reinforce hand washing.
S. When to call health care provider:
   1. Breathing difficulties.
   2. Irritability.
   3. No urine output in 12 hours.
   4. Seizures.
   5. Rash.
   6. Concerns.

BIBLIOGRAPHY

Behrman RE, Kliegman RM: *Nelson essentials of pediatrics,* ed 4, Philadelphia, 2002, WB Saunders.
Burns CE et al: *Pediatric primary care: a handbook for nurse practitioners,* ed 3, Philadelphia, 2004, WB Saunders.
Colyar MR: *Well-child assessment for primary care providers,* Philadelphia, 2003, FA Davis.
Dixon SD, Stein MT: *Encounters with children: pediatric behavior and development,* St Louis, 2000, Mosby.
Fox J, editor: *Primary health care of infants, children, and adolescents,* ed 2, St Louis, 2002, Mosby.
Green M, Palfrey J, editors: *Bright futures: guidelines for health supervision of infants, children, and adolescents,* ed 2 rev, Arlington, VA, 2002, National Center for Education in Maternal and Child Health.
Recommendations for using fluoride to prevent and control dental caries in the United States, *MMWR* 50:RR-14, August 2001.
Recommended childhood immunization schedule, United States, January-December 2004, *MMWR* 53:01, 2004.

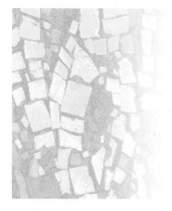

CHAPTER 11

9-Month Visit

PATRICIA CLINTON

Breathing difficulties, 786.09	Rash, 782.1
Irritability, 799.2	Seizures, 780.39
No urine output in 12 hours, 788.20	Separation anxiety, 309.21

I. General impression
  A. 9-Month-old infant is exploring, yet separating from parents is difficult.
  B. Rapidly gaining new motor/cognitive skills; 9-month-olds present new challenges to parents.

II. Nutrition
  A. Caloric needs: 98–100 kcal/kg/day.
  B. Breastfeeding/formula feeding.
    1. Infant receiving most nutrients from solid foods.
    2. Continue to encourage breastfeeding through first year.
    3. If using formula, continue with iron-fortified product.
    4. Avoid cow's milk until after first year.
  C. Assess for risk factors, screen for iron-deficiency anemia if necessary.
    1. Watch for use of cow's milk, low-iron formulas, low intake of iron-rich foods.
    2. Supplement as necessary (see Chapter 32).
  D. Solids.
    1. Infant should be eating table food with family.
    2. Finely chopped meats may be introduced.
    3. Finger foods appropriate at this time as fine pincer grasp has developed.
    4. Offer liquids from cup.
    5. Limit juice to 4–6 ounces per day.
    6. No honey or corn syrup (Karo) until after first year.

III. Elimination
  A. Voiding pattern.
    1. Stays dry for longer periods.
    2. Usually voids after naps.

63

   B. Stooling pattern.
      1. Stools usually firm, dark.
      2. Individual pattern established between 9 and 12 months.
      3. Generally 1–2 stools per day (but may vary considerably between infants).

IV. Sleep
   A. Requirements.
      1. Total sleep in 24 hours between 11 and 13 hours.
      2. Night awakenings common but should be able to put self back to sleep.
      3. Continues to nap in morning and afternoon.
   B. Environment.
      1. Bedtime rituals well established.
      2. Room should remain dim and not overly warm.
   C. Safety.
      1. Avoid bottles in bed.
      2. Lower crib mattress.
      3. Remind parents about removing blind or drapery cords, hanging objects, small objects in cribs.

V. Growth and development
   A. Physical.
      1. Growth is slower in second half of first year.
      2. Weight gains average 1 pound per month and length 1 inch per month.
      3. Growth should be steady but pattern may vary from early infancy; growth spurts more common.
   B. Motor.
      1. Fine.
         a. Pincer grasp developed. Able to pick up small objects.
         b. Begins to poke with index finger.
         c. Can drop, bang, throw objects.
         d. Can self-feed.
      2. Gross.
         a. Sits well.
         b. Creeping/crawling.
         c. May begin to pull up on furniture.
         d. Weight bearing when pulled to stand.
      3. Infant reflexes.
         a. Primitive reflexes should be absent.
         b. Parachute reflex emerges.
   C. Cognitive.
      1. Object permanence more prominently developed.
      2. May look for objects and go after them.
   D. Language.
      1. Combines syllables.
      2. Imitates speech sounds. Uses intonations.
      3. *Dada* and *mama* are nonspecific.
      4. Responds to name.

VI. Social development
A. Relationships.
 1. Beginning to indicate wants.
 2. May begin to wave bye-bye.
B. Environment: conditions that foster trust and development of positive psychosocial feelings. Separation anxiety emerges. Stranger anxiety apparent.

VII. Immunizations (see Appendix A)
A. No specific immunizations. Make up for missed immunizations.

VIII. Safety
A. Infant care activities.
 1. Always check bath water temperature.
 2. Never leave infant alone in tub, changing table, highchair.
 3. Use sunscreen; avoid prolonged sun exposure.
B. Environment
 1. Use car seat consistently.
 2. Never leave infant alone in car.
 3. Avoid use of walkers.
 4. Reinforce "baby proofing": outlet covers, door drawer latches, safety gates. Remove cords, wires, string, small objects, plastic bags from baby's environment.
 5. Keep sharp objects out of reach.
 6. Maintain smoke-free environment; use smoke alarms.
 7. Do not leave alone in room with pets or young children. Keep litter boxes away from infant's environment. Feed pets in area away from infant; do not allow infant near pet when eating.
 8. Avoid tablecloths or remove heavy/hot objects from tables with tablecloths.
 9. Keep toilet lid down, remove buckets with water.
 10. Use protective enclosures around swimming pools, hot tubs, other water sites (ponds, fountains).
 11. Provide poison control number (to be placed by telephone); syrup of ipecac no longer recommended.
 12. Keep houseplants out of reach; remove any poisonous plants.

IX. Anticipatory guidance
A. Nutrition.
 1. Stress importance of eating with family.
 2. Atmosphere should be relaxed, pleasant. Expect a mess!
 3. Avoid foods that may cause choking: grapes, raisins, peanuts/peanut butter, popcorn, hard candy, carrots, celery, other hard vegetables/fruits.
 4. Encourage infant to self-feed; provide infant with spoon.
 5. Watch for infant cues to signal satiation.
B. Parent–infant interaction.
 1. Continue to encourage floor time for infant to provide opportunities to explore.

2. Talk with infant while engaging in other activities (e.g., grocery shopping).
3. Continue singing and movement activities with infant. Play games such as "peek-a-boo."
4. Encourage reading activities with picture books, infant board books.
5. Discuss appropriate discipline measures aimed primarily at protecting infant from injury such as physical removal from danger, distraction, limited use of word "no." Begin to think about rules: keep them few and simple. Consistency is key to discipline.
6. Foster infant's ability to self-soothe with transitional objects such as blanket, stuffed toy.

C. Oral hygiene.
   1. No bottles in bed.
   2. Use soft toothbrush without toothpaste to clean teeth. Assess fluoride source and supplement as necessary (see Appendix B).

D. Illness prevention.
   1. Review illness symptoms/interventions.
   2. Reinforce importance of hand washing.
   3. Use cool mist vaporizer only.

E. When to call health care provider.
   1. Breathing difficulties.
   2. Seizures.
   3. Irritability.
   4. No urine output in 12 hours.
   5. Rash.
   6. Concerns.

BIBLIOGRAPHY

Behrman RE, Kliegman RM: *Nelson essentials of pediatrics,* ed 4, Philadelphia, 2002, WB Saunders.

Burns CE et al: *Pediatric primary care: a handbook for nurse practitioners,* ed 3, Philadelphia, 2004, WB Saunders.

Colyar MR: *Well-child assessment for primary care providers,* Philadelphia, 2003, FA Davis.

Dixon SD, Stein MT: *Encounters with children: pediatric behavior and development,* St Louis, 2000, Mosby.

Fox J, editor: *Primary health care of infants, children, and adolescents,* ed 2, St Louis, 2002, Mosby.

Green M, Palfrey J, editors: *Bright futures: guidelines for health supervision of infants, children, and adolescents,* ed 2 rev, Arlington, VA, 2002, National Center for Education in Maternal and Child Health.

Hay WW et al: *Current pediatric diagnosis and treatment,* New York, 2003, Lange/McGraw-Hill.

Meister K: *Feeding baby safely: facts, fads, and fallacies,* New York, 1997, ACSH Publications.

Mindell JA, Owens JA: *A clinical guide to pediatric sleep: diagnosis and management of sleep problems,* Philadelphia, 2003, Lippincott Williams, & Wilkins.

Recommended childhood immunization schedule, United States, January-December 2004, *MMWR* 53:01, 2004.

Recommendations for using fluoride to prevent and control dental caries in the United States, *MMWR* 50:RR-14, August 2001.

Samour PQ, Helm KK, Lang CE: *Handbook of pediatric nutrition,* ed 2, Gaithersburg, MD, 2004, Aspen.

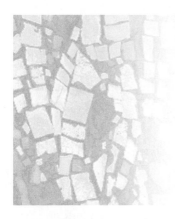

12-Month Visit

PATRICIA CLINTON

Anemia, 280.9	No urine output in 12 hours, **788.20**
Breathing difficulties, 786.09	Rash, **782.1**
Irritability, 799.2	Seizures, **780.39**

I. General impression
   A. 12-Month visit heralds onset of toddlerhood.
   B. Toddler's increasing mobility opens new worlds to explore and requires close supervision to prevent injuries.

II. Nutrition
   A. Caloric needs: 98–100 kcal/kg/day.
   B. Breastfeeding/formula feeding.
     1. Breastfeeding may continue, but toddler is getting majority of nutrients from table food.
     2. If formula feeding, discuss switching to whole cow's milk.
   C. Assess for risk factors, screen for iron-deficiency anemia if necessary.
     1. Birth weight <1500 grams, result of use of cow's milk or low-iron formulas during first year, low intake of iron-rich foods, low socioeconomic status.
     2. Supplement as necessary (see Chapter 32).
   D. Solids.
     1. Offer infant variety of foods from all food groups. Offer liquids from cup.
     2. Limit juice to 4–6 oz/day. Limit whole milk to 16–24 oz/day.

III. Elimination
   A. Voiding and stooling pattern.
     1. Regular patterns may be established but these continue to be involuntary.
     2. Discourage toilet training until closer to 24 months; toilet training dependent on complete myelinization of pyramidal tracts in spinal cord.

IV. Sleep
   A. Requirements.
     1. 12–13 Hours total/day.
     2. 1–2 Naps/day.

B. Environment.
   1. Continue bedtime rituals; consistency is key.
   2. Transitional objects continue to be important.
   3. Bedtime resistance and nightwakings are common.
   4. Avoid naps late in day that may interfere with nighttime sleeping.
C. Safety.
   1. Mattress should be in lowest position to prevent climbing out of crib.
   2. No bottles in bed.
   3. All cords, small objects, plastic bags, latex balloons removed.

V. Growth and development

A. Physical.
   1. Most toddlers will have tripled birth weight.
   2. Overall growth slows; typically will gain 3–3.5 kg (6–8 pounds) in next year and gain about 12 cm (5 inches) in length.
   3. Head circumference averages about 47 cm (18 inches); brain weight doubles its birth weight in first year.
B. Motor.
   1. Fine.
      a. Pincer grasp well developed.
      b. Puts block in cup.
   2. Gross.
      a. Stands alone for a few seconds. May take some free steps.
      b. Cruising around furniture.
C. Cognitive.
   1. Continues in Piaget's sensorimotor stage; actions more intentional.
   2. Increasing mobility fosters exploration of environment.
   3. Toddler observes other's actions, listens, touches/mouths objects.
D. Language.
   1. Uses 1–2 words.
   2. *Dada* and *mama* specific.
   3. Imitates sounds.
   4. Begins to respond to simple commands.
   5. Understands "no."

VI. Social development

A. Relationships.
   1. Anxious around strangers.
   2. Emotions emerge such as anger, affection.
B. Environment: conditions that foster trust and development of positive psychosocial feelings.
   1. Waves bye-bye.
   2. Plays games such as pat-a-cake.
   3. Indicates wants.
   4. Imitates activity of others.

VII. Immunizations (see Appendix A)

A. HepB #3 if necessary.

    B. Hib #4 between 12 and 18 months.

    C. IPV #3 if necessary.

    D. MMR between 12 and 15 months.

    E. Varicella at 12 months or after.

    F. PCV 12–15 months.

VIII. Safety

    A. Toddler care activities.

        1. Always check bath water temperature; make sure hot water thermostat <120°F (48.9°C).

        2. Never leave toddler alone in tub, changing table, highchair.

        3. Use sunscreen, avoid prolonged sun exposure.

    B. Environment.

        1. Switch to toddler car seat. Never leave toddler alone in car.

        2. Never leave toddler alone outside.

        3. Reexamine "baby proofing" from toddler walking perspective: outlet covers, door/drawer latches, safety gates. Remove cords, wires, string, small objects, plastic bags from toddler's environment.

        4. Climbing follows walking; anticipate dangers on counters, tables, stairs.

        5. Keep sharp objects out of reach.

        6. Maintain smoke-free environment; use smoke alarms.

        7. Do not leave alone in room with pets or young children. Feed pets in area away from toddler. Do not allow infant near pet when eating. Keep litter boxes away from toddler's environment.

        8. Avoid tablecloths or remove heavy or hot objects from tables with tablecloths.

        9. Keep toilet lid down, remove buckets with water.

      10. Protective enclosures around swimming pools, hot tubs, other water sites (ponds, fountains).

      11. Provide poison control number (to be placed by telephone). Syrup of ipecac no longer recommended.

      12. Keep houseplants out of reach; remove any poisonous plants.

IX. Anticipatory guidance

    A. Nutrition.

        1. Reinforce mealtime as family time.

        2. Three meals and 2 snacks per day appropriate; rule of thumb for serving size is 1 tablespoon per year.

        3. Toddler's attention span limits ability to sit for long periods.

        4. Foods should be chopped into small pieces. Avoid foods that may cause choking: grapes, raisins, peanuts, popcorn, raw vegetables.

        5. Limit juice to 4–6 ounces daily offered only in a cup.

        6. Encourage toddler to self-feed with spoon, cup.

        7. If breastfeeding, discuss interest in weaning to cup.

        8. If bottle feeding, weaning to cup should be started.

        9. Change from formula to whole cow's milk.

    10. Reassure parents that toddlers' eating patterns are inconsistent from meal to meal; think in terms of several days when reviewing recommended servings of foods.

B. Parent–toddler interaction.
   1. Continue to talk, sing, tell stories to toddler.
   2. Parent should make it a habit to describe what she/he is doing with toddler (e.g., this is how we put on socks).
   3. Play games such as naming things, body parts, people.
   4. Encourage reading activities with picture books, infant board books.
   5. Discuss appropriate discipline measures aimed primarily at protecting infant from injury such as physical removal from danger, distraction, limited use of word "no." Occasionally gentle physical restraint (holding toddler) may be necessary to prevent injury.
   6. Decide on a few important rules and be consistent about enforcing them.
   7. Limit TV to 1 hour or preferably less per day.
   8. Toddlers explore, this includes genital area.

C. Oral hygiene.
   1. No bottles in bed.
   2. Assess for bottle mouth caries.
   3. Use soft toothbrush, small pea size amount of fluoridated toothpaste. Assess fluoride source, supplement as necessary (see Appendix B).
   4. Make appointment for first dental visit.

D. Illness prevention.
   1. Review illness symptoms and interventions.
   2. Reinforce importance of immunizations.
   3. Reinforce importance of hand washing.
   4. Use only cool mist vaporizer in bedrooms.

E. When to call health care provider.
   1. Breathing difficulties.
   2. Seizures.
   3. Irritability.
   4. No urine output in 12 hours.
   5. Rash.
   6. Concerns.

BIBLIOGRAPHY

Behrman RE, Kliegman RM: *Nelson essentials of pediatrics,* ed 4, Philadelphia, 2002, WB Saunders.

Burns CE et al: *Pediatric primary care: a handbook for nurse practitioners,* ed 3, Philadelphia, 2004, WB Saunders.

Colyar MR: *Well-child assessment for primary care providers,* Philadelphia, 2003, FA Davis.

Dixon SD, Stein MT: *Encounters with children: pediatric behavior and development,* St Louis, 2000, Mosby.

Fox J, editor: *Primary health care of infants, children, and adolescents,* ed 2, St Louis, 2002, Mosby.

Green M, Palfrey J, editors: *Bright futures: guidelines for health supervision of infants, children, and adolescents,* ed 2 rev, Arlington, VA, 2002, National Center for Education in Maternal and Child Health.

Hay WW et al: *Current pediatric diagnosis and treatment,* New York, 2003, Lange/McGraw-Hill.

Meister K: *Feeding baby safely: facts, fads, and fallacies,* New York, 1997, ACSH Publications.

Mindell JA, Owens JA: *A clinical guide to pediatric sleep: diagnosis and management of sleep problems,* Philadelphia, 2003, Lippincott Williams, & Wilkins.

Recommended childhood immunization schedule, United States, January-December 2004, *MMWR* 53:01, 2004.

Recommendations for using fluoride to prevent and control dental caries in the United States, *MMWR* 50:RR-14, August 2001.

Samour PQ, Helm KK, Lang CE: *Handbook of pediatric nutrition,* ed 2, Gaithersburg, MD, 2004, Aspen.

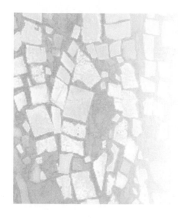

15- to 18-Month Visit

SUSAN G. RAINS

I. General impression
  A. Toddler is no longer an infant.
  B. World forever changed by new ability to move, explore, and control environment.

II. Nutrition
  A. Requirements.
    1. Growth slows in toddlerhood, decreasing energy needs to 102 kcal/kg/day, 1.2 g of protein/kg/day, fluids to 15 mL/kg/day; growth may average only 4½ lb/year.
    2. Servings should be 1 Tbsp of each food for each year of life or about ¼–⅓ of adult servings.
    3. Milk (whole milk until age 2) should be limited to <24 oz/day due to lack of iron and interference with intake of other nutrients.
    4. Limit fat to <30% of diet; protein to 15–20%, carbohydrates to 55%.
  B. Eating habits.
    1. Understanding toddlers.
      a. Lifelong eating habits, food preferences, activity level have roots in early self-feeding experiences.
      b. Able to recognize themselves as separate from others, need to explore independence by testing limits, including feeding limits.
      c. Recognize newness/difference of foods and also crave comfort of rituals.
    2. Promoting good habits.
      a. Eat meals as a family, without TV, at regularly scheduled times.

  b. Provide nutritious snacks 2–3 times per day, not as reward; limit sugar.
  c. Allow choices and experimentation, do not force.
  d. Allow toddler to self-feed with hands or utensils. Use cup, not bottle.
  e. Limit fruit juice to 4–6 oz/day.
  f. Serve appropriately sized portions, examples:
    • ½ Piece of fresh or ¼ cup canned fruit.
    • 2 Tbsp cooked vegetables.
    • 1 Tbsp smooth peanut butter (thinly spread on cracker or bread).
    • ½ Egg, 2 Tbsp ground meat.
    • ⅓ Cup yogurt, ½ cup milk.
    • 1–2 Crackers, ¼–½ slice of bread.
  3. Promoting safe eating.
    a. Sit when eating.
    b. Avoid screaming, fighting, tickling while eating.
    c. Avoid foods that can cause choking: popcorn, hot dogs/chunks of meat, globs of peanut butter with or without bread, seeds, nuts (or foods containing), hard candy/jelly beans, raw vegetables, whole grapes.

III. Elimination

  A. Attempting to toilet train child under 24 months of age is generally inadvisable.
    1. However, parents are encouraged to watch for signs of readiness:
      a. Child is dry at least 2 hours at a time during day or is dry after naps.
      b. Bowel movements become regular, predictable.
      c. Facial expressions, posture, words reveal child is about to urinate or have bowel movement.
      d. Child asks to wear grown-up underwear.
      e. Child asks to use the potty chair or toilet.
      f. Child seems uncomfortable with soiled diapers, wants to be changed.
      g. Child is able to follow simple directions.
      h. Child is able to walk to and from bathroom and help with undressing.
    2. Parents are encouraged to introduce children to "business" of toileting: allow child to observe older children/parents when appropriate; obtain potty chair, allow to sit on it; allow to flush toilet.
    3. Discourage parents from considering toilet training if child is under stress, such as new sibling arriving, moving houses, family crisis such as death, major illness, etc.

IV. Sleep

  A. Requirements.
    1. Averages 12 hours total/day.
    2. 1–2 Naps/day; may have difficulty combining morning and afternoon naps.
  B. Difficulty with sleep.
    1. Common, especially going to sleep and falling asleep.
    2. May be due to separation anxiety and independence issues.

C. Strategies to assist sleep.
 1. Bedtime rituals: standard sleep time, snack, quiet activity.
 2. Utilizing transitional objects such as special toy, blanket.
 3. Place child in bed while *awake.*
 4. Check on child at progressively longer intervals.
 5. Comfort, but do not feed, rock, place in bed with parent.
 6. Ideally, institute above strategies prior to child being able to climb out of crib.

V. Growth and development

A. Growth.
 1. Average increases in second year of life: weight, 5 lbs; height, 3 inches; occipital frontal circumference (OFC), 1 inch.
 2. Anterior fontanelle closes by 18 months.
 3. Head is smaller in proportion to body.
 4. Physique duck-like: lordotic, pot-bellied, bow-legged.
 5. Vision binocular (true strabismus should be referred).
 6. 14 Teeth on average by 18 months.
 7. Immune system much better developed, but passive immunities from mother gone (especially if not breastfed).

B. Development.
 1. Push and carry large objects.
 2. Put themselves into spaces such as boxes, cabinets, under tables.
 3. Delight in repetitive throwing and retrieving; scribbling. Handedness is established.
 4. By 15 months: says 3–6 words; can point to a body part; understands simple commands; walks well; stoops; climbs stairs; stacks 2 blocks; feeds self with fingers; drinks from cup; listens to story; tells what he/she wants by pulling, pointing, grunting.
 5. By 18 months: walks backwards; throws ball; says 15–20 words; imitate words; uses 2-word phrases; pulls a toy along the ground; stacks 3 blocks; uses a spoon and cup; listens to a story, looks at pictures and names objects; shows affection; kisses; follows simple directions; points to some body parts; scribbles.
 6. Understands much of language spoken to him/her, but commands very few words.
 7. Beginning to develop a memory.
 8. Starting to see objects symbolically.
 9. Imagination begins.

VI. Social development

A. Toddlers strive for independence (i.e., autonomy), looking for admiration/positive reinforcement of newly found skills.
B. Separation anxiety still present.
C. Beginning body image development.
D. Negativism is part of individualization.
E. May be becoming aware of gender.

F. Appropriate toys for toddler: swing sets, sandboxes, play kitchens, play tools, musical/talking toys (especially interactive ones), riding toys (especially without pedals), push toys, balls, containers, telephones, mirrors, dolls/puppets, large crayons, books.

G. Developmental delay. Possible referral if not present by 18 months:
  1. Walks upstairs with assistance.
  2. Self-feeds with spoon at times.
  3. Mimics actions of others.
  4. Uses at least 6 words.

H. Discipline.
  1. The toddler's new mobility and drive for autonomy make discipline challenging for parent/caregiver. Appropriate discipline guidelines include:
    a. Offering choices when available, including following a no with a yes.
    b. Keeping rules simple and few.
    c. Removing objects about which there is constant disagreement.
    d. "Catching the child being good," rewarding positive behaviors with verbal praise, physical affection.
    e. Time-out is not appropriate until 2½–3 years.
    f. Never spank a child <18 months due to increased risk of physical injury and child's inability to connect spanking and undesirable behavior.
  2. Parents should be encouraged to help child learn to express emotions such as joy, fear, anger, sadness, frustration.

VII. Immunizations (see Appendix A)
  A. Hib #4 (if not previously given).
  B. PCV #4.
  C. IPV #3.
  D. MMR #1 (if missed at 12 months, may be moved to 15 months to increase immunogenicity).
  E. Varivax (if missed at 12 months, may be moved to 15 months to increase immunogenicity).

VIII. Safety
  A. Motor vehicles.
    1. Use federally approved car seat in backseat of vehicle. May face forward if >1 year and >20 lbs.
    2. Never in front seat if airbag present.
  B. Poisoning.
    1. Childproof caps on medications; keep medications/household poisons (including plants) out of reach or locked.
    2. Keep poison control number readily available for all caregivers.
    3. Never tell children medication is candy.
  C. Burns.
    1. Use caution in kitchen when young children present.
    2. Turn handles of cooking utensils away from outer edge of stove.

3. Adjust hot water heater to <120°F.
4. Keep matches/candles out of reach.
5. Use sunscreen SPF 15+ when children are exposed to sunlight.
6. Keep sockets covered, cords out of sight.

E. Drowning.
1. Supervise closely near any water, including buckets.
2. Fence swimming pools.
3. Close bathroom doors and put lid down on toilet.
4. Utilize life preservers in addition to above.

F. Choking and suffocation.
1. Do not give danger foods listed in nutrition section (includes nuts, hot dogs, gum, hard candy).
2. Only allow play with appropriate-aged items (no small pieces).
3. Discard old appliances/furniture or remove doors.
4. Keep automatic garage door opener inaccessible.
5. Select safe toy chests without heavy, hinged lid.

G. Falls.
1. Confine play to fenced areas. Lock windows, screens, doors.
2. Supervise all climbing play.
3. Place gates at top and bottom of stairs.
4. Keep crib rails up and mattress at lowest level. Keep bumper pads, large stuffed animals out of crib or playpen (child may climb on top).
5. Dress in safe clothing that will not catch or drag.

H. Other injuries/dangers.
1. Never leave children alone in car or at home.
2. Do not allow play near any machinery.
3. Do not allow running with sharp objects or with anything in mouth.
4. Teach children to avoid strange animals, especially when eating.
5. Avoid personalized clothing in a public place.
6. Use safety glass and decals on large windows/doors.
7. Remove guns from house.

IX. Anticipatory guidance

A. Pediatric nurse practitioner's primary responsibility is to assist parents in understanding and parenting this emerging person—toddler's thoughts, behaviors, and needs—and attending to parents' needs.

B. Social competence.
1. Give individual attention; create opportunities for exploration, physical activity.
2. Encourage self-care, self-expression, choices.
3. Limit number of rules, but consistently enforce them.
4. Suggest acceptable alternatives.
5. Keep discipline brief.
6. Allow assertiveness within limits, but no hitting, biting, aggressive behavior.
7. Reassure once negative behavior has stopped.

   8. Delay toilet training.
   9. Expect genital curiosity.
C. Family relationships.
   1. Parent needs to take time for himself/herself and with partner.
   2. Pick up toddler, hold/cuddle, show affection. Help child express emotions.
   3. Listen; show respect and interest in activities.
   4. Encourage all family members to spend time playing with toddler. Keep family outings short.
   5. Do not expect child to share all toys. Help siblings resolve conflicts. Allow older children own space/things.
   6. Serve as role model for healthy habits and care.
D. Health promotion.
   1. Nutrition.
      a. Eat meals as family.
      b. Allow toddler to self-feed with hands, utensils. Drink from cup not bottle.
      c. Provide healthy choices, allow experimentation; do not force eating.
      d. Give 2–3 snacks per day, not as a reward; limit sugar.
      e. Avoid choking foods.
   2. Oral health.
      a. Never put baby to bed with a bottle.
      b. Brush teeth (allow imitation, but parent must do the job well). Investigate level of fluoride in child's water, supplement if necessary (see Appendix B).
      c. Encourage making appointment with dentist.
   3. Injury prevention (expanded list in safety section).
      a. Maintain smoke-free environment.
      b. Check smoke and carbon monoxide detectors.
      c. Check car seat use.
      d. Reexamine home to ensure it is childproof.
      e. Supervise toddler closely, especially near dogs, lawnmowers, streets/driveways.
      f. Ensure water safety.
      g. Use sunscreen.
      h. Discuss first aid procedures.
E. Community interaction.
   1. Assess needs of family for appropriate referrals: financial assistance, Medicaid, housing, transportation.
   2. Refer child for appropriate developmental, physical, behavioral problems.
   3. Refer parent to support group if appropriate.
   4. Review child care.
   5. Maintain community involvement by attending local activities.
F. When to call health care provider.
   1. Breathing difficulties.

2. Seizures.
3. Irritability.
4. No urine output in 12 hours.
5. Rash.
6. Concerns.

BIBLIOGRAPHY

American Academy of Pediatrics Committee on Injury, Violence, and Poison Prevention: Poison treatment in the home, *Pediatrics* 112:1182-5, 2003.

Burns C et al: *Pediatric primary care,* ed 3, Philadelphia, 2004, WB Saunders.

Centers for Disease Control and Prevention: Recommended childhood and adolescent immunization schedule, *MMWR* 52:Q1-4, 2003.

Fox J, editor: *Primary health care of infants, children, and adolescents,* ed 2, St Louis, 2002, Mosby.

Gottesman MM: Helping toddlers eat well, *J Pediatr Health Care* 16:92-96, 2002.

Gottesman MM: Nurturing the social and emotional development of children, a.k.a. discipline, *J Pediatr Health Care* 14:81-84, 2000.

Green M, Palfrey J, editors: *Bright futures: guidelines for health supervision of infants, children, and adolescents,* ed 2 rev, Arlington, VA, 2002, National Center for Education in Maternal and Child Health.

Green M et al: *Ambulatory pediatrics,* ed 5, Philadelphia, 1999, WB Saunders.

Haslam R: Screening scheme for developmental delay. In Behrman RE et al, editors: *Nelson textbook of pediatrics,* ed 17, Philadelphia, 2004, WB Saunders.

Reach out and read, 2004, retrieved from *www.reachoutandread.org* (for information in setting up literacy promotion programs in clinics and offices).

Vazquez M et al: Effectiveness over time of varicella vaccine, *JAMA* 291:851-855, 2004.

CHAPTER 14

2-Year Visit

FRANCES K. PORCHER

Breathing difficulties, 786.09

Fever, 780.6

No urine output in 12 hours, 788.20

Rashes, 782.1

Seizures, 780.39

Temper tantrums, 312.1

I. General impression

A. 2-Year-old is very active, has good vocabulary, and is integral part of family.

II. Nutrition

A. Quadruples birth weight by age 2 years.

B. Average 2-year-old weighs 12.5–13.5 kg (26–28 lb), is 85–90 cm (34–35 inches) tall, has head circumference of 48–50 cm (19–19½ inches).

C. Requires approximately 102 kcal/kg.

D. Needs approximately 1.2 g/kg of protein, 500–800 mg of calcium, 10 mg iron.

E. Fluoride supplement is necessary if water supply contains <0.3 ppm fluoridation (see Appendix B).

F. Requires 2–3 servings of protein, 2–4 servings of fruit, 3–5 servings of vegetables, 6–11 servings of grains, and 2 servings of milk each day.

G. Limit juice to 4–6 ounces per day. Offer skim, 1%, 2% milk versus whole milk.

H. Offer 5–6 smaller nutritious meal or snacks each day.

I. Start limiting fat intake to ≤30% of daily calories.

J. Child's serving is about ⅔ of a standard adult serving.

K. Needs structured mealtime environment.

L. Has unpredictable eating habits (likes one food one day but not next day).

M. Usually eats only 1–2 foods at meal.

N. Feeds self, loves finger foods.

O. Complete set of 20 primary teeth (second molars may not erupt until age 3 years).

P. Assess child's risk for hyperlipidemia.

III. Elimination

A. Regular elimination pattern is usually established with soft, formed stool daily or every other day and several urinations/day.

  B. Toilet training is major developmental task between ages $2\frac{1}{2}$ and $3\frac{1}{2}$ years.

  C. Ready for toilet training if bowel movements are regular; child interested in toileting.

IV. Sleep

  A. Should be able to sleep all night and maintain one day nap.

  B. Important to have pleasant bedtime routine.

  C. Not uncommon to experience nighttime sleep awakenings, bedtime difficulties.

  D. May sleep in crib or small bed depending on child's size, climbing skills.

V. Growth and development

  A. Age of autonomy, egocentrism, negativism.

  B. Gains $4\frac{1}{2}$–$6\frac{1}{2}$ pounds and $2\frac{1}{2}$–$3\frac{1}{2}$ inches per year from ages 2–5 years.

  C. Gross motor: runs without falling; kicks large ball; jumps; walks up/down stairs one step at a time.

  D. Fine motor: stacks 5–6 blocks; makes/imitates horizontal/circular strokes with crayon/large pencil; manipulates/solves single piece puzzle; can unravel, undo, untie.

  E. Language: 50% of speech is understandable by stranger; has at least a 20-word vocabulary; uses 2-word phrases; understands more than says; understands and uses "I" and "you"; clearly verbalizes wants; follows 2-step commands.

  F. Fears bodily harm (limit intrusive procedures, approaches).

  G. Increasingly independent, loves to explore.

  H. Negativity, temper tantrums often become an issue (hence, the "terrible twos").

  I. Time-out measures (no longer than 2 minutes per episode) recommended rather than hitting or spanking for discipline.

  J. Consistency with discipline measures important (discipline for same behavior tomorrow as today).

  K. Lots of love, reassurance needed.

VI. Social development

  A. Increasingly independent, curious (exploring, climbing, hiding).

  B. Active and delightful but testy and frustrating at times as child learns to become social.

  C. Frustration manifested as temper tantrums.

  D. Differentiates self from others but still needs frequent parental reassurance.

  E. Common to experience stranger anxiety (will hide head in parent's arms/behind legs).

  F. Engages in parallel play (plays alongside peers, not with them).

  G. Imitates adult activities/tasks (sweeping, dusting, shaving, combing hair).

  H. Often develops fears (fear of going down toilet with flushing).

  I. Needs positive behavior reinforced frequently (praise good behaviors).

VII. Immunizations (see Appendix A)

  A. Bring up to date.

    B. Consider varicella vaccine if no reliable history of disease or if not previously given.

    C. Consider hepatitis A vaccine if indicated by geographical area of residence.

    D. Consider tuberculin skin test (PPD) if meets risk criteria.

VIII. Safety

    A. Install and periodically check smoke alarms.

    B. Ensure crib slats are no more than $2\frac{3}{8}$ inches apart.

    C. Avoid crib mobiles due to risk of strangulation or choking.

    D. With small bed, ensure mattress is close to floor to minimize injury if child falls out of bed.

    E. Encourage use of potty chair that sits directly on floor rather than toilet.

    F. Remove dangling objects such as blind cords, curtain draws.

    G. Supervise play and do not allow toys with small or sharp parts.

    H. Supervise eating: do not allow foods that may lead to choking (popcorn, peanuts, marshmallows, wieners, raw vegetables).

    I. Use childproof lids on all medications, store medications in locked cabinet.

    J. Keep household cleaning products out of reach.

    K. Use gates and fences where appropriate to prevent falls.

    L. Supervise in kitchen (turn pot handles away from edge of stove, store knives out of sight).

    M. Supervise around water; set hot water thermostat to <120°F (48.9°C).

    N. Use child-approved sunscreen with at least SPF 15.

    O. Use child safety seats approved for child's weight at all times in motor vehicles. (If weighs at least 20 pounds, use forward-facing car seat in middle of backseat; never place car seat in front seat of vehicle with a passenger airbag.)

    P. Teach stranger safety.

IX. Anticipatory guidance

    A. Nutrition.

        1. Will eat variety of all food groups. Will eat larger servings.

        2. Still likes finger foods, but can use child-sized fork, spoon.

        3. Continues to drink skim, 1%, 2% milk (no more than 2–3 cups/day). Avoid flavored milk and soda.

        4. Encourage to drink water especially if playing outside in heat.

        5. Encourage to wash hands before eating.

        6. Brushes teeth with fluoridated toothpaste and parents' assistance.

        7. Needs dental check-up.

    B. Elimination.

        1. Daytime and nighttime bowel movement control established by age 3 years.

        2. Daytime urine control established by age 3 years. May still experience nighttime urination.

        3. Needs to be encouraged to wash hands after toileting and blowing nose.

C. Sleep.
   1. Continues to need regular bedtime routine.
   2. Needs 10–12 hours of sleep at night (does usually awaken).
   3. Usually continues to have one daytime nap.
   4. Should sleep in own bed.
   5. May experience nightmares.
D. Growth and development.
   1. Rate of growth slowing down.
   2. Gross motor: jumps in place, kicks ball, throws ball overhand, rides tricycle, climbs everything.
   3. Fine motor: copies circle and cross, dresses self, feeds self using small fork, washes and dries hands, can put on T-shirt, may be able to dress self without help.
   4. Language: at least 50% of speech is understandable, uses sentences, can carry on a conversation of 2–3 sentences, uses prepositions, may use adjectives, may be able to identify 4 colors, identifies friend by naming, identifies 4 pictures by naming, knows own name, age, gender.
E. Social.
   1. Parallel play still prevails; unlikely to share toys.
   2. Should not view more than 1 hour television/video per day.
   3. Needs daily physical activities (outdoors if possible).
   4. Curious about body parts, may start exploring (use correct terms for body parts).
   5. Needs positive reinforcement of good behaviors.
F. Safety.
   1. Needs supervision while playing, eating, when around water.
   2. Continues to need child safety seat or restraint appropriate to child's weight.
   3. May be able to learn own telephone number.
G. Immunizations: if current, should not need any until age 4 years.
H. When to call health care provider:
   1. Breathing difficulties.
   2. Seizures.
   3. No urine output in 12 hours.
   4. Rashes.
   5. Fever.
   6. Concerns.

BIBLIOGRAPHY

Green M, Palfrey J, editors: *Bright futures: guidelines for health supervision of infants, children, and adolescents*, ed 2 rev, Arlington, VA, 2002, National Center for Education in Maternal and Child Health.

Story M, Holt K, Sofka D, editors: *Bright futures in practice: nutrition*, ed 2, Arlington, VA, 2002, National Center for Education in Maternal and Child Health.

3-Year Visit (Preschool)

BETSY ATKINSON JOYCE

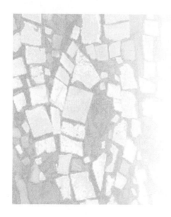

I. General impression

A. Preschooler can behave one moment and want to please the parent, but can also be unreasonable and resistant to being examined.

B. Pay attention to evidence of tooth cavities, eye alignment, evidence of bruising or other injuries that may indicate neglect, inadequate supervision, or abuse.

II. Nutrition

A. Needs 1000–1100 calories per day or 100 cal/kg/day.

B. 3 Small meals, 2 snacks, 16–24 ounces of milk.

C. 7 Grains, 3 vegetables, 2 fruits, 2 meats.

D. Eats with a fork or spoon.

III. Elimination

A. Toilet trained for daytime, occasional accidents.

B. Regular pattern for bowel movements.

IV. Sleep

A. Requires 10–12 hours of sleep a night.

B. 1 Nap/day (usually).

C. Arouses several times a night.

D. May have night terrors or nightmares.

   1. Night terrors: occur early after going to bed.

      a. Partial arousal from very deep sleep, screams, thrashes during the terror, returns to sleep without fully awakening.

      b. Will have no memory of incident in morning.

   2. Nightmares: occur usually during the second half of night.

      a. Scary dream followed by complete awakening, crying and fearful after awakening; parent should reassure child.

   b. May have trouble falling back to sleep.

   c. Remembers and may talk about it in the morning.

V. Growth and development

   A. Continues to follow individual growth chart curve.

   B. Pelvis straightens.

   C. Graceful and agile with good posture.

   D. Physical.

   1. Height: grow 2–4 inches per year.

   2. Weight: gain 4–6 pounds.

   3. Head: grows about 1 inch per year.

   4. Blood pressure averages 100/60.

   5. Heart rate range is 73–137.

   6. 20 Primary teeth; growth is mainly under the gums.

   E. Gross motor.

   1. Alternates feet when going up stairs.

   2. Rides tricycle.

   3. Dresses self, may need help with buttons.

   4. Puts on shoes.

   5. Climbs, jumps, hops.

   F. Fine motor.

   1. Holds crayon with fingers.

   2. Copies circle and cross.

   G. Language.

   1. Approximately 900 words by age 3; up to 1500 by age 4.

   2. 85–90% of speech understandable by people outside the family.

   3. Knows name, gender, age.

   4. Longer sentences.

   5. Uses plurals, pronouns, some prepositions (under, on, in, out).

   6. Understands concepts of big/little, up/down.

   7. Can tell you some colors.

VI. Social development

   A. Can separate easily from parents if they want to.

   B. Can take turns.

   C. Helps with simple chores.

   D. Needs other children to play with in order to learn socialization.

   E. Discipline method: continue with time-out.

VII. Immunizations (see Appendix A)

   A. No scheduled immunizations at this visit.

   B. Check for currency, only need if immunizations were delayed.

VIII. Safety/anticipatory guidance

   A. Share meals as family if possible, but otherwise child should eat first and get down from table.

   B. Do not get in food fights. Offer food; if does not eat, child gets down and no food or milk until next meal.

C. Improve (if necessary) nutritional quality of meals and snacks; limit fast food to less than once a week.
D. Promote toilet training if not already accomplished.
E. Limit TV viewing to 1–2 hours/day.
F. Promote active play. Indoors: have imagination station with safe active toys; outdoor: play with balls, jump ropes, games, etc.
G. Consistent discipline: use as a way to learn rules, not just punishment; set limits because if child knows limits, she/he can relax.
H. Find ways to praise child.
I. Encourage choices; link with consequences.
J. Realize need for constant vigilance, supervision, patience.
K. Safety-proof house (if not already done); reinforce safety issues.
L. Use car seat.
M. Practice water safety.
N. Use sunscreen of SPF 15 or higher.
O. Wear helmet when riding tricycles, scooters, or other toys with wheels.
P. Teach gun safety. Keep guns out of reach, locked, unloaded. Store ammunition and guns separately.
Q. Teach about "good touch/bad touch."

BIBLIOGRAPHY

Burns CE et al: *Pediatric primary care: a handbook for nurse practitioners,* ed 3, Philadelphia, 2004, WB Saunders.
Dixon SD, Stein MT: *Encounters with children: pediatric behavior and development,* St Louis, 2000, Mosby.
Green M, Palfrey J, editors: *Bright futures: guidelines for health supervision of infants, children, and adolescents,* ed 2 rev, Arlington, VA, 2002, National Center for Education in Maternal and Child Health.
Hoekelman R, editor: *Primary pediatric care,* ed 4, St Louis, 2001, Mosby.
Robinson D, Kidd P, Rogers K: *Primary care across the lifespan,* St. Louis, 2000, Mosby.
Sothern, MS: Putting research into practice, *J Pediatr Nutr Develop* 104, Fall 2002.

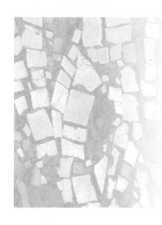

CHAPTER 16

6-Year Visit (School Readiness)

PAMELA MEADOR NICKELL

ADD, 314.00
ADHD, 314.01
Behavioral problems, 312.9
Bowel incontinence, 787.6
Emotional immaturity 300.9

Night terrors, 307.46
Nightmares, 307.47
School phobia, 300.23
Urinary incontinence, 788.39

I. General impression
   A. 6-Year-old will be attending school perhaps for first time and is quite excited about it and is becoming much more independent.

II. Nutrition
   A. Caloric and nutrient needs.
      1. 90 kcal/kg/day divided into 3 meals with 2 nutritious snacks.
      2. Limit junk food, nonnutritious foods.
      3. Refer to Food Guide Pyramid plus for serving size, food group recommendations (see Appendix E).
      4. Encourage family meals as often as possible.
   B. Oral hygiene.
      1. Semiannual dental visits.
      2. Regular tooth brushing twice/day.
      3. Fluoride supplement in diet or drinking water (see Appendix B).
      4. Discourage thumb sucking.

III. Elimination
   A. Most 6-year-olds are toilet trained but may have occasional accidents.
   B. Frequency of bowel movements varies. Obtain parental input for what is normal for child; 1–3 times/day to 1 time every 2–3 days is acceptable.
   C. Normal urine volume should be similar to adult: 650–1500 mL/day.
   D. Urination frequency approximately 5–6 times/day.
   E. Approximately 5–7% have problematic enuresis.
   F. Occasional incontinence due to miscues/deep sleep not uncommon.

IV. Sleep
   A. 8–12 Hours/night.
   B. Encourage consistent bedtime routine.
   C. Occasional nightmares are normal.
   D. Night terrors/sleepwalking may emerge.
V. Growth and development
   A. Average weight gain per year: 1.8–2.7 kg (4–6 lbs) for both boys and girls.
   B. Average linear growth per year: 5 cm for both boys and girls.
   C. Well-established vocabulary.
   D. Can follow 3-step directions.
   E. Moving from magical thinking to concrete operations.
   F. Mastered skills.
      1. Personal.
         a. Independent in dressing, hygiene; feeds self, monitoring only as needed.
         b. Can recite address, phone number.
      2. Fine motor.
         a. Can draw/copy shapes.
         b. Can draw a man with 6 parts.
         c. Can print some letters, numbers.
      3. Language.
         a. Can articulate needs but semantics may be incorrect.
         b. Recognizes most letters of alphabet.
         c. Can define at least 7 words.
         d. Can identify some opposites.
      4. Gross motor.
         a. Can balance each foot for 6 seconds.
         b. Can heel-toe walk forward and backward.
         c. Rides tricycle without problems.
VI. Social development
   A. The child is beginning to move from family relationships as primary focus to peer relationships as primary focus.
   B. Continues to use play to develop skills competencies and learn about his world.
   C. Social cooperation, morality, critical thinking, and self-concept are developing.
   D. Demonstrates cooperative play.
   E. Team/group activities encouraged (arts programs, organized clubs/sports, etc.); regular exercise encouraged.
   F. Making friends is primary social goal; developing "best friends."
   G. Developing conflict resolution skills.
VII. Immunizations (see Appendix A)
   A. Recommended.
      1. DTaP #5 if not done previously.
      2. IPV #4 if not done previously.
      3. MMR #2 if not done previously.

        4. PPD #1 if not done previously.

        5. Influenza annually.

    B. Catch-up.

        1. Hepatitis B series.

        2. Varicella.

        3. Pneumococcal vaccine.

    C. High-risk children.

        1. Influenza (yearly).

        2. Hepatitis A series.

        3. Pneumococcal pneumonia vaccine.

        4. PPD (yearly).

VIII. Safety

    A. Motor vehicle.

        1. Consistent use of appropriate safety restraints in motor vehicles.

        2. Knows appropriate pedestrian safety rules.

        3. Consistent helmet use when passenger on motorcycle. Riding a motorcycle is discouraged.

    B. Sports/recreation.

        1. Consistent use of appropriate protective equipment for all activities (biking, roller-blading, sports, boating, etc.).

        2. Ensure appropriate safety instruction provided for all activities.

        3. Obtain swim lessons.

        4. Ensure safety of sports/play areas and proper supervision provided.

        5. Use sunscreen of SPF 15 or higher.

        6. Discourage use of mini-bikes and ATVs.

    C. Household.

        1. Never leave child without appropriate supervision.

        2. Teach appliance safety and monitor use.

        3. Teach hazardous materials safety. Keep out of reach and monitor use.

        4. Teach fire safety. Develop family plan.

        5. Teach gun safety. Keep guns out of reach, locked, unloaded. Store ammunition and guns separately.

    D. Social.

        1. Teach phone number, address.

        2. Teach use of 911.

        3. Teach stranger safety.

        4. Teach about "good touch/bad touch."

IX. Anticipatory guidance

    A. Preventive care.

        1. Annual physical.

        2. Twice/year dental visits.

        3. Immunizations on schedule.

    B. Home.

        1. Establish family rules and remain consistent in enforcement.

        2. Avoid corporal punishment for breaking rules.

      3. Limit TV viewing to 1 hour/day.
      4. Enforce good personal hygiene.
      5. Avoid punishment for urinary or bowel incontinence.
      6. Encourage family meals.
      7. Encourage continued reading to and with child.
      8. If parents work, ensure appropriate, safe supervision is provided before and after school.
      9. Encourage responsibility for age-appropriate chores.
    10. Develop fire safety plan for home.

  C. Family/community.
      1. Encourage and praise school activity, accomplishments.
      2. Encourage socialization with peer groups in organized and unorganized activities.
      3. Encourage consistent exercise; ensure proper supervision provided with all activities.
      4. Discourage "hurried child syndrome"; no more than 1–2 activities/week.
      5. Reinforce school/bus rules; encourage parents to become actively involved in school/community parent groups.
      6. Encourage parents to teach/model moral behavior, good citizenship ("Do unto others as you would have them do unto you").

  D. Safety.
      1. Ensure proper motor vehicle restraints consistently used.
      2. Encourage swim lessons.
      3. Reinforce proper bicycle use, rules, and use of helmet.
      4. Reinforce use of proper safety equipment for all activities including sunscreen SPF 15 or higher applied 30 minutes before going outdoors.
      5. Reinforce proper pedestrian rules.
      6. Reinforce proper gun safety and storing of ammunition separately.
      7. Reinforce "good touch/bad touch" concepts.
      8. Teach "just say no" concepts.
      9. Reinforce how to use telephone to call 911 in an emergency.
    10. Ensure child knows address and phone number.
    11. Reinforce age-appropriate child-proofing in residence and use of smoke detectors.
    12. Reinforce fire safety; ensure family has plan for evacuation.
    13. Don't leave child without proper supervision.
    14. Discourage mini-bike and ATV use.

X. School readiness
  A. Physical readiness.
      1. Has met developmental milestones in cognitive, gross and fine motor areas.
      2. Cognitive, visual, hearing deficits addressed.
  B. Emotional readiness.
      1. Able to separate easily from parent.
      2. Dresses without supervision.

3. Toilet trained.
4. Follows instructions.
C. Screening and assessment tools.
1. Physical exam including full neurologic evaluation.
2. Vision and hearing screening.
3. Developmental testing (draw a man and Denver II recommended for ease of administration).
D. Anticipatory guidance.
1. Encourage and reinforce positive parental attitudes regarding school.
2. Prepare parent and child for separation, change in routine.
3. Have parent obtain list of school/classroom rules and review.
4. Tour school and meet teacher prior to first day of school.
5. Prepare parent for child's potential fear/anxiety.
6. Prepare family to advocate for child in positive, supportive manner.
E. Potential concerns.
1. School phobia.
2. Lack of expected intellectual ability/progress.
3. ADD/ADHD.
4. Emotional immaturity.
5. Behavioral problems related to classroom.

BIBLIOGRAPHY

Burns CE et al: *Pediatric primary care: a handbook for nurse practitioners,* ed 3, Philadelphia, 2004, WB Saunders.

Burns CE et al: *Pocket reference for pediatric primary care,* Philadelphia, 2001, WB Saunders.

Dixon SD, Stein MT: *Encounters with children: pediatric behavior and development,* St Louis, 2000, Mosby.

Green M, Palfrey J, editors: *Bright futures: guidelines for health supervision of infants, children, and adolescents,* ed 2 rev, Arlington, VA, 2002, National Center for Education in Maternal and Child Health.

Pulcini J: Assessing school readiness. In Fox J, editor: *Pediatric health care of infants, children adolescents,* ed 2, St Louis, 2002, Mosby.

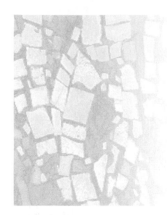

CHAPTER 17

7- to 10-Year Visit (School Age)

ELIZABETH GODFREY TERRY

I. Overall impression

    A. Early school-agers are in routine of being in school, learning; now gaining skills to get along with many different personalities.

II. Nutrition

    A. 3 Full meals and 2–3 snacks a day.

    B. Willing to try variety of foods from major food groups.

    C. Appetite varies according to growth, activity.

    D. May have big appetite during growth spurt and then cut back.

    E. Good internal cues regarding appetite.

F. Beginning steps toward obesity may start if child is not allowed to listen to internal cues.

G. About 15% of 6- to 11-year-old children are obese.

H. Consumes 1600–2400 calories per day:
1. Bread, cereal, pasta: 6–11 servings.
2. Fruits: 2–4 servings, $1/2$ cup of sliced fruit, medium-size whole fruit.
3. Dairy: 2–3 servings/day; 1 cup low-fat milk or yogurt, or $1^1/2$ ounces cheese.
4. Protein foods: 2–3 servings; 2–3 ounces cooked lean meat, poultry, or fish.
5. Vegetables: 3–5 servings.

I. Daily children's multivitamin if child is not consuming enough servings to get essential nutrients.

III. Elimination
A. Enuresis occurs in 10% of 6-year-olds, 5% of 10-year-olds, 3% of 12-year-olds.
1. Children with this condition should receive complete exam to rule out underlying conditions such as urinary tract infections.
2. Children with sleep apnea at greater risk for enuresis.
B. Encopresis affects 1.5% of young school children.

IV. Sleep
A. Need 10–11 hours per night.
B. Occasional nightmares or sleep disturbances such as night terrors, sleepwalking.
C. May have fear of dark or of being alone (separation anxiety).
D. Emotional disturbances such as stress, anxiety leading to insomnia.
E. Difficult bedtime behavior may develop.

V. Growth and development
A. Musculoskeletal.
1. Development not as rapid.
2. As body size increases, body fat relatively stable, giving slimmer appearance than preschool years.
3. Average height increase: a little over 2 inches per year.
4. The closer to puberty, greater the chances for increased growth.
5. Tends to be an increased growth rate between 6 and 8 years of age that may be accompanied by appearance of small amount of pubic hair.
6. If unusually short/tall for age, may need to consider possibility of growth disorder.
7. Appetite tends to vary due to growth fluctuations, but child should not be losing weight.
8. Orthopedic problems of this age group:
   a. Fractures, sprains, strains.
   b. Epiphyseal separations, dislocations.
   c. Scoliosis.
   d. Avascular necrosing lesions of epiphysis.
      • Legg-Perthes disease.
      • Osgood-Schlatter disease.
9. Motor skills improve in strength, balance, coordination.

B. Skin.
   1. Hair may become little darker, skin becomes more adult like.
   2. Scabies, impetigo, ringworm can be problems at this age.
C. Teeth.
   1. Should be able to brush teeth by themselves, may still require some assistance.
   2. Brush with fluoride toothpaste after each meal but at least twice a day; floss once a day.
   3. Water supply should contain adequate fluoride, if not, consider fluoride supplement (see Appendix B).
   4. Eruption of permanent teeth occurs in order in which primary teeth are lost.
   5. Dental visits twice a year for exams, cleanings.
   6. Sealants as recommended.
   7. Problems with dental decay can peak during these years as well as periodontal diseases, often due to poor hygiene.
D. Eyes: visual acuity of 20/20 although about age 8 may begin to have myopia with no overt signs except school difficulty.
   1. Annual eye screening exam by health care provider or eye specialist is recommended.
   2. Children who have difficulty learning to read despite passing standard vision screenings should be referred to reading specialists such as educational psychologists for language-processing-disorder evaluation.
E. Ears: problems decrease due to further development of eustachian tubes and nasopharynx, although ear infections can still be frequent in younger school-ager.
   1. Consider hearing screening if history of frequent ear infections or concerns about speech development.
F. Throat: tonsillar tissue continues to enlarge, reaching its peak from 8–12 years when it levels off, begins to recess.
G. Immune system: continues to mature; allergic conditions more common.
H. Hematopoietic system: abnormal hemoglobin/hematocrit levels should not be attributed to dietary intake. Etiology should be established for any hemoglobin below 11.5 g.
I. Heart.
   1. Murmurs are often heard in these years.
   2. Any doubt of etiology requires referral to pediatric cardiologist.
   3. Circulation.
      a. Average pulse rate:
         • Age 8: 78.
         • Age 10: 74.
      b. Average blood pressure:
         • Age 8: 105/60.
         • Age 10: 111/66.

J. Respiration rate.
   1. Age 8: 22 breaths/minute.
   2. Age 10: 20 breaths/minute.
K. Gastrointestinal system.
   1. Liver function is mature but still growing in size.
   2. Appendix: open lumen and increased size increases risk of blockage, inflammatory reaction (appendicitis).
L. Genitourinary system.
   1. Urinary tract infections can be common, especially in girls; often asymptomatic at this age.
M. Nervous system: essentially mature by age 10.
   1. Begins puberty.
      a. Girls.
         • Breast budding can begin as early as age 8; others not until 13, with the average being around age 10.
         • Puberty before age 8: girl should be evaluated for precocious puberty (twice as frequent in females as in males).
         • Peak growth period (height, weight, muscle mass, etc.) occurs 1 year after puberty has begun.
         • Menstruation usually begins 2 years after onset of puberty, on average just before age 13.
      b. Boys.
         • Peak growth period occurs about 2 years after onset of puberty.
         • Begins puberty about 1 year later than girls.
         • First sign of puberty in boys is enlargement of testes, thinning and reddening of scrotum. This occurs on average at age 11, but may occur anytime between 9 and 14 years of age.
         • Puberty before 9: boy should be evaluated for precocious puberty.
   2. Secondary sex characteristics.
      a. Girls.
         • Breast enlargement: 8–13 years.
         • Axillary hair: 11–13 years.
         • Pubic hair: 10–12 years.
         • Menarche: 10–16 years.
      b. Boys.
         • Genitalia enlargement: 9–13 years.
         • Axillary hair: 12–14 years.
         • Facial hair: 11–14 years.
         • Pubic hair: 12–15 years.
N. Language.
   1. Although better able to express emotions and ideas, may talk in abstract terms without fully comprehending meaning of such speech.
   2. Learning to communicate clearly with friends.
VI. Social development
A. Needs to master balance of feelings in dealing with successes, failures.

      1. Self-concept (body self, social self, cognitive self) affects child's ability to be successful.

  B. Successful accomplishments are of high priority for child in order to build positive self-image. Should feel successful with most day-to-day skills, activities.

  C. Making friends is one of most important mid-childhood tasks.

      1. Average number of friends: about 5.

      2. Sibling friendships may replace outside friends or need for them.

      3. Selects friends of similar temperament, interests.

      4. Often focus on "best friend" relationship, which can be more satisfying than large group.

  D. Increasingly seeks peer for companionship.

  E. Cliques may begin to form.

  F. Parents and teachers are important significant others and will influence behavior, self-concept.

  G. School issues.

      1. School phobia.

      2. Learning disorders.

      3. Attention deficit hyperactivity disorder.

VII. Immunizations (see Appendix A)

  A. Influenza vaccine.

      1. Annual fall flu shots are recommended for children ≥6 months of age.

      2. Especially recommended for children with chronic or immune disorders such as asthma, cystic fibrosis, heart disease, sickle cell anemia.

      3. Live-attenuated influenza vaccine, such as found in Flumist nasal form, is acceptable alternative to inactivated influenza vaccine for healthy persons 5–49 years of age.

  B. Varicella vaccine: children ≤13 who have not had chickenpox and who were never vaccinated should have single dose of vaccine.

  C. Measles, mumps, rubella (MMR): second dose recommended routinely at 4–6 years, may be given during any visit if at least 4 weeks passed since first dose and both doses given beginning at/after 12 months of age. Second dose should be completed by 11–12 years of age.

  D. Hepatitis A vaccine: recommended for children in selected states, regions and in high-risk groups; can begin vaccine at any visit with the 2 doses being given at least 6 months apart.

VIII. Safety/anticipatory guidance

  A. Nutrition.

      1. Need at least 800–1200 mg of calcium/day.

      2. Child may need multivitamin if not eating enough to get essential nutrients.

      3. Some children may still be picky eaters at this age; may eat more at snack times than at regular meals.

    4. Healthy snacks 1–2 times a day can include:
      a. Fresh, canned, frozen vegetables or fruits.
      b. Low-fat yogurt or cheese, low-fat string cheese.
      c. Air-popped popcorn.
      d. Baked tortillas or pretzels with salsa.
      e. Low-fat chocolate milk.
      f. Frozen yogurt, fruit sorbet, fruit juice bars, Popsicles.
      g. Whole-grain crackers, bread.
      h. Whole-grain cereals with low-fat/skim milk.
    5. No snacking in front of TV.
    6. Stress importance of offering variety of nutritious foods of all types; if child sees parent eating variety of nutritious foods, more likely to want them.

B. Sleep.
    1. Stay consistent in routine activities such as daily mealtimes, playtimes, bedtime, wake-up time.
    2. Avoid caffeine/other stimulants; limit food, drink before bedtime.
    3. An hour or so before bedtime, begin a relaxing routine such as warm bath, then a story in quiet bedroom.
    4. Bed should only be used for sleeping, not for watching TV or homework.
    5. Children who are overtired/have interrupted sleep may be more likely to have sleep disturbances such as night terrors.

C. Growth and development.
    1. Musculoskeletal.
      a. Need variety of age-appropriate daily physical activities including team/individual sports, family activities, free play, walking, bicycling, chores, walking up and down stairs.
      b. Limit the amount of TV, computer activities to <2 hours a day.
      c. As they approach puberty, children tend to put on a little more weight, which is normal.
      d. For children who are more than 40% overweight for age and height, diet closely supervised by health care provider may be considered.
      e. Because fractures are common in this age group, children should wear appropriate protective sports gear but also consume adequate calcium to decrease risk of fractures.
    2. Skin.
      a. 15–20 Minutes before going outside, thickly apply broad-spectrum UVA-UVB sunscreen with SPF 15+ to every exposed area, including ears, nose, forehead, neck.
      b. Reapply sunscreen every 2 hours or so after swimming or sweating heavily, regardless of whether sunscreen is waterproof.
    3. Teeth.
      a. Dental visits twice a year for exams, cleaning.
      b. Brush teeth at least twice a day with tartar-control, fluoride toothpaste; floss once a day.

  c. Still may need some help with brushing.

  d. Verify water source for adequate fluoride.

  e. Discuss importance of wearing mouth guards, helmets while playing sports.

 4. Eyes.

  a. Wear sunglasses with UVA-UVB protection whenever outside, in car.

  b. Wear appropriate protective eyewear while engaged in high-risk activities such as sports (basketball, baseball, hockey, etc.) or when around yard debris.

  c. Warn about dangers of fireworks to eyes; enjoy fireworks displays put on by professionals.

 5. Puberty.

  a. Encourage honest, age-appropriate discussions about sex with child using accurate terminology and listening carefully to child's questions so parent only gives as much information as child requires.

  b. Concerns of girls about puberty:
- Menstruation.
- Breast development.

  c. Concerns of boys about puberty:
- Voice change.
- Wet dreams.
- Involuntary erections.
- Breast enlargement.
- One testicle lower than other.

 6. Cognitive and social development.

  a. Very sensitive to views of others.

  b. Appreciate having rules.

  c. Begin to have strong internal gauge of right and wrong.

  d. Friendship and teamwork are important parts of this stage of development.

  e. Eager for more independence but frustrated by what cannot accomplish since they are still in process of mastering skills. Important to have sense of achievement, accomplishment to build strong self-esteem.

D. Safety.

 1. Auto.

  a. Children should be properly secured at all times while traveling in car.

  b. Children who are 4 feet, 9 inches before 8th birthday may be ready for adult safety belts. Can move to safety belt when child can place his/her back firmly against vehicle seat back cushion with knees bent over vehicle seat cushion. Lap belt must fit low and tight across upper thighs. Belt should rest over shoulder and across chest.

  c. Shoulder belt should never be placed under arm or behind child's back.

    d. Children ≤ 12 should never ride in front seat.

    e. Keep all doors locked while in motion.

    f. Never leave young children alone in car.

    g. Children should not ride in truck beds or any other area of vehicle that does not have seat and seat belt.

    h. Children lack judgment, coordination, reflexes to drive other motorized vehicles such as mopeds, snowmobiles, mini-bikes, ATVs.

  2. Bicycle safety. Children who ride bikes should:

    a. Wear helmets at all times.

    b. Know basic road rules such as obey all traffic signs/lights, stop and look both ways at intersecting points such as driveways/streets, ride in single file or on bike paths, ride in same direction as traffic.

    c. Not wear loose-fitting clothing, strings, ties that could get caught in bike chain or parts.

    d. Wear shoes with laces tied.

    e. Not wear earphones while riding.

  3. Skateboard safety: children should always wear helmet and never ride near traffic.

  4. Water safety.

    a. Never allow children to swim alone or play unsupervised by water.

    b. Child should take lessons from qualified instructor.

    c. Backyard swimming pools should be enclosed with high, locked fence on all sides.

    d. Diving should not be allowed until underwater depth has been determined and checked for hazards.

    e. No swimming near boats, fisherman, unsupervised open water.

  5. Fire and burn accidents.

    a. Install smoke detectors, particularly in or near sleeping areas.

    b. Keep fire extinguishers in kitchen, other areas where fire could start.

    c. Have family fire plan in place; practice regular fire drills.

    d. Discourage playing with matches, etc.

    e. To avoid scalding burns from water, heaters should never be set >120°F (48.9°C).

  6. Home alone: parents need to make sure child is comfortable with safety, security, emergency guidelines before leaving home alone.

  7. Gun safety: guns, ammunition need to be stored and locked separately.

  8. Bullying: children of this age can sometimes be the target of bullies.

  9. Sexual abuse.

    a. Most sexual abuse occurs between the ages of 8 and 12.

    b. In 80% of these cases, abuser is known to child.

 10. Substance abuse.

    a. Begins with experimentation and casual use, often under peer pressure.

b. Problem drinking often begins in grade school.

c. Prevention of substance abuse needs to begin before adolescence.

d. Secondhand smoke is a serious health hazard for children. Increases their risk of developing asthma, bronchitis, middle-ear disease, pneumonia, wheezing and coughing spells, behavioral/ cognitive problems.

e. Children whose parents smoke are more than twice as likely to smoke themselves than are children of nonsmokers.

BIBLIOGRAPHY

American Academy of Ophthalmology: Policy statement: vision screening for infants and children, revised and approved, September 1996, retrieved from *www.aao.org/member/ policy/children.cfm*.

American Academy of Pediatrics: Policy statement: prevention of pediatric overweight and obesity, 2003.

American Academy of Pediatrics: Policy statement: recommended childhood and adolescent immunization schedule, United States, January-June 2004.

Brooks LJ, Topol HI: Children with sleep apnea at higher risk for bedwetting, *J Pediatr* May 2003.

Dietz WH, editor: *American Academy of Pediatrics guide to your child's nutrition*, New York, 1999, Random House.

National Association for Sport and Physical Education; see information at *www.naspeinfo.org*.

National Highway Transportation Safety Association: Best practices for promoting booster seat use—know the facts about booster seats, retrieved from *www.nhtsa.dot.gov/CPS/ promote/know.htm*.

National Sleep Foundation: Sleep in America, retrieved from *www.sleepfloundation.org*.

Position of the American Dietetic Association: total diet approach to communicating food and nutrition information, *J Am Dietetic Assoc* 102 (1):100-108, January 2002.

Schor EL, Stern L, editors: *American Academy of Pediatrics, caring for your school-age child, ages five to twelve*, New York, 1995, Bantam Books.

NOTES

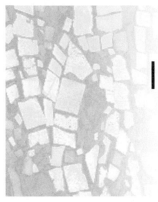

CHAPTER 18

11- to 13-Year Visit (Preadolescent)

MARY J. ALVARADO

Acne, 706.1	HIV, 042.
Coronary artery disease, 414.00	Peripheral vascular disease, 443.9
Depression, 311.	Physical abuse, 995.54
Emotional abuse, 995.51	Scoliosis, 737.30
Goiter, 240.9	Sexual abuse, 995.53

I. General impression
   A. Preadolescence is time of rapid change and emotional turbulence.
   B. Need support, understanding, caring from adults in particular, which is not usually what they receive.

II. Nutrition
   A. Nutritional requirements.
      1. Increased energy and protein requirement due to rapid growth.
      2. Require 2200–3000 calories/day.
      3. To meet increased need, increase milk and dairy products to 4 servings/day, bread group servings to 9/day.
      4. $\frac{1}{4}$ of daily calories are typically consumed in snacks; encourage fruit, cheese, milk beverages, raw vegetables, nuts.
      5. Diet should consist of 10–15% protein, 25–30% fat, 50–60% carbohydrates.
      6. Needs 8–15 mg of iron/day; iron is most commonly deficient nutrient.
      7. A well-balanced diet does not require supplementation; irregular eating patterns and/or high-calorie/low-nutrient snacking may lead to deficiencies requiring multivitamin.
   B. Nutritional assessment.
      1. Calculate and plot body mass index (BMI) (see Appendix D).
      2. Evaluate 24-hour recall.
      3. Examine intake, eating patterns; ask about special diets or supplements.
      4. Assess for eating disorders.

  5. Monitor athletes' increased need for calories; advise on appropriate dietary changes.
  6. Provide guidance about nutrition annually.
  7. Refer to nutritionist if indicated.

III. Elimination

  A. Expect consistent pattern of elimination.
  B. Changes may occur with irregular eating patterns, illness, diets, stress, eating disorders.
  C. Check understanding of normal elimination and methods employed to deal with problems.

IV. Sleep

  A. Question about amount of sleep; at least 8 hours per night.
  B. Age and activity level.
  C. Monitor for any difficulties, ability to cope.
  D. Advise on sleep hygiene if necessary.

V. Growth and development

  A. Physical.
  1. Early adolescence is marked by rapid physical change. Tempo of adolescent development is variable and may be influenced by gender, health, socioeconomic status, genetics. Predictable sequence of events occurs over 2–6 years from onset, which on average is age 9–11 for girls and age 10–12 for boys. The preadolescent may prefer to be examined with parent out of the room.
  2. Perform complete physical exam with attention to the following:
     a. Document height, weight, and BMI annually (see Appendix D).
     b. Assess and document Tanner stage of pubertal development annually.
     c. Monitor blood pressure annually.
     d. Screen cholesterol once in this age group if following risk factors exist:
        • Parent with serum cholesterol >240.
        • Family history unknown.
        • Parent/grandparent with stroke, peripheral vascular disease, coronary artery disease, sudden cardiac death <55 years.
     e. Palpate thyroid gland; goiter may present in this age-group.
     f. Examine spine for development/progression of scoliosis during rapid growth.
     g. Assess for presence/severity of acne.
     h. Ask about sexual activity; screen sexually active teens for sexually transmitted infections (STIs), evaluate risk for acquiring HIV.
  B. Emotional.
  1. Rapid physical changes of early adolescence lead to increased self-consciousness and focus on external characteristics.
  2. Adolescent feels everyone is looking at him/her and questions if he/she is normal.
  3. Reassure about normal findings in the physical exam.

4. Explain that each individual progresses through physical changes of adolescence in same sequence but at his/her own pace.
5. Ask about friends, family, school. Is there a best friend? A supportive adult? Monitor self-esteem.
6. Ask about moods. Emotional lability is normal. Assess for excessive stress or depression.
7. Ask about physical, emotional, or sexual abuse.

C. Intellectual.
1. Adolescent begins to transition from concrete to abstract thinking; timing is variable. Some develop higher level thinking in early adolescence, some later or not at all. Individual may be able to think abstractly about algebra but not about decision making regarding risky behaviors. Abstract thinking gives adolescent better ability to reason and see other points of view.
2. How is school performance? Ask about academic, sport, personal goals. May still have impractical/unrealistic ideas.
3. What are responsibilities at home? Early adolescents should be encouraged to take on new responsibilities with supervision.
4. Ask about extracurricular activities. Encourage involvement in groups that interest him/her. Increasing communication skills help with problem solving. Group discussions help adolescents learn to express themselves.
5. Advise to keep TV viewing, computer time, video games to <2 hours per day. These activities interfere with opportunities to engage in communication with peers, family.

VI. Social development
A. Early adolescents begin to develop greater independence from parents, family.
B. Establishment of reliable relationships with peers, other adults is important developmental task.
C. New peer group, which is usually same sex, provides opportunity to test, evaluate values/behaviors. It allows for sense of belonging, self-worth and affords opportunity to build social competence.
D. Recognize that hairstyles, clothing, music preferences, piercing are expressions of individuality; often mirror others in peer group.
E. Preoccupation with own appearance is typical. Help parents anticipate greater privacy need.
F. Encourage variety of school/community activities to allow wider exposure to peers/interests.
G. Testing authority may occur. Encourage families to clearly establish and enforce guidelines for appropriate behavior. Identify consistent caring adult with whom adolescent is comfortable communicating.
H. Question about friends, peer groups, adult role models. Social isolation is not normal.
I. As with other areas of development, individuals progress at variable rates and often oscillate between dependence/independence.

VII. Immunizations

A. Immunizations should be given according to recommended childhood immunization schedule (see Appendix A):
1. Hepatitis B: complete or initiate series.
2. MMR: give second dose now if not already administered.
3. Tetanus toxoid (Td): recommended at age 11–12 if at least 5 years since last dose. Subsequent doses every 10 years throughout adulthood.
4. Varicella: give if not previously immunized or unreliable history of disease. If 13 years or older, give 2 doses 4 weeks apart.

VIII. Safety

A. Unintentional injury is main cause of death and disability in this age group.
1. Counsel about accident prevention: seat belts, helmets, proper sports equipment, water safety instruction, CPR.
2. Instruct that firearms should be locked up, ammunition kept separate.
3. Educate about dangers of drug use, both ingested and inhaled. Provide strategies to resist negative peer pressure.
4. Discuss date rape prevention.
5. Assess for depression. Adolescents at high risk for suicide: those with chronic illness or extreme stress (i.e., overachievers), athletes, those who feel unwanted.
6. Assess for physical, emotional, sexual abuse.

IX. Anticipatory guidance

A. Promotion of health.
1. Review pubertal development of same and opposite sex.
2. Explain menstruation and its management to female clients.
3. Advise to get 8 hours of sleep every night.
4. Encourage moderate to vigorous exercise for 30–60 minutes at least 3 times a week.
5. Instruct to eat 3 nutritious meals per day. Snack on healthy foods such as fruits, vegetable, nuts, low-fat dairy. Choose foods rich in calcium, iron.
6. Encourage maintaining healthy weight through exercise, appropriate eating habits.
7. Remind to schedule dental exam every 6 months. Brush teeth twice a day. Floss daily.
8. Educate about acne management.
9. Provide safety instruction, avoidance of substance abuse and gang involvement.

B. Social development.
1. Encourage participation in school activities.
2. Advise to take on new responsibilities in home, school, community.
3. Clarify parental limits, consequences of unacceptable behavior.

C. Mental health.
1. Encourage teens to consider their strengths and talents.

2. Recommend talking with trusted adult/health professional if teen feels sad or helpless often.
3. Advise against alcohol, drug use. Discuss strategies to resist negative peer pressure.
4. Evaluate for potential abuse, counsel on avoiding date rape, gang involvement, abusive relationships.
 D. Sexuality.
1. Counsel on sexual abstinence. Encourage to identify supportive adult to provide accurate information. Invite adolescent to call the office for advice/information as needed. Explain confidentiality policy.
2. If sexually active, discuss contraceptive methods, STI prevention. Counsel on abstinence.
3. Educate about protection against STIs and pregnancy as indicated.

BIBLIOGRAPHY

Elster A, Kuznets N: *Guidelines for adolescent preventive services,* Baltimore, 1994, Williams & Wilkins.

Fisher J, Wildey L: Developmental management of adolescents. In Burns C et al, editors: *Pediatric primary care: a handbook for nurse practitioners,* ed 3, Philadelphia, 2004, WB Saunders.

Fox J, editor: *Primary health care of infants, children, and adolescents,* ed 2, St Louis, 2002, Mosby.

Green M, Palfrey J, editors: *Bright futures: guidelines for health supervision of infants, children, and adolescents,* ed 2 rev, Arlington, VA, 2002, National Center for Education in Maternal and Child Health.

Neinstein L: *Adolescent health care: a practical guide,* ed 4, Philadelphia, 2002, Lippincott Williams & Wilkins.

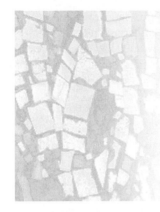

CHAPTER 19

14- to 18-Year Visit (Adolescent)

MARY LOU C. ROSENBLATT

Abdominal pain, **789.00**	Hallucinations, **780.1**
Acunthosis nigricans, **701.2**	Hyperlipidemia, **272.4**
Anemia, **285.9**	Hypertension, **401.9**
Anxiety, **300.00**	Insomnias, **780.52**
Catalepsy, **300.1**	Iron-deficiency anemia, **280.9**
Constipation, **564.00**	Narcolepsy, **347.**
Delayed sleep phase syndrome, **780.50**	Obesity, **278.00**
Depression, **311.**	Obesity, morbid, **278.01**
Diabetes, **250.00**	Peristalsis of colon, **787.4**
Diabetes, family history of, **V18.0**	Poor nutrition, **269.9**
Drug abuse, **305.90**	Sleep apnea, **780.57**
Dysmenorrhea, **625.3**	Sleep deprivation, **780.50**
Eating disorders, **307.50**	Snoring, **786.09**
Enlarged tonsils, **474.11**	Thyroid disease, **246.9**

I. General impression

   A. This well visit is opportunity to provide health care for individual who is faced with many developmental challenges on road to adulthood.

   B. Introduce yourself and your role to teen and parent. Explain that you need information from both parent and teen and will spend some time just with teen to check on his/her concerns.

   C. Be knowledgeable of your state's confidentiality and consent statutes and explain how that will be handled in practice. Assure both teen and parent that your first goal is well-being of teen.

   D. Listening skills are especially important with teens. Show interest in their concerns and address them. "Hear" pauses, hesitation, body language and validate your understanding of meaning of nonverbals with teen.

   E. Be nonjudgmental and gather information before giving advice.

   F. Have supply of well-written and informative handouts on variety of issues.

G. Involve parents by finding out what advice they give on sensitive subjects, such as substance abuse and sex. Interaction between parent and teen will give feedback on what is discussed in home and how open they are with each other. Encourage both parent and teen to talk about these subjects together.

H. Ask responsibilities teen has at home. Many parents advance privileges based on teen's ability to take care of his/her chores. This can also support fair negotiations that take place in family.

I. Use tool such as HEADS assessment to take snapshot of teen's life and identify problem areas to focus on during acute visits. HEADS assessment: ask open-ended questions about Home, Education, Activities, Drug use and depression, Sexuality.

J. Have resources available if issues such as drug abuse, school problems, physical/sexual abuse, depression, sexual activity, pregnancy are present.

K. If an undesired behavior, which is identified through screening, can be dealt with during primary care office visit, state desired behavior, offer health information detailing risks of undesired behavior, benefit of change, and alternatives. If teen can commit to change, set goal and time frame, offer support and resources, set up follow-up time.

II. Nutrition

A. History.
1. Ask for 24-hour diet recall.
2. Are any foods/food groups avoided and why?
3. Is milk consumed? Skim, 2%, whole?
4. Is meat eaten? What types?
5. What fruits, vegetables does teen eat? How much juice is consumed?
6. Trying to gain or lose weight? How?
7. Are meals skipped? Is breakfast eaten?
8. Are meals eaten on run or sitting down with family?
9. What types of "junk" foods are consumed? How much?
10. How often does he/she eat at fast-food restaurants? What foods?
11. Does teen watch TV and snack?
12. How much soda is consumed? Regular or diet?
13. What types of exercise is teen involved in?
14. Does teen spend time thinking about how to be thin?
15. Has he/she tried dieting, diet pills, laxatives, vomiting to control weight?
16. Does teen ever eat in secret?
17. Is teen dieting to fit into weight class for sports?
18. Are any nutritional supplements taken?

B. Teaching.
1. Use Food Guide Pyramid (see Appendix E) to encourage healthy eating practices, daily requirements of protein, calcium, vitamins, fiber.
2. Recognize that teen is likely making more choices on own, can start to read labels, becomes conscious of nutritional value.
3. Skipping breakfast may make it harder to concentrate in school and lead to more hunger after school, possibly poor nutritional choices.

   4. Skipping meals may lead to more hunger, poor food choices.
   5. Encourage teen to talk with parent about planning meals, snacks.
   6. Encourage trying new foods.
   7. When limiting soda, drink more water, avoid excessive calories from juice products.
   8. Discuss sources of calcium.
   9. 5–8% of teen girls have iron-deficiency anemia.
  10. Teens risk dental decay with high-sugar diets, poor dental hygiene.
  11. 13–15% of children and adolescents are estimated to be overweight.
  12. Teach behavioral techniques for weight management, such as goal setting, self-monitoring, positive reinforcement, problem solving, social support.
  13. Incidence of eating disorders has increased and is estimated to affect 7% of male adolescents and 13% of female adolescents. Eating disorders can be associated with depression, substance abuse, low self-esteem.
  14. Discourage rapid weight gain/loss to fit into weight class for sports.
  15. Discourage major weight/dietary restrictions during growth spurt.
C. Physical exam.
   1. Chart height, weight, body mass index (BMI); review growth curves with teen.
   2. BMI at or above 95th percentile is considered overweight/obese. For obese teens, BMI is objective measure that is useful in motivating them to recognize their risks of developing heart disease, diabetes.
D. Labs.
   1. Screen hematocrit at first visit/at end of puberty or both to check for anemia due to rapid growth, poor nutrition, menstrual losses.
   2. Glucose if there is family history of diabetes, symptoms of diabetes, or obesity and *Acanthosis nigricans.*
   3. Cholesterol for adolescents with heart disease, hypertension, diabetes or if there is family history of heart disease or hyperlipidemia
E. Treatment plan.
   1. Encourage healthy eating practices.
   2. Encourage good exercise habits.
   3. For teens just starting to exercise, start slow, for example, walking for 20 minutes 3 times per week, so they can build up their exercise tolerance.
   4. For teens with special diets, such as vegetarian diets, be prepared to assess dietary content, give advice/referral resource to offer nutritional guidance, support.
   5. For obese teens, offer support and encouragement. When motivated, they may be ready for weight loss program. Suggest starting by keeping daily food diary to look for problem areas in diet. Behavioral techniques, mentioned above, may be enough for some teens to get started with healthier eating practices. In supportive environment, family involvement may help to cut down excess intake. Some teens benefit from professional weight loss programs. Refer morbidly obese patients to medical weight loss program.

6. When eating disorders are suspected, careful assessment and monitoring are needed. Denial is common and should not offer reassurance. Patients require nutritional, medical management as well as mental health assessment and referral. Referral to eating disorder program will offer comprehensive approach to assessment and management.

III. Elimination

A. Teens are normally independent in their elimination practices.
B. Constipation.
1. Infrequent and/or difficult passage of feces.
2. Common cause of abdominal pain.
C. History.
1. What are bowel habits?
2. When was last bowel movement? Hard and dry? Any abdominal pain?
3. How long has constipation been a problem?
4. Is fiber present in teen's diet?
5. What is fluid intake?
6. Does teen avoid public or school restrooms?
7. Does schedule allow time to use bathroom?
8. Have laxatives or stool softeners been tried? How often?
9. Ask about other signs of thyroid disease, such as menstrual disorder, dry skin, brittle hair, lethargy, and weight gain.
D. Teaching.
1. Describe gastrocolic reflex (peristalsis of colon induced by entrance of food into empty stomach).
2. Describe bowel function and need for fluid and fiber to keep stool moist and moving through GI tract.
E. Physical exam.
1. Firm loops of bowel may be palpable on thin patients.
2. Rectum is typically filled with hard stool.
3. Passage of hard stool may cause anorectal pain or bleeding.
F. Labs.
1. Abdominal film may be needed in case of abdominal pain, after ruling out other systems as sources of pain.
2. Make sure female patients are not pregnant before sending for x-ray.
G. Treatment plan.
1. Encourage drinking plenty of water.
2. Help teen plan on how to add fiber to diet.
3. Encourage good toilet habits, such as right after meals.
4. Consider use of stool softener.
5. In addition to the above, sitz baths may help anal fissure heal.
6. Follow up in 1-2 weeks.

IV. Sleep

A. Teenagers need 9–10 hours of sleep per night. Most teens do not get it.
B. Sleep history.
1. Does teen feel rested or tired?
2. What are concerns about sleep? Frequency? Duration?

3. What are usual bedtimes and wake-up times?
4. Are naps taken? If so, do they interfere with sleep later that night?
5. Has family complained about teen's snoring?
6. Does teen fall asleep in class? Other times?
7. What are school hours?
8. What are after-school activities?
9. Does teen have job? How many hours?
10. How many hours are spent on homework?
11. Does teen care for child or have other household responsibilities?
12. Is there family history of sleep disorders?
13. Is teen depressed, sad, moody?
14. Are stimulants (coffee, tea, soda, OTC medications, illicit drugs) used to stay awake longer?
15. Does teen have TV, radio/stereo, computer, phone in bedroom? Are these in use when trying to go to sleep and delaying bedtime?

C. Teaching.
1. Insomnias are most frequent sleep disorder during adolescence.
2. Insomnias involve problems falling asleep, staying asleep, waking too early.
3. Delayed sleep phase syndrome is inability to fall asleep at appropriate time, but if left to fall asleep naturally would fall asleep late, get up late. These teens will be sleepy if awakened to attend school.
4. Teens may be motivated to stay up late, sleep late. If teen can awaken by his/her own motivation but not for school, this may be form of school refusal.
5. Insomnia may occur due to stress, anxiety, poor sleep habits.
6. Excessive daytime sleepiness can be caused by chronic sleep deprivation, usually due to busy schedule.
7. Sleep apnea may be associated with obesity and symptoms include snoring, apneic periods during sleep, nighttime waking, and daytime sleeping.
8. Narcolepsy is uncommon disorder that has an onset of 10–25 years of age. Components include sleep attacks, catalepsy, sleep paralysis, and/or hallucinations. There is evidence of genetic component.

D. Physical.
1. Does teen appear alert?
2. Does teen appear sad or depressed?
3. Note blood pressure and pulse.
4. Is teen obese?
5. Is teen comfortable and able to breathe through both nostrils?
6. Are tonsils enlarged?

E. Lab.
1. To rule out sleep apnea, consider sleep study if teen/family reports snoring, frequent wake-ups, apneic periods, daytime sleep.

F. Treatment plan.
1. Have teen track sleep patterns for 1–2 weeks.
2. Any question of depression needs assessment.

3. Have teen/parent look at schedule and commitments. Are there ways to decrease workload for overloaded teen?
4. Cut down on caffeine products, including OTC stimulants.
5. Cut out nap time.
6. Use bedroom for sleep only and put TV, computer, etc., elsewhere.
7. Teach relaxation techniques.
8. Identify stressors and write them down. If stressors are complex, consider counseling.
9. Stick to regular schedule of bedtime and waking up.
10. Encourage weight loss for obese teens.
11. Refer teens with nasal breathing problems/enlarged tonsils to ENT specialist.
12. Refer teens with difficult sleep problems, including those who do not do well with above plan, to sleep clinic.

V. Growth and development

A. While some teens are able to state concerns, others may hope you will mention possible concerns for them, such as height, weight, pubertal development. Comfortable way to start such conversation may be "Some teens worry about being shorter (or taller, heavier, thinner) than their friends. I wonder if you have any concerns about this...."
B. Use growth charts to help see progress over time, relate their parameters to their blood relatives or point out what future growth is likely.
C. Tanner or sexual maturity rating (SMR) also may be reassuring.
D. For development outside of expected range, evaluate for medical cause.
E. Height.
   1. 33–60% of adult bone growth occurs during adolescence.
   2. 20–25% of final adult height occurs in puberty.
F. Weight: 50% of ideal adult body weight is gained during adolescence.
G. SMR: By middle adolescence most teens are in latter classes of Tanner or SMR scales. Spermarche occurs at about SMR 2.5. Menarche usually occurs at SMR 3 or 4. Using SMR can help teen to see where he/she is in puberty and what can be expected without having to compare him/herself to friends.
   1. Menstrual history.
      a. Age at menarche?
      b. Frequency, duration, quantity of menstrual periods?
      c. Last menstrual period (LMP)?
      d. Dysmenorrhea and treatments used?
H. Psychosocial developmental tasks.
   1. Increased independence from parents, inviting conflicts over control.
   2. Peer group involvement intensifies. Conformity with peer values. Less time for family. Teams, clubs, gangs may become important.
   3. Interest in dating, sexual experimentation. Preoccupation with romantic fantasy. Sexual orientation more evident to peers.
   4. Identity and individuality grow. Increased acceptance of body image, more established ego and sexual identity. Increased intellectual abilities, emotional feelings. Vocational ideas more realistic.

5. Sense of omnipotence and immortality that may lead to high-risk behaviors.
6. Improved ability with abstract thought.

VI. Social development

A. Family.
 1. Who are family members living with teen?
 2. What is level of communication between members?
 3. What are supports? Conflicts?
 4. What are house rules? Who makes them?
 5. What are teen's responsibilities?
 6. Is there a curfew?
 7. Does teen drive family car? What supervision is given?

B. School.
 1. What is teen's school performance? Any recent changes?
 2. What does teen like or dislike about school?
 3. How does teen relate to classmates? To teachers?
 4. Are there learning problems? Has teen been evaluated by school?
 5. Are there behavior problems? How have those been addressed?
 6. What is educational/vocational plan?
 7. Has teen dropped out of school?
 8. Is he/she planning to get a GED?
 9. If chronic illness, is there teaching plan in place for missed days?

C. Peers.
 1. Who are teen's friends?
 2. Is there a best friend?
 3. Is there a trusted adult to talk to?
 4. Does teen prefer to be with friends or alone?
 5. What are interests and activities of peer group?
 6. Does parent know teen's friends?

D. Interests.
 1. What are teen's activities? Hobbies?
 2. Does teen have a job? How many hours? Safety hazards on job?
 3. Does teen like to read?
 4. Does teen enjoy sports? Exercise?

E. Dating.
 1. What are house rules about dating?
 2. What advice have parents given about dating?
 3. Is teen thinking about dating?
 4. Does he/she have romantic feelings about anyone?
  a. Is this person male or female?
  b. If these feelings are for same-sex person, does teen feel support from parents? Friends? Community?

F. Sexual history.
 1. Is teen thinking about sexual relationship or has he/she had sexual relations.
 2. Able to talk with parent about being sexually active?

3. Aware of risks of sexual activity (emotional, sexually transmitted infections [STIs], pregnancy)?
4. Vulnerable to these risks?
5. Reason for being sexually active? Does teen feel pressured?
6. Specific sexual behaviors (vaginal/anal intercourse or oral-genital sex)?
7. Teen's age at first intercourse?
8. Number of lifetime partners?
9. How old is current partner? Is there more than one partner now?
10. Are condoms used? Hormonal contraception? Spermacides?
11. Does teen know how to use male/female condom?
12. Does teen know about emergency contraception (EC)? Does teen who only uses condoms have prescription for EC?
13. Any history of or current symptoms of STIs?
14. Any history of pregnancy? Pregnancy scares? LMP?
15. History of pregnancy termination? If so, how is teen coping?
16. For teen parents, what are stresses? Support?
17. Does teen feel safe in current relationship?
18. In dating situations, has teen been hit or pushed? What did she/he do?

G. Substance use.
1. Does teen know risks of substance use?
2. Do any friends smoke cigarettes, drink alcohol, use inhalants, marijuana, other drugs?
3. Does teen smoke cigarettes, drink alcohol, use inhalants, marijuana, other drugs?
4. If teen does use substances, use screen such as CAGE to obtain more information (have resource available to teen who needs substance abuse treatment):

   C: Do you think you should cut down your use of...?

   A: Do you get angry or annoyed when people tell you that you should cut down your use of ...?

   G: Do you feel guilty about your use of ...?

   E: Do you use this substance as eye-opener to get going in morning?
5. Does teen drink alcohol or use other drugs when driving?
6. Does teen attend parties where alcohol is served?
7. What plans are there to get home safely? Does teen have to deal with parents for this type of situation?

H. Antisocial behavior.
1. Does teen skip school?
2. Has he/she had trouble with the law?
3. Does teen belong to or associate with a gang?

VII. Immunizations (see Appendix A)

A. May not have completed recommended vaccinations.
B. Immunization status can be reviewed at each visit.
1. TD: booster usually given between 11 and 12 years but before 16 years, then every 10 years.

2. MMR: 2 doses needed before school entry.
3. Hepatitis B: recommended for all adolescents, especially those at risk (sexually active, injection drug abusers, work-related exposure to blood/body fluids). Routine vaccination of infants began in 1991; may be in need of immunization. 2-dose regimen for 11- to 15-year-olds; 3 dose regimen for others.
4. Varicella: needed if there is no history of varicella disease. If history is unclear, vaccine is well tolerated, more cost effective than serologic testing in most cases. 2 doses given more than 4 weeks apart needed if ≥13 years of age.
5. Influenza: recommended for teens with chronic illness (i.e., asthma, sickle cell disease, HIV, etc.) or those living with persons with impaired immunity. Can be given to others who want immunity. Cannot be given to individuals with egg allergy.
6. Hepatitis A: vaccination recommended for those living in high-risk areas; 2 doses needed, at least 6 months apart.
7. *Neisseria meningitidis:* vaccination recommended in many states for college freshmen living in dormitories.

VIII. Safety

A. Self-protection.
 1. Does teen have any self-defense skills?
 2. Is teen aware of surroundings when in public?
 3. Does teen travel with friends?
 4. Has teen been victim of any attack in past? Any fear of someone threatening harm currently? Are parents/authorities aware?
 5. Does teen feel safe in school?
 6. Can teen walk away from conflict if she/he feels fear/anger?
 7. Does teen get into fights regularly?
 8. Is teen exposed to violence in home, community, media?
 9. Does teen have access to gun? What are rules for gun safety?
 10. Does teen carry a weapon? Why?
B. Injury prevention.
 1. Does teen wear seat belts?
 2. Does teen wear a helmet?
 3. Does teen plan to take driver's education classes?
 4. Does teen drive at night or with friends?
 5. Does teen use alcohol/other drugs?
 6. Does teen routinely take risks?
 7. Has teen had injuries in past?
 8. Does teen use power tools/lawn equipment?
C. Suicide prevention.
 1. Does teen or family worry about teen being depressed?
 2. Has teen lost pleasure in usual interests?
 3. Weight loss or gain?
 4. Sleep problem: too much or too little?
 5. Increased/decreased activity level?

6. Daily fatigue?
7. Feelings of worthlessness, excessive/inappropriate guilt?
8. Decreased concentration or ability to make decisions?
9. Asking teen about mood can be done at every visit and is especially important if teen visits frequently or if physical complaints do not seem to make sense.
10. Recurrent thoughts of death or suicide? (If teen is suicidal, have resources, such as ability to escort to emergency department for psychiatric evaluation, immediately available.)

IX. Anticipatory guidance
A. Many opportunities to give advice exist during history and physical exam.
B. Giving information in nonjudgmental way allows teen to make up his/her own mind about how to improve his/her health.
C. Puberty: acknowledge where individual is regarding pubertal development and how development is likely to proceed.
D. Health care:
   1. Have yearly physical exam.
   2. See dentist twice/year, practice good dental hygiene.
   3. Keep up with routine vision care.
   4. Discuss use of sunscreen and skin cancer prevention.
E. Injury prevention.
   1. Wear seat belt when traveling in car.
   2. Wear helmet when riding bike, skates, scooter, motor bike/cycle.
   3. Wear appropriate protection when engaging in sports.
   4. Drowning prevention includes learning how to swim, not swimming alone, never abusing substances while doing water activities, entering unknown depths feet first.
   5. When operating equipment such as power tools, lawn mowers, tractors, know safety rules and use appropriate safety equipment.
   6. Leading causes of death and injury of young drivers are inexperience, risk taking (speeding, dares), distraction (driving with friends, talking on cell phones), driving at night. Parents who recognize these risks can outline safety plan (curfew, supervision, no driving with peers until parent feels teen is ready, contracting for no substance abuse) for young driver going through "rite of passage."
   7. Ask parents to remove guns from home. If not an option, guns/ammunition need to be stored separately, in locked boxes. Especially important for parents of depressed teens to realize risk guns pose to their teen.
   8. Learn CPR.
F. Self-exam:
   1. Teach females self breast exam. Use breast model to show how lumps may feel. Reassure teen that most lumps in her age group are not cancer.
   2. Teach males self testes exam. Reinforce that concerns are okay to talk about. Teach warning signs for testicular tumors, torsion, and epididymitis.
G. Nutrition.
   1. Eat breakfast.

   2. Eat a low-fat diet.
   3. Watch junk food, soda consumption.
   4. Use Food Guide Pyramid (see Appendix E) to evaluate diet.
   5. Encourage maintenance of healthy weight.
H. Exercise.
   1. Do aerobic exercise 3 times per week.
   2. Look for ways to increase exercise opportunities in daily life.
I. Peer pressure and self-esteem.
   1. Pick good friends who are interested in positive activities.
   2. Look at best qualities you have and feel good about them.
   3. Participate in activities because you want to, not because everyone else is doing so.
   4. Figure out goals important to you, make sure friends won't get you off track.
J. Body modification: tattoos and piercings:
   1. Reasons for getting a tattoo range from expressing independence to being part of a group. Some teens may be self-described "risk takers" who may also engage in drug use and sexual activity.
   2. Parental consent may be required in some locales.
   3. Advise teens that tattoos should be considered permanent because removal is expensive, time consuming, and may leave a scar.
   4. Tattoos and piercings may become infected. Advise teens to research sterile practices of the tattoo/piercing establishment. Postcare hygiene needs to be strictly followed.
   5. Teens should not get a tattoo or piercing if they are upset or intoxicated.
   6. Alternatives such as temporary tattoos or magnetic piercing look-a-likes may satisfy a passing need.
K. Stress reduction.
   1. Encourage setting aside time for yourself to rest and gather thoughts.
   2. Get plenty of sleep at night.
   3. Eat varied, nutritious diet.
   4. Encourage physical activity.
   5. Teach deep breathing and counting to 10 if feeling stressed or angry.
   6. Keep lines of communication open with parent/guardian.
   7. Get help from adult in your life if you have much stress.
   8. Try to keep open communication with family.
   9. Have resources available for depressed teens.
   10. Arrange emergency evaluation for suicidal intent/severe depression.
L. Substance abuse.
   1. Do not smoke cigarettes or marijuana.
   2. Do not drink alcohol, use inhalants, other drugs.
   3. Do not drive if intoxicated. Have teen make plan with parents about what to do if out and driver providing ride becomes intoxicated.
   4. Point out risks of substance use including health consequences, accidents, school performance, impact on family/friends, legal implications, gateway to other drug use.
   5. Make sure athletes are aware of risks of performance enhancing drugs.

M. Sex.

1. Consider benefits of abstinence, such as ability to focus on personal and academic goals, less complicated breakups, STI prevention.
2. Consider risks of sexual activity, such as emotional stress, pregnancy, STIs.
3. Discuss how to deal with issues important to individual teen: sex drive, peer pressure, older partners, partners who refuse to use protection, desire to have baby.
4. If teen decides sexual activity is right for him/her, advise use of condoms and make sure teen knows how to leave room at top of male condom for ejaculate and that female condoms can cover part of external genitalia.
5. Be frank about risks of STIs, especially HIV and other viral infections.
6. Educate about all types of appropriate birth control.
7. Make sure teens are aware of emergency contraception and how to obtain it.
8. For sexually active teens, screen for STIs.
9. For sexually active females, perform yearly Pap smear.
10. Encourage teen to talk with adult in his/her life about sex if able.
11. If teen identifies as minority sexual identity (gay, lesbian, bisexual, transgendered) make sure teen has resources, support.
12. If teen is pregnant, outline options and encourage parental involvement.

BIBLIOGRAPHY

Behrman RE, Kleigman RM, Jenson HB: *Nelson textbook of pediatrics,* ed 17, Philadelphia, 2004, WB Saunders.

Dixon SD, Stein MT: *Encounters with children: pediatric behavior and development,* St Louis, 2000, Mosby.

Goldenring JM, Cohen E: Getting into adolescent heads, *Contemp Pediatr* 5:75-90, 1998.

Gotlieb EM, editor: *Practicing adolescent medicine: a collection of resources,* Elk Grove Village, IL, 1994, American Academy of Pediatrics.

Jellinek M, Patel BP, Froehle MC, editors: *Bright futures in practice: mental health, vol I, practice guide,* Arlington, VA, 2002, National Center for Education in Maternal and Child Health.

Joffe A, Blythe MJ, editors: *Handbook of adolescent medicine,* Philadelphia, 2003, Hanley and Belfus.

Kaplan DW, et al: American Academy of Pediatrics: Identifying and treating eating disorders, *Pediatrics* 111 (1), 204-211, January 2003.

Krebs NF, et al: American Academy of Pediatrics: Prevention of pediatric overweight and obesity, *Pediatrics* 112 (2), 424-430, August 2003.

Melnyk BM, et al: Improving the mental/psychological health of US children and adolescents: Outcomes and implementation strategies from the National KySS Summit, *J Pediatr Health Care* 17 (6):S1-S23, November-December 2003.

Neinstein LS: *Adolescent health care, a practical guide,* ed 4, Baltimore, 2002, Williams and Wilkins.

Schwimmer JB: Managing overweight in older children and adolescents, *Pediatr Ann* 33 (1):39-44, January 2004.

Sheehan K: Intentional injury and violence prevention, *Clin Pediatr Emerg Med* 4(1), March 2003.

Song EH, Martel S, Anderson JE: Decorating the "human canvas": Body art and your patients, *Contemp Pediatr* 19(8), 86-102, August 2002.

Common Childhood Disorders

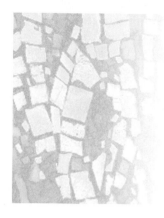

CHAPTER 20

Dermatologic Disorders

PEGGY VERNON

ACNE

Acne, 706.1	Papule, 709.8
Blackhead, 706.1	Pustules, 686.9
Comedone, 706.1	Skin nodule, 782.2
Hyperpigmentation, 709.00	Whitehead, 706.2

I. Etiology
  A. Disorder of pilosebaceous follicles.
  B. Hormonal stimulation increases inflammation.

II. Occurrence
  A. 40% of children 8–10 years of age will develop early lesions.
  B. Highest incidence during adolescent years; 85% of all adolescents experience some form of acne.
  C. 10% of adults in 30s, 40s, 50s continue to experience acne.
  D. Familial tendency.

III. Clinical manifestations
  A. Primary lesions are open and closed comedones.
    1. Open comedone, or blackhead: obstruction of follicle that is filled with stratum corneum cells, black color due to compacted melanocytes.
    2. Closed comedone, or whitehead: result of swelling of follicular duct below epidermis.
  B. Accumulation of sebum, keratin cause follicle wall to rupture into dermis, causing inflammatory acne/papules/pustules; inflammatory reaction to sebum, fatty acids, bacteria.
    1. *Propionibacterium acnes* distends follicle, causing leakage around comedone.
    2. Lesions developing in lower portion of follicle create warm, tender nodules and cysts. Lesions may result in scars, which can develop into keloids.

3. Inflammatory acne lesions may resolve with postinflammatory hyperpigmentation, which usually clears after several months.

IV. Physical findings
A. Highest concentration of sebaceous glands occurs on face, chest, back, shoulders.
B. Variety of lesions appear simultaneously, presenting with variety of comedones, papules, pustules, nodules.
C. Acne appears more severe in winter months; females report premenstrual hormonal correlation.
D. Severity determined by quantity, type, distribution of lesions (Table 20-1).

V. Diagnostic tests
A. Visual diagnosis.
B. History to include family history, other medical disorders, duration of acne, products used, previous treatments (both over-the-counter as well as prescription).
C. Physical examination includes grade of acne according to type, location of lesions.
D. Laboratory testing indicated only if adrenal/gonadal function are in question.

VI. Differential diagnosis

Flat warts, 078.10	Nevus comedonicus, 757.33
Miliaria, 705.1	Tuberous sclerosis, 759.5
Molluscum contagiosum, 078.0	

A. Tuberous sclerosis.
B. Nevus comedonicus.
C. Miliaria of newborn.
D. Flat warts.
E. Molluscum contagiosum.

TABLE 20-1 • Grading scale for acne severity

Scale	Definition
0	None: skin is clear
1	Few comedones
2	Mild comedones, few papules, minimal erythema
3	Comedones, papules, pustules, erythema
4	Moderate comedones, greater number of papules, pustules extending over wider area of face, chest, shoulders, back, increasing erythema
5	Comedones, increasing number of papules, pustules, nodules with erythema
6	Comedones, papules, pustules, nodules, cysts; scarring may or may not be present with hyperpigmentation

From Burns C, et al: *Pediatric primary care: a handbook for nurse practitioners,* ed 3, St Louis, 2004, Mosby, p. 1013.

VII. Treatment
  A. Goals of treatment: altering keratinization, counteract excess sebum production, decrease production of *P. acnes,* minimize scarring.
  B. Treatment choices (Table 20-2) depend on the severity of acne.

VIII. Follow-up
  A. Evaluate every 3–6 months for compliance, treatment progress, worsening symptoms.
  B. Monthly monitoring of patients treated with isotretinoin (Accutane).

IX. Complications

Antisocial, 301.7
Depression, 311.

  A. Lack of patient motivation, inappropriate treatments, inappropriate expectations complicate acne treatment.
  B. Psychologic effects of acne include poor self-esteem, depression, problems with interpersonal relationships.

TABLE 20-2 • Treatment of acne

Types of acne	Lesions	Initial treatment	If not improving
Comedonal (706.1)	Open or closed comedones	Benzoyl peroxide 5% gel qd (if mild) *OR* tretinoin (Retin A) 0.025% cream qd (if moderate) *OR* adapalene 0.1% gel	Combine benzoyl peroxide with tretinoin *OR* increase strength to 0.05%.
Mild papulo (709.8), pustular (686.9)	Red papules, few pustules	Benzoyl peroxide 5–10% qd *OR* adapalene 0.1% gel *OR* azelaic acid bid (if mild) *OR* topical antibiotic bid *OR* erythromycin 3% with 5% benzoyl peroxide qd–bid (if moderate) *OR* clindamycin 1% with 5% benzoyl peroxide qd–bid.	Increase benzoyl peroxide to bid *OR* combine benzoyl peroxide with tretinoin (for comedones). Substitute topical antibiotic bid (for inflammatory).
Moderate to severe papulo (709.8), pustular (686.9)	Red papules, many pustules	Benzoyl peroxide 5% *AND* tretinoin 0.025% *OR* adapalene 0.1% gel *OR* azelaic acid (if comedonal) *OR* topical antibiotic bid (if not comedones) *AND* oral antibiotic bid	Increase strength of treatment or refer to dermatologist.
Nodulocystic, scarring, or unresponsive (709.2)	Red pustules, cysts, and nodules	Oral antibiotics bid *AND* tretinoin 0.05% qd *OR* adapalene 0.1% gel *AND* benzoyl peroxide 10% gel bid (if comedonal)	Refer to dermatologist for oral isotretinoin.

Abbreviations: bid, twice a day; qd, every day.
From Burns C, et al: *Pediatric primary care: a handbook for nurse practitioners,* ed 3, St Louis, 2004, Mosby, p. 1014.

C. Resistance to treatment, especially oral antibiotics, also complicates treatment.

X. Education

A. Proper use of medications, cleansers, moisturizers, makeup are important to encourage compliance.

B. Although no evidence indicates dietary restrictions are helpful, well-balanced diet including adequate intake of water is important in treatment.

C. It takes weeks to months to treat acne; occasionally disorder will worsen with treatment. Compliance is crucial.

ANIMAL BITES

Animal bite, E906.5	*Staphylococcus aureus,* 041.11
Cellulitis, 682.9	Streptococcal, 041.00

I. Etiology

A. May be provoked or unprovoked.

II. Occurrence

A. Cat and dog bites, other animal bites are common injuries.

III. Clinical manifestations

A. May be infected with *Staphylococcus aureus,* streptococci, other oral flora bacteria.

B. About $1/3$ of animal bites contain anaerobic bacteria.

C. Difficult to predict which wounds will become infected.

IV. Physical findings

A. Injuries include lacerations; crushing injuries; deep puncture wounds; bone, tendon, muscle, neurovascular tissue damage from deep bites.

B. Secondary infection can lead to cellulitis.

V. Diagnostic tests

A. Wound cultures identify infectious agents.

B. X-ray and MRI studies reveal bone, vascular, nerve damage.

VI. Differential diagnosis

A. Identify laceration and puncture wounds from other sources.

VII. Treatment

A. Culture wounds before cleansing and debridement.

B. Antibiotics for infected wounds; management of bone, tendon, nerve, vascular wounds by appropriate specialists.

C. If suturing, observe closely for infection.

D. Hospitalization, reconstructive surgery as indicated.

E. Tetanus booster if indicated. Rabies prophylaxis if indicated.

F. Psychologic management.

VIII. Follow-up

A. Call family within 24 hours for update on condition, see as needed.

IX. Complications

Crushing injury, 929.9

A. Lacerations.

    B. Crushing injuries.

    C. Deep puncture wounds.

    D. Secondary infections.

X. Education

    A. Teach children not to provoke any animal.

    B. Provide adequate adult supervision of children.

    C. Report stray animals to animal control officials.

HUMAN BITES

Haemophilus influenzae, 041.5

Human bite, E928.3

Staphylococcus aureus, 041.11

I. Etiology

    A. May be provoked or unprovoked.

II. Occurrence

    A. Many occur in day care centers and should be considered high risk for infection.

III. Clinical manifestations

    A. Human bite wounds harbor both anaerobic and aerobic bacteria, as well as *S. aureus* and *Haemophilus,* with higher incidence of infections and complications than other bites.

    B. Human bites include occlusional wounds when teeth are sunk into skin and clenched-fist injuries when tooth penetrates joint or bone.

IV. Physical findings

    A. Assess for type, size, extent of injury.

    B. If on extremity, assess for movement.

V. Diagnostic tests

    A. Radiographic and surgical evaluation if joint or bone is penetrated.

    B. Bacterial cultures for anaerobic and aerobic bacteria.

VI. Differential diagnosis

    A. Lacerations and puncture wounds from other causes.

VII. Treatment

    A. Irrigation decreases risk of infection.

    B. Debridement of wound edges, broad-spectrum antibiotics (Augmentin, erythromycin) should be used for all human, cat, rat, most dog puncture bites.

    C. Immunocompromised children also receive antibiotic treatment.

VIII. Follow-up

    A. Call family within 24 hours for update on condition, see as needed.

IX. Complications

Abscess, 682.9

Osteomyelitis, 730.20

Stiffness of joint, 719.50

Tendonitis, 726.90

    A. Residual disability frequent after clenched-fist injuries; includes abscess, osteomyelitis, tendonitis, tendon rupture, stiffness of joint.

X. Education
   A. Teach family how to care for wound.
   B. Use time-out for those children who are known to bite.

ATOPIC DERMATITIS/ECZEMA

Atopic dermatitis, 691.8	Lichenification, 698.3
Crusts, 782.8	Papules, 709.8
Dry skin, 701.1	Pruritus, 698.9
Eczema, 692.9	Scale, 782.8
Erythema, 695.9	Skin disorder, 709.9
Excoriations, 919.8	Skin vesicle, 709.8

 I. Etiology
   A. Chronic disorder characterized by exacerbations, remissions.
   B. Strong family history of allergies, asthma.
 II. Occurrence
   A. Most common skin disorder seen in children, affecting 10–15% of all children.
   B. 30–80% continue to experience flares during lifetime.
 III. Clinical manifestations
   A. Usually begins with dry skin, then itch, scratch cycle begins.
   B. Redness, papules, vesicle, crusts.
 IV. Physical findings
   A. Characterized by intense pruritus, erythema, scale, excoriations. Borders are diffuse.
   B. Crusting, oozing common in infants.
   C. Thickened skin (lichenification) from persistent scratching, rubbing may be present.
   D. Distribution: scalp, face, extensors in infants, neck and flexor folds in children, hands and feet in adolescents and adults.
 V. Diagnostic tests
   A. Clinical diagnosis based on careful history and clinical examination.
   B. A potassium hydroxide (KOH) scraping will exclude fungal infections.
 VI. Differential diagnosis

Molluscum contagiosum, 078.0	Seborrheic dermatitis, 690.10
Psoriasis, 696.1	Tinea, 110.9
Scabies, 133.0	

   A. Tinea.
   B. Seborrheic dermatitis, psoriasis, scabies.
   C. Molluscum contagiosum.
 VII. Treatment
   A. Goals of treatment include controlling itching with antihistamines, hydrating skin with lukewarm tub soaks followed by application of emollient moisturizers, such as Cetaphil or Aquaphor.

B. Inflammation is alleviated with topical corticosteroids.
   1. Low-potency steroids are used for face, armpit, groin; medium potency steroids for other body parts.
   2. Steroids should be applied 1–2 times daily for no longer than 2 weeks.
C. Maintain remission with immunomodulators such as Elidel and Protopic applied twice daily.
D. Treat secondary bacterial infections with appropriate topical and systemic antibiotics.
   1. Bactroban or Polysporin are appropriate topically.
   2. Cephalosporins and erythromycin are appropriate systemically.

VIII. Follow-up
A. Refer to dermatology specialist for phototherapy if fail to respond to treatment.
B. Refer to allergist.

IX. Complications

Group A beta-hemolytic streptococci, **041.01**	Molluscum contagiosum, **078.0**
Herpes simplex, **054.9**	*Staphylococcus aureus,* **041.11**
	Warts, **078.10**

A. Secondary bacterial infections from excoriations include Group A beta-hemolytic streptococci and staphylococci.
B. Patients have higher incidence of viral infections including herpes simplex, molluscum contagiosum, warts.

X. Education
A. No cure for atopic dermatitis.
B. Characterized by exacerbations and remissions.
C. Teach proper use of antihistamines, topical corticosteroids, immunomodulators, as well as bathing followed by application of moisturizers.
D. Identify aggravating factors such as stress, allergies, weather change, infections.

BURNS

Burns, **949.0**

I. Etiology
A. Can be caused by thermal, chemical, or electrical agents.

II. Occurrence
A. Majority are thermal; minority are chemical.
B. Most burns are minor, can be managed on outpatient basis.

III. Clinical manifestations
A. Burns are classified by depth of injury.
   1. Superficial or first-degree burns involve only epidermis.
   2. Partial-thickness or second-degree burns involve damage to epidermis and varying depths of dermis.

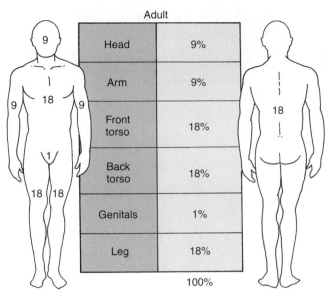

FIGURE 20-1 • Rule of nines. (From Buttaro TM, et al.: *Primary care: a collaborative practice,* ed 2, St. Louis, 2003, Mosby.)

    3. Full-thickness or third-degree burns are painless and involve epidermis, dermis, subcutaneous fat.

  B. Size of burn measured by percent of total body surface area (TBSA) involved. Rule of nines estimates TBSA (Figure 20-1).

IV. Physical findings

  A. Includes TBSA, distribution, depth of involvement.

V. Diagnostic tests

  A. Bacterial cultures for suspected infection.

  B. Laboratory evaluation for serious burns includes CBC, serum electrolytes, serum glucose, BUN, creatinine, urinalysis.

VI. Differential diagnosis

Ritter's disease, 695.81
Scalded skin syndrome, 695.1

  A. Careful history will determine type of injury, degree of burn.

  B. Other diseases include scalded skin syndrome, Ritter's disease.

VII. Treatment

  A. Management depends on classification of burn.

  B. Electrical, chemical burns usually require hospital observation.

  C. Injuries with associated upper airway injury, fractures, abuse, or severe pain also should be hospitalized.

  D. Outpatient treatment includes maintenance of proper nutrition.

  E. Superficial burns: treat with cool compresses and pain management.

    F. Partial-thickness burns: treat with daily cleansing; debridement of devitalized tissue; application of silver sulfadiazine cream, bacitracin, or gentamicin ointment; thin gauze dressing; appropriate pain management.

VIII. Follow-up
    A. Treatment should continue for 1–2 weeks or until wounds are healed.

    B. Assessment for infection should continue.

IX. Complications

Neurologic disturbance, 094.84

Vascular disturbance, 459.9

    A. Local infection and inflammation, neurologic and vascular compromise.

X. Education
    A. Home and environmental safety issues should be addressed, first aid measures, proper use of sunscreen to prevent sunburn of affected areas.

    B. Extent of scarring difficult to predict; depends on severity/extent of burn, whether grafting was needed, skin color.

DIAPER DERMATITIS

Candida albicans, 112.9

Diaper dermatitis, 691.0

Impetigo, 684.

Skin disorder, 709.9

Staphylococcus aureus, 041.11

Streptococcus, 041.00

I. Etiology
    A. Inflammation of skin in diaper area due to breakdown of skin's natural barrier.

II. Occurrence
    A. Most common skin disorder seen in infants <2 years of age.

    B. If not properly controlled, can recur regularly until toilet training is complete.

III. Clinical manifestations
    A. Causes include irritant secondary to prolonged contact with urine and feces, Candida albicans, bacterial infections including impetigo secondary to staphylococci or streptococci.

IV. Physical findings
    A. Most prevalent form is irritant dermatitis.

        1. Usually confined to buttocks, perineal area, medial thighs, sparing intertriginous areas.

        2. Contributing factors: prolonged time between diaper changes, harsh soaps, improper moisturization, use of barrier ointments, excessive heat in warm climates.

    B. Candidal diaper dermatitis suspected when diaper rash does not respond to topical treatments.

        1. Common occurrence with use of oral antibiotics.

        2. Characterized by erythema on buttocks, suprapubic area, medial thighs with raised edges with sharply demarcated margins with pinpoint satellite lesions surrounding borders.

    C. Impetigo characterized by flaccid vesicles and bullae on lower abdomen, medial thighs, buttocks.

V. Diagnostic tests

    A. Microscopic examination with potassium hydroxide (KOH) will reveal budding yeasts with hyphae in candidal infections.

    B. Bacterial culture of vesicle or crust will diagnose bacterial infection.

VI. Differential diagnosis

Atopic dermatitis, 691.8	Monilial infection, 112.9
Bacterial infection, 041.9	Seborrhea, 706.3
Contact dermatitis, 692.9	Viral infection, 079.99

    A. Contact dermatitis, atopic dermatitis, seborrhea.

    B. Bacterial, monilial, viral infections.

VII. Treatment

    A. Irritant diaper dermatitis: treat with frequent diaper changes, cleansing skin with mild cleanser, drying skin, applying barrier such as petrolatum. Air drying between changes is also helpful.

    B. Candidal rashes: treat with topical antifungal medications.

        1. Avoid topical corticosteroid ointments, including combination antifungal and corticosteroid medications such as Lotrisone and Mycolog to reduce possibility of atrophy in occluded area.

        2. Resistant infections: treat with appropriate oral antifungal medications.

    C. Bacterial infections: treat with appropriate antibiotics. Infections including large proportion of diaper area are best treated orally. Isolated areas may be treated appropriately with topical antibiotics, such as mupirocin (Table 20-3).

VIII. Follow-up

    A. Have parents call within 2 days for update.

    B. If not better in 1 week, see again.

IX. Complications

    A. Resistant infections.

X. Education

    A. Parents should be taught proper skin cleansing, frequent diaper changes, proper use of barriers to prevent contact of urine, stool with skin.

INFESTATIONS: PEDICULOSIS (LICE)

Body lice, 132.1	Pediculosis, 132.9
Crusts, 782.8	Pubis lice, 132.2
Head lice, 132.0	Skin lesion, 709.9
Papules, 709.8	Skin ulcerations, 707.9

  I. Etiology

    A. Caused by *Pediculus humanus* (head and body) or by *Phthirus pubis* (pubic).

 II. Occurrence

    A. Spread from human to human; epidemics common in schoolchildren.

TABLE 20-3 • Diagnosis and treatment of diaper dermatitis (691.0)

Type	Cause	Presentation and location	Other characteristics	Treatment
Irritant contact dermatitis (692.9)	Related to wearing diapers; contact with urine and feces	Chapped, shiny, erythematous, parchment-like skin with possible erosions on convex surfaces; creases spared	Peak at 9–12 mo; may progress to involve creases; skin may be dry	Frequent diaper changes, gentle cleansing; greasy lubricant; sitz bath, air dry; hydrocortisone for inflammation
Candidiasis (112.9)	Related to wearing diapers; a superinfection with *Candida*	Shallow pustules, - fiery-red	Satellite lesions, oral thrush; recent antibiotic or diarrhea; occurs at any age	Antifungal cream plus same measures as for contact dermatitis
Miliaria (705.1) or intertrigo (695.89)	Related to wearing diapers; due to heat and occlusion	Discrete vesicles or papules (miliaria); erythematous, scaly, maceration in skin folds	Sweat retention or friction associated	Self-limited (miliaria); avoid precipitation factors; care as for contact dermatitis
Seborrhea (706.3)	Exaggerated by wearing diapers; overgrowth of *Malassezia* yeast in areas of sebaceous gland activity	Greasy, erythematous scales; well circumscribed in creases of skin, groin; spared convex surfaces	Onset at 3–4 weeks of age also occurs on face or body; often superinfected with *Candida*	Ketoconazole is treatment of choice, or hydrocortisone

Continued

TABLE 20-3 • Diagnosis and treatment of diaper dermatitis (691.0)—cont'd

Type	Cause	Presentation and location	Other characteristics	Treatment
Atopic dermatitis (AD) (691.8)	Exaggerated by wearing diapers; exact cause unknown	Increased numbers of lines in skin; areas of excoriation in folds and convex surfaces and buttocks; less widespread	AD in other areas; usually begins in first year of life; scratches skin with diaper change; hyperlinear skin folds with diffuse borders	Skin care as for contact dermatitis and as indicated for AD; antibiotics for bacterial infection
Psoriasis (696.1)	Exaggerated by wearing diapers; psoriasis evolves as response to chronic trauma	Erythematous, well-defined sharp, scaly plaques on convex surfaces and inguinal folds; less widespread	Psoriasis affects other places; rare occurrence, if found, usually at 6–18 mo	Treatment often required for weeks or until toilet trained; steroids, ketoconazole if *Candida* present
Bacterial dermatitis (692.9)	Usually due to staphylococcal or streptococcal infection	Red, denuded areas of fragile blisters; crusting, and pustules in suprapubic area and periumbilicus	Usually in newborn, can occur anywhere	Econazole/ketoconazole cream if yeast present as well; mupirocin if minimal; cephalexin, amoxicillin, erythromycin if extensive

From Burns C, et al: *Pediatric primary care: a handbook for nurse practitioners*, ed 3, St Louis, 2004, Mosby, p. 1018.

B. *Pediculosis corporis* often found in crowded living conditions, areas of poor personal hygiene.

III. Clinical manifestations

A. Nits (louse eggs) are found in hair on scalp.

IV. Physical findings

A. Pediculosis corporis begins as small papules with secondary lesions developing from scratching, resulting in crusted papules, ulcerations.

V. Diagnostic tests

A. White nits are obvious on hair shaft. Hair may be plucked and microscopic examination will reveal nits.

B. *Pediculosis corporis:* diagnosed by examining seams of clothing, which reveal louse.

VI. Differential diagnosis

Atopic dermatitis, 691.8
Eczema, 692.9
Scabies, 133.0

A. Atopic dermatitis or other eczematous dermatitis.
B. Scabies.

VII. Treatment

A. Remove nits with fine-toothed comb after soaking in vinegar or OTC products such as Nix Crème Rinse, Rid, Acticin.
B. Second application of these agents recommended in 7–10 days.
C. Shaving affected area is not necessary.

VIII. Follow-up

A. Daily and weekly checks at home for lice and nits.
B. Can see in 2 weeks to ensure infestation is cleared.

IX. Complications

Atopic dermatitis, 691.8
Pruritus, 698.9

A. Atopic dermatitis secondary to pruritus and reaction to nits and eggs.
B. Treat with appropriate topical corticosteroids and antihistamines.

X. Education

A. Proper use of topical medications and nit comb.
B. Application of gasoline is not accepted treatment, must be avoided.

SCABIES

Erythema, unspecified, 695.9   Skin lesion, 709.9
Pruritus, 698.9   Skin vesicles, 709.8
Scabies, 133.0

I. Etiology

A. Infestation caused by *Sarcoptes scabiei.*

B. Usually spread by skin-to-skin contact among household members and by sexual contact.

C. Fertilized female mite burrows in stratum corneum, laying eggs and feces, which create irritation, pruritus.

II. Occurrence
A. All age groups and socioeconomic groups.

III. Clinical manifestations
A. Itching usually worse at night; becomes more intense.

IV. Physical findings
A. Pinpoint vesicles and erythematous papules in S-shaped pattern.

B. Common sites of lesions: finger webs, flexor wrists, areolae, umbilicus, waistband area, groin, axilla.

C. Children, adults rarely have lesions above neck. Infants can manifest lesions on palms, soles.

D. Incubation from infestation to onset of symptoms is usually 1 month, with nocturnal itching most intense.

V. Diagnostic tests
A. Mineral oil applied to vesicle, scraped with No. 15 blade, placed on slide with cover slip reveals mites, eggs, or feces on microscopy.

VI. Differential diagnosis

Atopic dermatitis, 691.8
Drug eruptions, 693.0
Insect bites, 989.5

A. Insect bites.

B. Atopic dermatitis.

C. Drug eruptions.

VII. Treatment
A. Permethrin is treatment of choice, but not proven safe in infants <2 months of age; in pregnant/lactating women, use precipitated sulfur ointment for 3 nights.

B. Treat all household contacts.

C. Treat pruritus with appropriate antihistamines such as Zyrtec, Claritin, Benadryl; secondary dermatitis with appropriate low to midpotency corticosteroids.

VIII. Follow-up
A. None needed unless complications.

IX. Complications

Atopic dermatitis, 691.8
Bacterial infection, 041.9

A. Secondary atopic dermatitis and bacterial infection.

B. Treatment failures usually secondary to noncompliance, improper application of scabicide.

C. Reinfection.

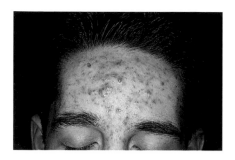

COLOR PLATE 1 • Acne vulgaris of the forehead. (From Callen JP, Greer KE, Paller AS, et al: *Color atlas of dermatology,* ed 2, Philadelphia, 2000, Saunders.)

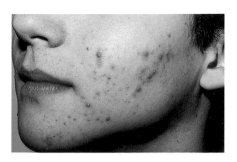

COLOR PLATE 2 • Acne vulgaris of the lower face. (From Callen JP, Greer KE, Paller AS, et al: *Color atlas of dermatology,* ed 2, Philadelphia, 2000, Saunders.)

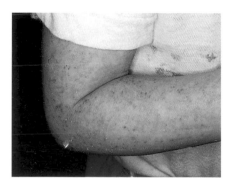

COLOR PLATE 3 • Atopic dermatitis. Minute excoriations with lichenification in the antecubital fossa seen. (From Callen JP, Greer KE, Paller AS, et al: *Color atlas of dermatology,* ed 2, Philadelphia, 2000, Saunders.)

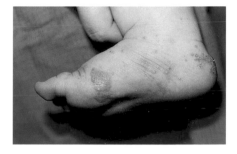

COLOR PLATE 4 • Impetiginized atopic dermatitis. (From Callen JP, Greer KE, Paller AS, et al: *Color atlas of dermatology,* ed 2, Philadelphia, 2000, Saunders.)

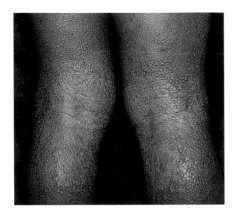

COLOR PLATE 5 • Flexural involvement of popliteal fossa in atopic dermatitis. (From Weston WL, Morelli JG, Lane A: *Color textbook of pediatric dermatology*, ed 3, St Louis, 2002, Mosby.)

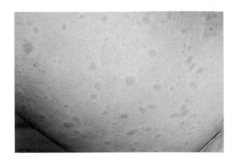

COLOR PLATE 6 • Urticaria. (From Callen JP, Greer KE, Paller AS, et al: *Color atlas of dermatology,* ed 2, Philadelphia, 2000, Saunders.)

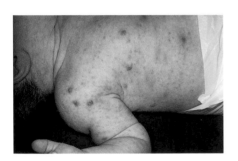

COLOR PLATE 7 • Scabies. (From Callen JP, Greer KE, Paller AS, et al: *Color atlas of dermatology,* ed 2, Philadelphia, 2000, Saunders.)

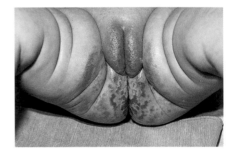

COLOR PLATE 8 • Irritant diaper dermatitis. (From Callen JP, Greer KE, Paller AS, et al: *Color atlas of dermatology,* ed 2, Philadelphia, 2000, Saunders.)

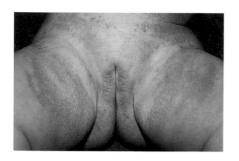

COLOR PLATE 9 • Chafing type of diaper dermatitis. (From Weston WL, Morelli JG, Lane A: *Color textbook of pediatric dermatology,* ed 3, St Louis, 2002, Mosby.)

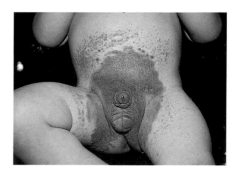

COLOR PLATE 10 • Candidiasis in the diaper area. A positive culture for Candida can be obtained from satellite pustules. (From Weston WL, Morelli JG, Lane A: *Color textbook of pediatric dermatology,* ed 3, St Louis, 2002, Mosby.)

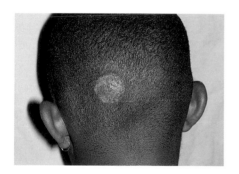

COLOR PLATE 11 • Inflammatory superficial fungal infection. (From Callen JP, Greer KE, Paller AS, et al: *Color atlas of dermatology,* ed 2, Philadelphia, 2000, Saunders.)

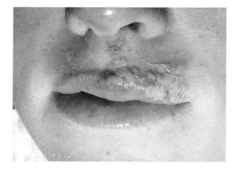

COLOR PLATE 12 • Recurrent herpes simplex. (From Callen JP, Greer KE, Paller AS, et al: *Color atlas of dermatology,* ed 2, Philadelphia, 2000, Saunders.)

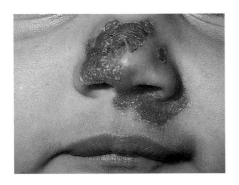

COLOR PLATE 13 • Impetigo. Spread of infection to top of nose from beneath the nose in an infant with impetigo. (From Weston WL, Morelli JG, Lane A: *Color textbook of pediatric dermatology,* ed 3, St Louis, 2002, Mosby.)

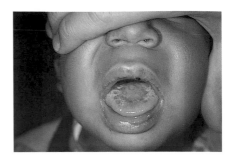

COLOR PLATE 14 • Infant with primary herpes gingivostomatitis. (From Weston WL, Morelli JG, Lane A: *Color textbook of pediatric dermatology,* ed 3, St Louis, 2002, Mosby.)

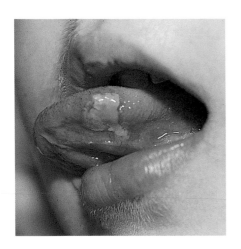

COLOR PLATE 15 • Erosion of the tongue in a child with hand-foot-and-mouth syndrome. (From Weston WL, Morelli JG, Lane A: *Color textbook of pediatric dermatology,* ed 3, St Louis, 2002, Mosby.)

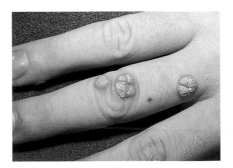

COLOR PLATE 16 • Common warts on a child's fingers. (From Weston WL, Morelli JG, Lane A: *Color textbook of pediatric dermatology,* ed 3, St Louis, 2002, Mosby.)

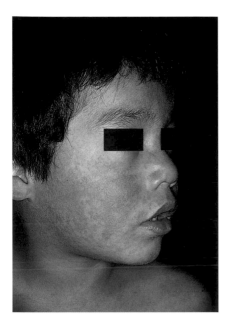

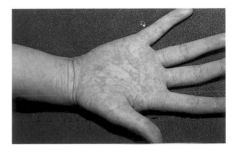

COLOR PLATE 17 • Slapped-cheek appearance of a child with parvovirus B19 infection (erythema infectiosum). (From Weston WL, Morelli JG, Lane A: *Color textbook of pediatric dermatology,* ed 3, St Louis, 2002, Mosby.)

COLOR PLATE 18 • Lacy pink eruption over the palms in erythema infectiosum. (From Weston WL, Morelli JG, Lane A: *Color textbook of pediatric dermatology,* ed 3, St Louis, 2002, Mosby.)

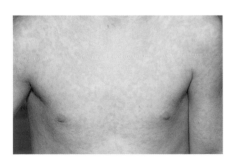

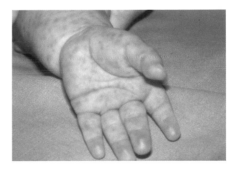

COLOR PLATE 19 • Lacy pink eruption of erythema infectiosum on chest and upper abdomen. (From Wes-ton WL, Morelli JG, Lane A: *Color textbook of pediatric dermatology,* ed 3, St Louis, 2002, Mosby.)

COLOR PLATE 20 • Rocky Mountain spotted fever. RMSF, acral dusky oval purpuric lesions. (Courtesy of Dr. Russell Steele. From Schachner LA, Hansen RC: *Pediatric dermatology,* ed 3, St Louis, 2003, Mosby.)

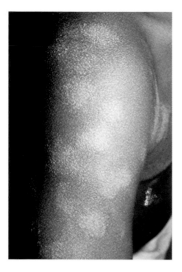

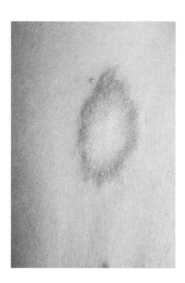

COLOR PLATE 21 • Pityriasis alba. In some atopic patients, subtle inflammation may result in poorly demarcated areas of hypopigmentation, known as pityriasis alba. Lesions are most prominent in darkly pigmented individuals. (From Cohen BA: *Pediatric dermatology*, ed 2, St Louis, 1999, Mosby.)

COLOR PLATE 22 • Pityriasis rosea. The large herald patch on the chest of this 10-year-old girl shows central clearing, which mimics tinea corporis. (From Cohen BA: *Pediatric dermatology*, ed 2, St Louis, 1999, Mosby.)

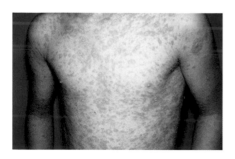

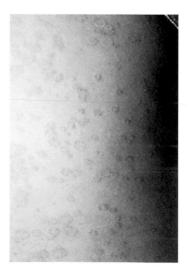

COLOR PLATE 23 • Pityriasis rosea. Numerous oval lesions on the chest of a Caucasian teenager. (From Cohen BA: *Pediatric dermatology*, ed 2, St Louis, 1999, Mosby.)

COLOR PLATE 24 • Tinea versicolor. The well-demarcated, scaly papules appear darker than surrounding skin on the back of a Caucasian adolescent. (From Cohen BA: *Pediatric dermatology*, ed 2, St Louis, 1999, Mosby.)

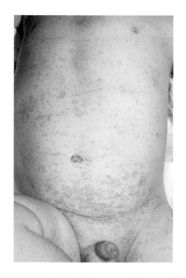

COLOR PLATE 25 • Roseola/exanthema subitum. A generalized, pink, maculopapular rash suddenly appeared on this infant after 3 days of high fever. (From Cohen BA: *Pediatric dermatology,* ed 2, St Louis, 1999, Mosby.)

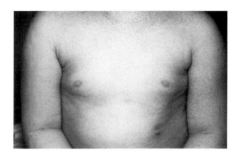

COLOR PLATE 26 • Scarlet fever. A generalized, bright red, sandpaper-like papular rash developed in a 7-year-old boy with a streptococcal pharyngitis. (From Cohen BA: *Pediatric dermatology,* ed 2, St Louis, 1999, Mosby.)

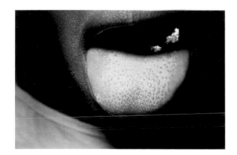

COLOR PLATE 27 • Scarlet fever. A white strawberry tongue precedes red-strawberry tongue. (From Cohen BA: *Pediatric dermatology,* ed 2, St Louis, 1999, Mosby.)

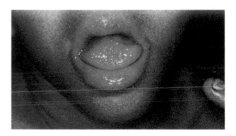

COLOR PLATE 28 • Scarlet fever. A red-strawberry tongue as the erythrotoxin-mediated enanthema evolves. (From Cohen BA: *Pediatric dermatology,* ed 2, St Louis, 1999, Mosby.)

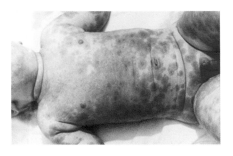

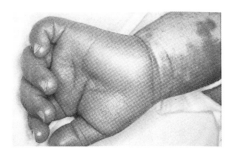

COLOR PLATE 29 • Kawasaki syndrome. A generalized, morbilliform, erythema multiforme-like rash is a characteristic clinical finding. (From Cohen BA: *Pediatric dermatology,* ed 2, St Louis, 1999, Mosby.)

COLOR PLATE 30 • Kawasaki syndrome. Palmar and plantar erythema with edema of the hands and feet is a characteristic clinical finding. (From Cohen BA: *Pediatric dermatology,* ed 2, St Louis, 1999, Mosby.)

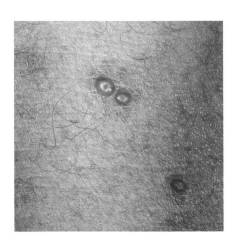

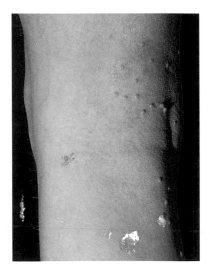

COLOR PLATE 31 • Molluscum contagiosum. Individual lesions are 2- to 5-mm, flesh-colored, dome-shaped umbilicated papules. (From Habif TP: *Clinical dermatology,* ed 4, St Louis, 2004, Mosby.)

COLOR PLATE 32 • Molluscum contagiosum spreads rapidly in eczematous skin. This patient has atopic dermatitis of the popliteal fossa. (From Habif TP: *Clinical dermatology,* ed 4, St Louis, 2004, Mosby.)

X. Education

A. Proper application of scabicide. Mites can survive for 2–5 days on inanimate objects such as clothing, stuffed animals. Proper laundering should be taught.

BITES: LYME DISEASE

Arthralgias, 719.4	Headache, 784.0
Borrelia burgdorferi, 101.	Lyme disease, 088.81
Chills, 780.99	Malaise, 780.79
Erythema annulare, 695.0	Papule, 709.8
Fever, 780.6	Rash, 782.1

I. Etiology

A. Systemic infection caused by spirochete, *Borrelia burgdorferi*. Successful transmission requires 48–72 hours.

II. Occurrence

A. Found in northeastern and midwestern US; can occur in any season, although most prevalent during warmer months.

III. Clinical manifestations

A. Flulike symptoms including malaise, arthralgias, headache, fever, chills precede development of rash.

IV. Physical findings

A. Red macule/papule at site of tick bite 2–30 days after infection.
B. Lesions expand to form annular erythematous lesions, generally with central clearing.
C. Center of lesion becomes darker, vesicular, hemorrhagic, or necrotic.
D. Common sites: thigh, groin, trunk, axilla.

V. Diagnostic tests

A. History including exposure to tick bite.
B. Enzyme-linked immunosorbent assay (ELISA) and Western blot analyses for *B. burgdorferi* recommended by US Centers for Disease Control and Prevention (CDC).

VI. Differential diagnosis

Erythema annulare, 695.0	Tinea corporis, 110.5
Granuloma annulare, 695.89	Urticaria, 708.9

A. Tinea corporis.
B. Urticaria.
C. Granuloma annulare.
D. Erythema annulare.

VII. Treatment

A. Amoxicillin 50 mg/kg/day in 2 doses for children <8 years of age.
B. Adults: 500 mg tid × 21 days, doxycycline 100 mg bid × 21 days, ceftriaxone 500 mg bid × 21 days.
C. Azithromycin or erythromycin: second-line treatments for pregnant patients or those unable to tolerate above treatments.

VIII. Follow-up
A. Call family 24 hours after treatment has started to assess how the child is doing, then follow up as needed.

IX. Complications

Arthralgias, 719.4
Headache, 784.0

A. Arthralgias.
B. Headaches may persist after treatment as other symptoms resolve.

X. Education
A. Educate patients on proper use of insect repellents (<10% DEET if <12 years of age; <30% if >12 years of age).
B. Inspect skin carefully in tick-infested areas and during tick season.
C. Spray permethrin on clothing before going outside, wear light-colored long pants tucked into shoes/boots, long sleeve shirt, hat.

ROCKY MOUNTAIN SPOTTED FEVER

Anorexia, 783.0	Muscle pain, 729.1
Chills, 780.99	Rash, 782.1
Diarrhea, 787.91	Rickettsial disease, 083.9
Edema, 782.3	Rocky Mountain spotted fever, 082.0
Fever, 780.6	Sweating, 780.8
Headache, 784.0	Tickborne fever, 066.1
Joint pain, 719.40	Vomiting, 787.03
Malaise, 780.79	

I. Etiology
A. Prototype for all tickborne spotted fevers, caused by *Rickettsia rickettsii*.

II. Occurrence
A. Occurs primarily in southeastern and south-central US.
B. All ages are susceptible; however, most common in children <15 years of age.
C. Incidence is highest in midsummer, lowest in winter.

III. Clinical manifestations
A. History of tick bite is common in over 80% of cases.
B. Prodrome of low-grade fever, headache, malaise, joint/muscle pain, anorexia may precede illness, which is sudden, consisting of sweating, chills, severe aches, vomiting, diarrhea.
C. Most common clinical findings: rash, edema, fever.

IV. Physical findings
A. Rash may appear soon after onset of symptoms, first on ankles and feet, spreading to wrists, hands, trunk, head.
B. Discrete, rose-colored macules, blanching on pressure, soon become papular or purpuric.
C. Resolving rash may desquamate with resulting hyperpigmentation.

    D. Nonpitting edema is frequent, with periorbital edema common in children.

    E. Conjunctivitis, pharyngitis, photophobia, CNS symptoms including confusion, delirium, seizures, coma are common (see color insert).

V. Diagnostic tests

    A. Generally no rise in antibody titer is detected until second week of disease.

    B. ELISA assay if immunoglobulin M (IgM) and immunoglobulin G (IgG) to *R. rickettsii* is sensitive and specificity is indicated.

    C. Tissue direct and indirect immunofluorescence may identify rickettsiae.

VI. Differential diagnosis

Disseminated gonococcal infection, 098.0	Varicella, 052.9
Drug eruptions, 693.0	Viral exanthems, 057.9
Lyme disease, 088.81	

    A. Viral exanthems.

    B. Drug eruption.

    C. Varicella.

    D. Disseminated gonococcal infection.

    E. Lyme disease.

VII. Treatment

    A. Doxycycline or tetracycline.

    B. Chloramphenicol is an alternative for those you can't treat with or are allergic to doxycycline or tetracycline.

    C. Supportive treatment for fever and myalgias.

VIII. Follow-up

    A. Close follow-up for complications persisting >1 year after acute infection for neurologic and nonneurologic disabilities.

IX. Complications

Bladder incontinence, 780.30	Hearing loss, 389.9
Bowel incontinence, 787.6	Language disorder, 315.31
Cerebral dysfunction, 348.30	Peripheral neuropathy, 356.9

    A. Death is associated with older patients, those with delay in treatment, or undiagnosed disease. Untreated disease death rate is 25%.

    B. Other complications: neurologic disorders including hearing loss, peripheral neuropathy, bladder and bowel incontinence, cerebellar dysfunction, language disorders.

X. Education

    A. Avoidance of tick bites, prompt removal of ticks. No vaccine is available.

MOLLUSCUM CONTAGIOSUM

Molluscum contagiosum, 078.0
Itching, 698.9
Papules, 709.8

I. **Etiology**
   A. Molluscum contagiosum is virus caused by poxvirus infecting epidermis, causing white papules.
   B. Center of lesions is filled with keratinous material.

II. **Occurrence**
   A. Molluscum contagiosum common in infants, toddlers; most adults are immune.

III. **Clinical manifestations**
   A. Itching.
   B. 1- to 6-mm discrete umbilicated papules usually seen in intertriginous areas.
   C. Occasionally, larger lesions up to 15 mm may be found.
   D. Incubation period is 2–7 weeks.
   E. Children are contagious as long as lesions are present.
   F. Lesions may resolve spontaneously, may take years (see color insert).

IV. **Physical findings**
   A. Axilla, face, trunk, genitalia are most commonly affected areas.

V. **Diagnostic tests**
   A. None.

VI. **Differential diagnosis**

Blisters, **709.8**
Epidermal cysts, **706.2**
Warts, **078.10**

   A. Warts, closed comedones, epidermal cysts.
   B. Blisters may be confused with molluscum contagiosum.
   C. In young children with genital lesions, must suspect child abuse.

VII. **Treatment**
   A. Papules may be removed by curette or incision and drainage; however, procedure is painful, may result in scarring.
   B. Treatment with liquid nitrogen, cantharidin, potassium hydroxide, podophyllin applied to central umbilication is less traumatic.
   C. Topical treatment at home with imiquimod cream is alternative.

VIII. **Complications**

Atopic dermitis, **691.8**
Impetigo, **684.**
Scarring, **709.2**

   A. Secondary impetigo.
   B. Atopic dermatitis.

IX. **Follow-up**
   A. Office visits every 2 weeks for treatment will control spread of lesions.

X. **Education**
   A. Lesions are benign but highly contagious.

WARTS

Human papillomavirus, 079.4
Papules, 709.8
Warts, 078.10

I. **Etiology**
  A. Warts are benign virus-induced tumors caused by human papillomavirus (HPV).
  B. More than 76 subtypes identified; associated with specific cutaneous and mucous membrane location.
II. **Occurrence**
  A. Transmission is by direct contact; infection can occur by autoinoculation, especially in intertriginous areas.
  B. Immunocompromised patients are at increased risk.
III. **Clinical manifestations**
  A. Verrucous papules appear as solitary lesions or may be grouped, confluent, flat, or pedunculated.
IV. **Physical findings**
  A. May appear anywhere on body, occur most often on extremities, interrupting dermal ridges.
V. **Diagnostic tests**
  A. No testing necessary.
VI. **Differential diagnosis**

Calluses, 592.9   Lichen planus, 697.0
Filiform warts, 078.10   Molluscum contagiosum, 078.0
Flat warts, 078.10   Plantar warts, 078.19

  A. Plantar warts differentiated from calluses by interruption of dermal ridges.
  B. Common and filiform warts present no diagnostic challenge.
  C. Flat warts are often confused with closed comedones, lichen planus, molluscum contagiosum.
VII. **Treatment**
  A. Multiple therapeutic modalities are available for treatment, including liquid nitrogen, cantharidin, electrodesiccation, laser therapy, candida and bleomycin injection, excision.
  B. Unlikely warts will resolve with single treatment except excision; recurrence is high.
  C. Warts frequently resolve spontaneously; exercise good clinical judgment when considering various therapies versus cautious observation.
  D. Multiple salicylic acid treatments available OTC, as well as prescription retinoids, podophyllin, imiquimod cream.
  E. Covering topical medications with nonporous tape (duct tape or athletic tape) suffocates virus. Leave in place for 6 days, remove tape, shave wart, reapply tape.

TABLE 20-4 • Treatment of viral warts

	Treatment		
Type of wart	First choice	Alternative	Response rate (%)
Common (078.10)	Cryotherapy	Salicylic acid paint	60–90
Periungual (078.10)	Imiquimod cream	Cantharidin	60
Flat (078.10)	Retinoic acid	Imiquimod cream	50
Filiform (078.10)	Surgery	Cryotherapy with forceps	50
Plantar (078.19)	Salicylic acid plaster	Imiquimod cream	60
Venereal (078.19)	Podophyllin or Condylox	Imiquimod cream	90

From Weston W, Lane A, Morelli J: *Color textbook of pediatric dermatology,* ed 3, St Louis, 2002, Mosby, p. 114.

   F. Cimetidine 30–40 mg/kg per day in combination with other
      treatment modalities is effective for resistant warts
      (Table 20-4).
VIII. Follow-up
   A. Close follow-up every 2 weeks.
   IX. Complications

Anxiety, **300.**
Genital warts, **078.19**
Skin pain, **782.0**

   A. Proliferation of warts, resulting in pain or difficulty with daily tasks.
   B. Social anxiety, isolation due to cosmetic embarrassment requires more
      aggressive treatment.
   X. Education
   A. Recalcitrant nature of warts should be emphasized, as well as need for
      multiple treatments.
   B. Genital warts in infants, toddlers: evaluate for possibility of sexual abuse.

FIFTH DISEASE (ERYTHEMA INFECTIOSUM)

Erythema infectiosum, **057.0**   Human papillomavirus, **079.4**
Fever, **780.6**   Malaise, **780.79**
Fifth disease, **057.0**   Myalgias, **729.1**
Headache, **784.0**

   I. Etiology
   A. Erythema infectiosum (fifth disease) is caused by human parvovirus B19.
   B. Spread by respiratory tract secretions.
   II. Occurrence
   A. Usually seen in 2- to 15-years-olds.
   B. Spread to household contacts is common.

III. Clinical manifestations
   A. Headache, malaise, mild fever, myalgias.
   B. Fifth disease begins with intense red cheeks (slapped cheeks), spreads to involve arms, legs, trunk with macular red lacy exanthem.
   C. Although initially lasting <1 week, with heat exposure exanthem can recur for up to 4 months.
IV. Physical findings
   A. May present with nonspecific symptoms: fever, malaise, myalgias, red cheeks or lacy rash (see color insert).
V. Diagnostic tests
   A. Serum obtained within 30 days of onset of rash will confirm presence of immunoglobulin M (IgM) human parovirus B19 antibodies.
VI. Differential diagnosis

Drug eruptions, 693.0

   A. Drug eruptions, other morbilliform eruptions differentiated by classic lacy rash of fifth disease.
VII. Treatment
   A. No specific treatment or specific control measures, other than avoid exposure to pregnant women and those who are immunocompromised.
   B. Disease no longer contagious once skin eruption occurs.
VIII. Follow-up
   A. None needed.
IX. Complications

Aplastic anemia, 284.9
Hydrops fetalis, 778.0

   A. Hydrops fetalis may result in pregnant women who have not developed antibodies.
   B. Immunocompromised children may develop persistent infection.
   C. Patients with transient anemias may develop aplastic crisis and severe anemia.
X. Education
   A. Inform of likelihood of recurrence with heat exposure, including exercise and sun exposure.
   B. Avoid pregnant women, immunocompromised individuals, those with chronic anemias.

BIBLIOGRAPHY

Burns C, et al: *Pediatric primary care: a handbook for nurse practitioners,* ed 3, St Louis, 2004, Mosby.
Buttaro T, et al: *Primary care: a collaborative approach,* St Louis, 1999, Mosby.
Fitzpatrick T, et al: *Color atlas & synopsis of clinical dermatology,* ed 4, New York, 2001, McGraw-Hill.

Goodheart H: *Goodheart's photoguide of common skin disorders,* Philadelphia, 2003, Lippincott Williams & Wilkins.

Habif T: *Clinical dermatology,* ed 3, St Louis, 1996, Mosby.

Schachner L, Hansen R: *Pediatric dermatology,* ed 3, St Louis, 2003, Mosby.

Weston W, Lane A, Morelli J: *Color textbook of pediatric dermatology,* ed 3, St Louis, 2002, Mosby.

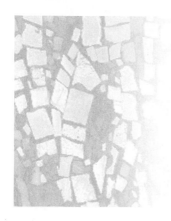

CHAPTER 21

Eye Disorders

FRANCES K. PORCHER

ALLERGIC CONJUNCTIVITIS

Allergic conjunctivitis, 372.14	Atopic dermatitis, 691.8
Allergic rhinitis, 477.9	Conjunctival hyperemia, 372.71
Allergic rhinitis due to other allergens, 477.8	Conjunctivitis, 372.30
Allergic rhinitis due to pollen (seasonal rhinitis), 477.0	Excessive tearing, 375.20
	Stringy, mucoid discharge, 372.89
Asthma, 493.90	Upper respiratory infection, 465.9

Conjunctivitis: inflammation or infection of bulbar and/or palpebral conjunctiva.

I. Etiology
   A. Allergens such as pollen, molds, animal dander, smoke, dust.

II. Occurrence
   A. Common in all age groups.
   B. Often seasonal.
   C. May have had recent upper respiratory infection.

III. Clinical manifestations
   A. Watery red eyes.
   B. Itching or burning bilaterally.
   C. Excessive tearing.

IV. Physical findings
   A. Diffuse conjunctival hyperemia.
   B. Boggy conjunctiva.
   C. Stringy, mucoid discharge.
   D. May see concurrent asthma, atopic dermatitis, or allergic rhinitis.

V. Diagnostic tests
   A. None.
   B. Culture if conjunctivitis is persistent or does not respond to treatment.

VI. Differential diagnosis

Conjunctivitis, bacterial, 372.30   Corneal abrasion, 918.1
Conjunctivitis, viral, 077.99   Nasolacrimal duct obstruction, 375.56

    A. Bacterial or viral conjunctivitis.
    B. Nasolacrimal duct obstruction.
    C. Corneal abrasion.

VII. Treatment

    A. Eliminate offending agent.
    B. Systemic oral antihistamine (Claritin, Zyrtec).
    C. Topical ophthalmic mast-cell stabilizer (Cromolyn, Alomide).
    D. Topical ophthalmic antihistamine/mast-cell stabilizer combination (Patanol).
    E. Artificial tears.
    F. Cool, wet compresses.

VIII. Follow-up

    A. Routine follow-up not necessary.
    B. Return if fails to improve in 2–3 days or worsens.

IX. Complications

Allergic reaction to medication, 995.5
Secondary bacterial infection, 041.9

    A. Allergic reaction to medication.
    B. Secondary bacterial infection.

X. Education

    A. Avoid rubbing eyes.
    B. Use meticulous hand washing.
    C. Avoid wearing eye makeup until resolved.
    D. Avoid use of contact lenses until resolved.
    E. Will last about 10–14 days.

BACTERIAL CONJUNCTIVITIS

Conjunctival hyperemia, 372.71
Conjunctivitis, bacterial, 372.30
Otitis media, 382.9

I. Etiology

    A. *Haemophilus influenzae.*
    B. *Streptococcus pneumoniae.*
    C. *Moraxella catarrhalis.*

II. Occurrence

    A. Common in school-age children.
    B. Accounts for 80% of pediatric acute conjunctivitis.

III. Clinical manifestations

    A. Red eyes.
    B. Purulent discharge, with matted eyelids on awakening.

    C. May complain of gritty sensation in eye.

    D. Usually starts unilaterally becoming bilateral.

IV. Physical findings

    A. Diffuse and marked conjunctival hyperemia.

    B. Purulent or mucopurulent discharge.

    C. May see concurrent otitis media (especially with *H. influenzae*).

V. Diagnostic tests

    A. Culture in infants <1 month of age, multiple cases in a day care/school; unless conjunctivitis is persistent or does not respond to treatment.

VI. Differential diagnosis

Blepharitis, 373.00	Corneal ulcer, 370.00
Chlamydial conjunctivitis, 077.98	Herpes simplex, 054.43
Conjunctivitis, viral, 077.99	Nasolacrimal duct obstruction, 375.56
Corneal abrasion, 918.1	*Neisseria gonorrhoeae* conjunctivitis, 098.40

    A. Viral conjunctivitis.

    B. Chlamydial conjunctivitis (refer to ophthalmologist).

    C. *Neisseria gonorrhoeae* conjunctivitis (refer to ophthalmologist).

    D. Nasolacrimal duct obstruction.

    E. Blepharitis.

    F. Corneal abrasion or ulcer (refer to ophthalmologist).

    G. Herpes simplex (refer to ophthalmologist).

VII. Treatment

    A. 1 Year of age, newer generation ophthalmic fluoroquinolones:

        1. Levofloxacin (Quixin).

        2. Moxifloxacin (Vigamox).

        3. Gatifloxacin (Zymar).

    B. <1 Year of age:

        1. Tobramycin (Tobrex) ophthalmic solution or ointment.

        2. Erythromycin ophthalmic ointment.

    C. Cool, wet compresses.

VIII. Follow-up

    A. No routine follow-up necessary.

    B. Recheck if fails to improve in 2–3 days or worsens.

IX. Complications

Blindness 369.00
Systemic infection 038.9

    A. Systemic infection.

    B. Blindness.

X. Education

    A. Continue treatment for at least 7 days or for at least 3 days after symptoms have resolved.

    B. Very contagious; meticulous hand washing and no sharing of linens.

C. No school or day care until antibiotic treatment for 24 hours.

D. Instillation of ophthalmic ointment will blur vision.

CHLAMYDIAL CONJUNCTIVITIS

Chlamydial conjunctivitis, 077.99	Pneumonia, 486.
Chlamydial pneumonia, 483.1	Rhinorrhea, 478.1
Cough, 786.2	Tachypnea, 786.06
Hyperemic conjunctiva, 372.71	

I. Etiology

  A. *Chlamydia trachomatis.*

II. Occurrence

  A. Neonatal occurrence, acquired from infected cervix during birth.

  B. Adult occurrence, acquired through sexual contact.

III. Clinical manifestations

  A. Purulent discharge.

  B. May occur in one or both eyes.

  C. Neonatal infection appears from day 2 to week 8.

IV. Physical findings

  A. Mucopurulent discharge.

  B. Hyperemic conjunctiva.

  C. May see *Chlamydia* pneumonia in infants.

V. Diagnostic tests

  A. Giemsa-stained epithelial cells from conjunctival scraping.

  B. Conjunctival culture from swab (requires special tissue culture techniques).

  C. Immunofluorescent staining of conjunctival scraping.

  D. Chlamydial antigen test.

VI. Differential diagnosis

Congenital glaucoma, 743.20	Conjunctivitis, viral, 077.99
Conjunctivitis, bacterial, 372.30	*Neisseria gonorrhoeae* conjunctivitis, 098.40

  A. *Neisseria gonorrhoeae* conjunctivitis (refer to ophthalmologist).

  B. Bacterial conjunctivitis.

  C. Viral conjunctivitis.

  D. Congenital glaucoma (refer to ophthalmologist).

VII. Treatment

  A. Refer all neonates for evaluation and treatment (systemic oral erythromycin).

  B. Refer mother and mother's sexual partner for evaluation and treatment.

  C. Report to appropriate authority (sexually transmitted infection).

VIII. Follow-up

  A. Return in 3 days to monitor eye infection.

  B. Return sooner if infant has signs of pneumonia or parental concerns.

IX. Complications

  A. Other sexually transmitted infections.

X. Education
   A. Review good hand washing with family.
   B. Mother and partner need treatment because disease is usually transmitted vaginally during birth.
   C. Eye infection can be associated with pneumonia that started during first 6 weeks with cough, rhinorrhea, tachypnea.
   D. Infant may need second round of erythromycin; efficacy is 80%.

VIRAL CONJUNCTIVITIS

Conjunctivitis, viral, 077.99	Pharyngitis, 462.
Diffuse conjunctival hyperemia, 372.71	Upper respiratory infection, 465.9

I. Etiology
   A. Adenovirus (most).
   B. Herpes simplex.
   C. Varicella-zoster.
   D. Coxsackie.

II. Occurrence
   A. Common in all age groups.
   B. Very contagious; 8-day incubation period.

III. Clinical manifestations
   A. Pinkish-red eyes.
   B. Watery or serous discharge, with crusty eyelids on awakening.
   C. May complain of gritty sensation in eye.
   D. May complain of sore throat, upper respiratory infection, flulike symptoms.
   E. One or both eyes involved.
   F. Vesicles on skin around eye (herpes).

IV. Physical findings
   A. Diffuse conjunctival hyperemia with follicles.
   B. Watery or serous discharge.
   C. Discomfort, not acute pain.
   D. Preauricular and submandibular adenopathy.
   E. May see concurrent pharyngitis and/or upper respiratory infection.
   F. Vesicular lesions on skin around eyes (herpes).
   G. Normal vision.

V. Diagnostic tests
   A. None.
   B. Culture if conjunctivitis is persistent or does not respond to treatment.

VI. Differential diagnosis

Blepharitis, 373.00	Corneal abrasion, 918.1
Conjunctivitis, allergic, 372.14	Corneal ulcer, 370.00
Conjunctivitis, bacterial, 372.30	Nasolacrimal duct obstruction, 375.56

   A. Bacterial conjunctivitis.
   B. Allergic conjunctivitis.

    C. Nasolacrimal duct obstruction.

    D. Blepharitis.

    E. Corneal abrasion or ulcer (refer to ophthalmologist).

VII. Treatment

    A. Antibiotics not indicated.

    B. Cool, wet compresses.

    C. Artificial tears.

    D. Refer if suspect conjunctivitis due to herpes.

VIII. Follow-up

    A. No routine follow-up necessary.

    B. Recheck if fails to improve in 10–14 days, or sooner if worsens.

IX. Complications

Secondary bacterial infection, **041.9**

    A. Secondary bacterial infection.

X. Education

    A. Very contagious; meticulous hand washing and no sharing of linens.

    B. Avoid touching eyes.

    C. Will last about 12–14 days.

    D. No school or day care until discharge is resolved.

CONGENITAL NASOLACRIMAL DUCT OBSTRUCTION (DACRYOSTENOSIS)

Congenital nasolacrimal duct obstruction (dacryostenosis), **375.56**

Defect of lacrimal drainage system resulting in blockage.

I. Etiology

    A. Imperforate membrane at distal end of nasolacrimal duct.

II. Occurrence

    A. Occurs in up to 6% of all newborn infants.

    B. Both eyes involved, 33%; one eye involved, 66%.

III. Clinical manifestations

    A. Persistent, excessively watery eyes.

    B. Mucopurulent discharge.

    C. Matted eyes on awakening.

IV. Physical findings

    A. Watery eyes, often overflowing onto cheek.

    B. Sclera clear.

    C. Reflux of mucopurulent discharge from punctum easily obtained with gentle pressure over nasolacrimal sac.

    D. May see concurrent erythema or irritation of skin around eyes.

V. Diagnostic tests

    A. Gentle pressure over nasolacrimal sac produces mucopurulent discharge from punctum.

VI. Differential diagnosis

Blepharitis, 373.00
Conjunctivitis, bacterial, 372.30
Conjunctivitis, viral, 077.99
Dacryocystitis, 375.30

    A. Viral conjunctivitis.
    B. Bacterial conjunctivitis.
    C. Blepharitis.
    D. Dacryocystitis.

VII. Treatment
    A. Massage lacrimal sac several times a day.
    B. If secondarily infected, treat with antiinfective (see Bacterial Conjunctivitis entry).
    C. Refer to ophthalmologist if not resolved by 12 months of age.

VIII. Follow-up
    A. Recheck at all well-baby exams and as needed.

  IX. Complications

Conjunctivitis, bacterial, 372.30
Dacryocystitis, 375.30
Periorbital or orbital cellulites, 376.01

    A. Bacterial conjunctivitis.
    B. Dacryocystitis.
    C. Periorbital or orbital cellulites.

  X. Education
    A. Wash hands before touching infant's eyes.
    B. Teach massage technique: place index finger over lacrimal sac, exert gentle downward pressure, and slide finger downward toward mouth.

BLEPHARITIS

Blepharitis, 373.00
Conjunctivitis, 372.30

Inflammation or infection of margins of eyelid.
  I. Etiology
    A. Seborrhea.
    B. Staphylococcal.
    C. *Pediculus pubis* or *P. capitis.*

  II. Occurrence
    A. Can occur in all age groups.

  III. Clinical manifestations
    A. Red eyelid margin.
    B. Itching or burning of eyelid margin.
    C. Crusting or scaling of eyelid margin.
    D. Commonly bilateral and chronic or recurrent.

IV. Physical findings
A. Seborrhea.
   1. Easy to remove yellow greasy scales along base of eyelashes.
   2. May see concurrent and similar scales on eyebrows, scalp, external ears.
B. Staphylococcal.
   1. Fibrinous, difficult to remove scales along base of eyelashes.
   2. Inflammation or ulceration of lid margins.
   3. Loss of eyelashes.
   4. May see concurrent conjunctivitis.
C. Pediculosis.
   1. Lice along lid margins.
   2. May see concurrent pubic or head lice.

V. Diagnostic tests
A. Culture of lid margin indicated only if fails to respond to treatment.

VI. Differential diagnosis

Conjunctivitis, allergic, 372.14	Dermatitis, contact, 692.9
Conjunctivitis, bacterial, 372.30	Nasolacrimal duct obstruction, 375.56
Conjunctivitis, viral, 077.99	Seborrheic dermatitis, 690.10
Dermatitis, atopic, 691.8	

A. Conjunctivitis (allergic, bacterial, or viral).
B. Nasolacrimal duct obstruction.
C. Atopic or contact dermatitis.
D. Seborrheic dermatitis.

VII. Treatment
A. Clean eyelid margins twice a day with dilute baby shampoo.
B. Seborrhea blepharitis: treat eyebrows, scalp, ears with selenium sulfide shampoo.
C. Staphylococcal blepharitis: apply topical anti-infective ointment (erythromycin ophthalmic ointment or bacitracin/polymyxin B ophthalmic ointment).
D. Pediculosis blepharitis: remove parasite by smothering with ophthalmic petrolatum along lid margins.

VIII. Follow-up
A. No routine follow-up necessary.
B. Recheck if fails to improve, or sooner if worsens.

IX. Complications

Conjunctivitis, 372.30
Hordeolum, external 373.11
Hordeolum, internal, 373.12

A. Loss of eyelashes.
B. Conjunctivitis.
C. Hordeolum or chalazion.

X. Education
    A. Frequent hand washing.
    B. Discourage rubbing of eyes.

HORDEOLUM

> Hordeolum, external 373.11
> Hordeolum, internal, 373.12

Infection of meibomian glands (internal hordeolum) or glands of Zeis or Moll (external hordeolum or stye) of eyelid.

I. Etiology
    A. Usually *Staphylococcal aureus.*

II. Occurrence
    A. Can occur at any age.

III. Clinical manifestations
    A. Internal: painful and tender eyelid, red eye, usually without pustule.
    B. External: painful and tender eyelid, red eye, usually with pustule.

IV. Physical findings
    A. Internal: large, erythematous, tender mound of one eyelid with associated mild conjunctival hyperemia.
    B. External: smaller, more superficial eyelid pustule with associated mild conjunctival hyperemia.

V. Diagnostic tests
    A. None indicated.

VI. Differential diagnosis

> Chalazion, 373.2
> Eyelid abscess, 373.13

    A. Chalazion.
    B. Eyelid abscess.

VII. Treatment
    A. Frequent, warm compresses.
    B. May use topical antiinfective ointment (erythromycin ophthalmic ointment or bacitracin/polymyxin B ophthalmic ointment).
    C. Refer if mass fails to disappear after several weeks (may need surgical incision and drainage).

VIII. Follow-up
    A. No routine follow-up necessary.
    B. Recheck if fails to resolve or worsens.

IX. Complications

> Orbital or eyelid cellulites, 376.01

      A. Orbital or eyelid cellulitis.
X. Education
      A. Frequent hand washing.
      B. Avoid rubbing eyes.

CHALAZION

Chalazion, 373.2

Inflammation of meibomian glands of eyelid.
    I. Etiology
      A. Granulomatous inflammation.
    II. Occurrence
      A. Can occur at any age.
    III. Clinical manifestations
      A. Hard mass in upper or lower eyelid.
      B. Not red or pustular.
      C. Chronic appearance.
    IV. Physical findings
      A. Firm, nontender nodule in upper or lower eyelid.
      B. Not erythematous or pustular.
      C. No eye discharge.
    V. Diagnostic tests
      A. None indicated.
    VI. Differential diagnosis

Dacryocystitis, 375.30   Hordeolum, internal, 373.12
Eyelid abscess, 373.13   Orbital cellulitis, 376.01
Hordeolum, external, 373.11

      A. Hordeolum (internal or external).
      B. Orbital cellulitis.
      C. Dacryocystitis (inflammation of the lacrimal sac).
      D. Eyelid abscess.
    VII. Treatment
      A. Most spontaneously subside without treatment.
      B. Surgical removal if size distorts vision.
    VIII. Follow-up
      A. No routine follow-up necessary.
      B. Recheck if fails to improve or worsens.
    IX. Complications

Distorted vision, 368.15

      A. Distorted vision secondary to size of lesion.
    X. Education
      A. Frequent hand washing.
      B. Avoid rubbing eyes.

OPHTHALMIC TRAUMA: CHEMICAL BURN

Burn of the eye, 940.9	Opacity of corneal tissue, 371.00
Eye pain, 379.91	Photophobia, 368.13
Eyelid burn, 940.9	Swollen corneas, 379.92

Instillation of alkali or acid solution or substance to eye. True emergency needs immediate referral to ophthalmologist.

I. Etiology
   A. Installation of alkali or acid solution or substance into eye.

II. Occurrence
   A. Boys > girls.
   B. 11- to 15-Year-olds have highest rate of injury.

III. Clinical manifestations
   A. Eye pain.
   B. Unable to open eye(s).

IV. Physical findings
   A. Eyelid burn.
   B. Opacity of corneal tissue, pale surrounding tissue.
   C. Photophobia.
   D. Tearing, swollen corneas.

V. Diagnostic tests
   A. None.

VI. Differential diagnosis

Eyelid injury, 921.1
Foreign body, eye, 930.0

   A. Foreign body.
   B. Type of chemical burn.
   C. Eyelid injury.

VII. Treatment
   A. Emergency treatment is immediate irrigation with copious amounts of water or saline.
   B. Emergency referral to ophthalmologist.

VIII. Follow-up
   A. Per ophthalmologist.

IX. Complications

Loss of vision, 369.9

   A. Loss of vision.

X. Education
   A. Prevention is most important.
   B. Need to know name of chemical in eye; acid burns affect cornea and anterior chamber of eye.
   C. Alkali burns can continue for days.

CORNEAL ABRASION (SUPERFICIAL)

Corneal abrasion (superficial), **918.1**
Decreased vision, **369.9**
Excessive tearing, **375.20**

Eye pain, **379.91**
Photophobia, **368.13**

Scratched, abraded, or denuded cornea.

I. Etiology
A. Usually due to accidental contact with object (fingernail, branches, bushes, paper, contact lens overwear).

II. Occurrence
A. Can occur at any age.

III. Clinical manifestations
A. Pain.
B. Excessive tearing.
C. Photophobia.
D. Decreased vision.

IV. Physical findings
A. May see uneven light reflection or cloudiness of cornea.
B. May see foreign body.
C. After staining with fluorescein and using cobalt-blue light or Wood's lamp, will see area of green staining (persists with blinking).
D. Decreased visual acuity.

V. Diagnostic tests
A. Fluorescein staining and cobalt-blue light or Wood's lamp.

VI. Differential diagnosis

Foreign body, eye, **930.0**

A. Foreign body.

VII. Treatment
A. Instill topical ophthalmic anti-infective ointment (erythromycin ophthalmic ointment or bacitracin/polymyxin B ophthalmic ointment).
B. Patching not recommended.

VIII. Follow-up
A. Recheck in 24–48 hours, or sooner if worsens.

IX. Complications

Impaired vision, **369.9**
Eye infection, **360.00**

A. Infection.
B. Impaired vision.

X. Education
A. Frequent hand washing.
B. Avoid use of contact lenses for at least 1 week following healing of abrasion.

FOREIGN BODY (CONJUNCTIVAL, CORNEAL)

Excessive tearing, 375.20
Foreign body, eye, 930.0

Photophobia, 368.13
Sensation that something is in eye, 368.9

Presence of abnormal substance or object in eye.
I. Etiology
   A. Usually object is airborne.
II. Occurrence
   A. Can occur at any age.
III. Clinical manifestations
   A. Excessive tearing.
   B. Photophobia.
   C. Sensation that something is in eye.
IV. Physical findings
   A. Excessive tearing.
   B. Use bright light or magnification to visualize corneal and conjunctival surfaces for foreign body.
   C. May need to evert upper eyelid to find foreign body.
V. Diagnostic tests
   A. None.
VI. Differential diagnosis

Eye infection, 360.00
Perforation of ocular globe, 370.06

   A. Infection.
   B. Perforation of ocular globe.
VII. Treatment
   A. Test visual acuity.
   B. Remove foreign body if possible with moistened, cotton-tipped applicator.
   C. After removal of foreign body, inspect for corneal abrasion using fluorescein.
   D. Refer to ophthalmologist if large abrasion or unable to find foreign body.
VIII. Follow-up
   A. Recheck in 24 hours or sooner if worsens.
IX. Complications
   A. Infection.
   B. Damage to cornea.
X. Education
   A. Avoid rubbing eyes.
   B. Teach prevention of eye injuries (protective eyewear).

HEMORRHAGE (SUBCONJUNCTIVAL)

Hemorrhage (subconjunctival), 372.72
Ruptured blood vessel in eye, 459.0

A ruptured blood vessel in conjunctiva.

I. **Etiology**
   A. Sudden increase in intrathoracic pressure (coughing, sneezing).
   B. Direct ocular trauma.
II. **Occurrence**
   A. Can occur at any age.
III. **Clinical manifestations**
   A. Ruptured blood vessel in eye.
IV. **Physical findings**
   A. Blotchy, bulbar erythema of conjunctiva.
V. **Diagnostic tests**
   A. None.
VI. **Differential diagnosis**
   A. Ocular trauma.
VII. **Treatment**
   A. None; will spontaneously resolve in 5–7 days.
   B. Refer to ophthalmologist if due to trauma.
VIII. **Follow-up**
   A. No routine follow-up necessary.
   B. Recheck if fails to disappear in 5–7 days, or worsens.
IX. **Complications**
   A. Usually none.
X. **Education**
   A. Teach measures to avoid increasing intrathoracic pressure.

HYPHEMA

Eye pain, **379.91**
Hyphema, **364.41**
Impaired vision, **369.9**

Blood in anterior chamber of eye.
I. **Etiology**
   A. Usually due to blunt or perforating trauma to eye.
II. **Occurrence**
   A. Variable.
III. **Clinical manifestations**
   A. Bright or dark red area near iris.
   B. Painful.
IV. **Physical findings**
   A. Bright or dark red fluid level between cornea and iris.
V. **Diagnostic tests**
   A. X-rays, CT scan for other injuries
VI. **Differential diagnosis**

Foreign body, conjunctival, **930.1**

   A. Type of foreign body.

VII. Treatment
 A. Immediate referral to ophthalmologist.
VIII. Follow-up
 A. Per ophthalmologist.
 IX. Complications

Impaired vision, 369.9

 A. More extensive ocular injury.
 B. Rebleeding, which may result in vision impairment.
 X. Education
 A. Children sometimes take weeks for vision to return to normal.
 B. Prevention is best.
 C. Encourage parents to continue follow-up as recommended by ophthalmologist.

OCULAR TRAUMA

Blurred vision, 368.8   Eye pain, 379.91
Decreased/impaired vision, 369.9   Eye redness, 379.93
Double vision, 368.2

Indirect or direct serious injury to eye.
 I. Etiology
 A. Fireworks, sticks, stones, BB shots.
 B. Sports related.
 II. Occurrence
 A. One-third of all causes of acquired blindness.
 B. Males > females 4:1.
 III. Clinical manifestations
 A. Double, blurred, or decreased vision.
 B. Eye pain or pain in surrounding area.
 C. Tearing.
 IV. Physical findings
 A. Unable to open eye.
 B. Tearing.
 C. Corneal redness.
 V. Diagnostic tests
 A. X-rays if orbital fracture or nasal fracture is suspected.
 VI. Differential diagnosis

Laceration to ocular globe or orbit, 871.4
Orbital wall fracture, 802.8
Perforation to ocular globe or orbit, 370.06

 A. Laceration to ocular globe or orbit.
 B. Perforation to ocular globe or orbit.
 C. Orbital wall fracture.

VII. Treatment
   A. Referral to ophthalmologist.
VIII. Follow-up
   A. Per ophthalmologist.
IX. Complications

Blindness, 369.00
Eye infection, 360.00

   A. Extensive ocular injury.
   B. Blindness.
   C. Infection.
X. Education
   A. Prevention: use of goggles or glasses when spraying.
   B. Do not instill any medication.
   C. Immediate referral to ophthalmologist.

PERIORBITAL CELLULITIS

Dental abscess, 522.5   Periorbital cellulitis, 376.01
Edematous, 782.3   Sinusitis, 473.9
Erythema, unspecified, 695.9   Swelling of the eye, 379.92
Fever, 780.6

Inflammation and infection of eyelids and periorbital tissue.
   I. Etiology
   A. *Staphylococcal aureus.*
   B. *Streptococcus pneumoniae.*
   C. *Streptococcus pyogenes.*
   D. *Haemophilus influenzae* type b.
   II. Occurrence
   A. Common in young children secondary to trauma, infected wound or insect bite, severe sinusitis, dental abscess.
   III. Clinical manifestations
   A. Red, painful swelling around eye.
   B. May or may not have fever.
   C. History of local trauma to area, insect bite, sinusitis, dental abscess.
   IV. Physical findings
   A. Erythematous, edematous, tender, warm area around eye.
   B. Regional adenopathy.
   V. Diagnostic tests
   A. CBC (will indicate leukocytosis in severe cases).
   B. Blood culture.
   C. Head CT scan (helps delineate extent of disease).

VI. Differential diagnosis

Conjunctivitis, 372.30

Contact dermatitis, 692.9

Neuroblastoma, 160.0

Retinoblastoma, 190.5

Rhabdomyosarcoma, 171.9

  A. Severe contact dermatitis.
  B. Severe conjunctivitis.
  C. Ophthalmic malignancy or tumor (retinoblastoma, rhabdomyosarcoma, neuroblastoma).

VII. Treatment

  A. Uncomplicated and >2 months of age: ceftriaxone then oral antibiotics, oral antiinfective (amoxicillin-clavulanate, cephalexin, or erythromycin).
  B. Complicated/extensive or <2 months of age: requires hospitalization and intravenous antibiotics.

VIII. Follow-up

  A. Daily follow-up is necessary to monitor for rapid improvement.

IX. Complications

Eyelid abscess, 373.13

Loss of vision, 369.9

  A. Spread of infection with possible abscess formation.
  B. Loss of vision.

X. Education

  A. Frequent hand washing.
  B. Teach prevention (avoid trauma, use insect repellent, cleanse wounds).

BIBLIOGRAPHY

Anthony M: Corneal abrasions: To patch or not to patch, *Clinician Rev* 13:10, 2003.

Behrman RE, Kliegman RM, Jenson HB: *Nelson textbook of pediatrics,* ed 17, Philadelphia, 2004, Saunders.

Gross RD: Differential diagnosis of conjunctivitis. In Brunell PA, editor: *Infectious diseases in children monograph: ocular infections in children—best practices in diagnosis and treatment,* Thorofare, NJ, 2004, Slack Incorporated.

Hunter A: Problems related to the head, eyes, ears, nose, throat or mouth. In Barnes K, editor: *Paediatrics—a clinical guide for nurse practitioners,* Philadelphia, 2003, Butterworth-Heinemann.

Lichtenstein SJ: Treatment options for pediatric conjunctivitis. In Brunnell PA, editor: *Infectious diseases in children monograph: ocular infections in children—best practices in diagnosis and treatment,* Thorofare, NJ, 2004, Slack Incorporated.

Trobe JD: *The physician's guide to eye care,* ed 2, San Francisco, 2001, The Foundation of the American Academy of Ophthalmology.

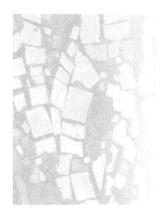

CHAPTER 22

Ear Disorders

JANE A. FOX

FOREIGN BODY

Decreased hearing, **389.9**

Discharge from ear, **388.60**

Foreign body, ear, **931.**

Otitis externa, **380.10**

Pain or itching, **388.70**

I. Etiology
A. Usually results from young children or their companions placing stones, erasers, vegetables (beans, peas, string beans), paper, jellybeans, toy parts, or small alkaline batteries in their ear(s).
B. Insects may become lodged in ear.
C. Chronic irritation or inflammation (e.g., otitis externa may result from putting objects in ear).

II. Occurrence
A. Most common between 2 and 4 years of age.

III. Clinical manifestations
A. Presenting complaints may include:
1. Pain or itching.
2. Decreased hearing.
3. Buzzing if insect is in ear canal.
4. Feeling of fullness in ear or pressure.
5. Discharge from ear.

IV. Physical findings
A. Foreign object or insect visualized on otoscopic exam.
B. Check all body orifices if foreign body found in one.
C. Carefully check ear after removal of foreign object for additional ones.

V. Diagnostic tests
A. Usually none.

VI. Differential diagnosis

Contact dermatitis and eczema, 692.9	Otitis media, 382.9
Impacted cerumen, 380.4	Psoriasis, 696.1
Otitis externa, 380.10	Trauma, 959.09

  A. Foreign body: object or insect is visualized on otoscopic exam.
  B. Otitis media (OM).
  C. Otitis externa.
  D. Trauma.
  E. Impacted cerumen.
  F. Dermatologic disorders (psoriasis or eczema).

VII. Treatment

  A. Remove foreign body. If bleeding occurs, object must be removed.
  B. Have child lie down, restrain head if needed.
  C. DO NOT IRRIGATE if foreign body is vegetable or wood and/or suspect perforation of tympanic membrane.
  D. Insect in ear: kill insect by filling ear canal with mineral oil or alcohol before removal. Ticks: dislodge ticks by filling canal with 70% alcohol and then remove.
  E. Removal of objects.
    1. Best: remove objects using an otoscope with an opening head for visualization.
    2. Objects that are soft and unwedged:
      a. Remove by irrigation with tepid water (body temperature) and water pik on low setting or an 18-gauge butterfly catheter with needle cut off. Pulsating water should help dislodge object.
      b. Insert pliable tubing into ear canal behind foreign body.
  F. If object does not completely occlude canal, can use ear loop, curette, forceps for removal.
  G. Refer to otolaryngologist if:
    1. Object is an alkaline battery.
    2. Object cannot be easily removed.
    3. Ear canal is swollen or bleeding.
    4. Object is tightly wedged in canal.
    5. Child is unable to cooperate.

VIII. Follow-up

  A. Generally none, well-child care.

IX. Complications

Perforation of tympanic membrane, 384.20

  A. Perforation of tympanic membrane (TM).

X. Education

  A. Advise parents not to attempt to remove foreign body.
  B. Tell parents some bleeding may occur after removal.
  C. Cleaning ear canal is not necessary.

HEARING LOSS: CONDUCTIVE, SENSORINEURAL

Allergies, 477.9
Anomalies of external ear, 744.3
Cholesteatoma, 385.30
Decreased hearing, 389.9
Delayed language development, 315.39
Foreign body, ear, 931.
Head and ear trauma, 959.09
Head anomalies, 756.0
Hearing loss, conductive, 389.00

Hearing loss, sensorineural, 389.10
Impacted cerumen, 380.4
Middle ear anomalies, 744.03
Middle ear effusions, 389.03
Neck anomalies, 744.9
Otitis externa, 380.10
Otitis media, 382.9
TM perforation, 384.20

I. Etiology
   A. Genetic or hereditary factors, environmental or acquired diseases, malformations.
   B. Trauma.
   C. Congenital perinatal infections.
   D. About ⅓ of cases of hearing impairment: cause unknown.

II. Occurrence
   A. About 15% of school-age children have significant conductive hearing losses.
   B. OM and its sequelae most common cause of conductive hearing losses during childhood.
   C. Acquired conductive hearing losses most common types of hearing loss in childhood.

III. Clinical manifestations
   A. *Conductive hearing loss* (middle ear hearing loss):
      1. Decreased hearing.
      2. May have history of middle ear effusions.
      3. OM and its sequelae.
      4. Foreign body and/or impacted cerumen.
      5. May report delayed language and speech development or parental concern about child's ability to hear.
      6. Allergies.
      7. Head or ear trauma.
      8. Middle ear anomalies.
      9. Cholesteatoma can cause hearing loss.
   B. *Sensorineural hearing loss* (perceptive or nerve deafness) may report distortion of sound and problems in discrimination of sounds. Hearing loss often involves high-range frequencies, speech difficulties.

IV. Physical findings
   A. *Conductive hearing loss* (middle ear hearing loss).
      1. Possible:
         a. Otitis externa.
         b. OM.

    c. Foreign body.

    d. Impacted cerumen.

    e. Growths or tumors, cholesteatomas.

    f. TM perforation.

  2. Rinne test on affected side; bone conduction (BC) > air conduction (AC).

  3. Weber test sound lateralized to involved side.

  4. Average hearing loss 27–31 dB (mild), may be intermittent, may occur in one or both ears.

B. *Sensorineural hearing loss* (perceptive or nerve deafness).

  1. Possible dysmorphic facial features suggesting presence of syndrome.

  2. Head and/or neck anomalies.

  3. Anomalies of pinnae and external ear canals.

  4. Weber test sounds louder in unaffected ear.

  5. Rinne test: in normal ear or ear with sensorineural hearing loss, AC > BC.

C. Audiometric testing: soft sounds not well perceived, loud sounds perceived almost normally. In older children, if normal in high and low frequencies but poor in middle frequencies, suspect congenital hearing loss.

D. Acquisition of language skills affected.

V. Diagnostic tests

A. Evoked otoacoustic emissions (EOAE) testing (can be performed on children of all ages): newer type of newborn screening, 10 minutes.

B. Automated auditory brainstem response (ABR): for newborn screening, 10 minutes.

C. Brainstem auditory evoked response (BAER): newborn screening, 90 minutes; often used in children of all ages who are unable to cooperate for audiometry testing.

D. Behavioral observation audiometry.

E. Pure tone audiometry for children >5 years of age.

F. Tympanometry identifies a middle ear effusion.

G. Impedance audiometry.

H. Language screening: Early Language Milestone Scale.

VI. Differential diagnosis

Hearing loss, conductive, **389.00**
Hearing loss, sensorineural, **389.10**
Mixed conductive sensorineural loss, **389.2**

A. Careful history and thorough physical examination, including screening and laboratory data, essential in identifying those at risk and in early detection of hearing losses.

B. Hearing disorders classified into 3 categories:

  1. Conductive hearing loss.

  2. Sensorineural hearing loss.

  3. Mixed conductive sensorineural loss.

VII. Treatment
  A. Refer for audiologic testing.
  B. Surgery for conductive hearing loss (usually bilateral myringotomy with tubes).
  C. Refer to multidisciplinary team, hearing center or ENT specialist if hearing impairment detected.
  D. For sensorineural loss:
    1. Amplification (hearing aids; bilateral is best) benefits most children.
    2. Cochlear implants with sensorineural loss, if done within 4 years of hearing loss.
    3. Clarion CII Bionic Ear System for deafness.
VIII. Follow-up
  A. Determined by type and cause of hearing loss.
  B. Well-child care.
 IX. Complications

Speech and language disorder, 315.39

  A. Speech and language disorders.
 X. Education
  A. Early detection imperative to minimize negative consequences for language, other development.
  B. Disease process, type of loss, causes. Conductive loss usually reversible, sensorineural loss often irreversible.
  C. To decrease incidence of communication disorder in child with middle ear disease:
    1. When speaking to child, turn off sources of background noise (e.g., dishwasher, television, radio, stereo, computer games, etc.).
    2. Make sure child is looking directly at speaker and that speaker has child's attention.
    3. Speak louder than normal.
    4. Child should sit in front of classroom (may need referral for full evaluation of hearing needs).
  D. Effects on child.
    1. Speech and language development.
    2. Social development.
    3. Learning process.
  E. Needs of child.
    1. Emotional.
    2. Social.
    3. Educational.
  F. Parents' role.
    1. Care and function of hearing aids, if indicated.
    2. Medic alert bracelet.
  G. Parent support groups.
  H. Support groups for the child.
  I. Prevention: limit exposure to loud noise.

OTITIS EXTERNA

Contact dermatitis and eczema, **692.9**   Psoriasis, **696.1**
Otitis externa, **381.10**   Seborrhea, **706.3**
Perforation of the tympanic
    membrane, **384.20**

I. Etiology
  A. Bacteria: *Pseudomonas aeruginosa* (most common); *Streptococcus* species, *Staphylococcus epidermidis*, *Proteus* species, *Mycoplasma* species.
  B. Fungi: *Aspergillus* species, *Candida* organisms.
  C. Excess cerumen or loss of protective cerumen from exposure to excess moisture.
  D. Trauma to the ear canal caused by overzealous cleaning with a cotton-tipped applicator or a foreign body.
  E. Allergic reaction to chemical or physical agents; contact dermatitis.
  F. Excessive wetness from swimming, bathing, or high humidity.
  G. Excessive dryness; child or family history of eczema, psoriasis, seborrhea.
  H. Purulent otitis media with perforation of the tympanic membrane and drainage may masquerade as otitis externa, usually painless with no swelling of the canal.

II. Occurrence
  A. Most common in hot, muggy weather, summer months.
  B. Persons who are swimmers or divers are more susceptible.
  C. Higher incidence in those with smaller ear canals.
  D. Male and females equally affected.
  E. Affects all ages.

III. Clinical manifestations
  A. Ear pain and itching (common in fungal infections) in the ear, especially when chewing or pressure on tragus.
  B. Feeling of fullness or obstruction of ear.
  C. Frequently, a history of exposure to water.
  D. Purulent discharge and hearing loss (conductive) possible.

IV. Physical findings
  A. Pain on movement of pinna or tragus.
  B. Periauricular adenitis may occur, but not necessary for diagnosis.
  C. External canal: gross edema and erythema of canal, accumulation of moist debris in canal. Patient may resist insertion of ear speculum.
  D. Tympanic membrane often difficult to visualize and may be mildly inflamed but is mobile on insufflation.

V. Diagnostic tests
  A. No tests specific to diagnosing of otitis externa.
  B. Gram stain and culture of discharge may be helpful, particularly when fungal cause is suspected.

VI. Differential diagnosis

Abscess of otitis externa, 380.10	Furuncle of otitis externa, **680.0**
Contact dermatitis and eczema, **692.9**	Mastoiditis, 389.3
Cyst of otitis externa, 382.00	Otitis externa, malignant, 160.1
Dental infection, 522.4	Otitis media with perforation, 384.00
Foreign body, ear, **931.**	Postauricular lymphadenopathy, 289.3

    A. Cyst, furuncle, or abscess.
    B. Foreign body.
    C. Otitis media with perforation.
    D. Dental infection.
    E. Mastoiditis.
    F. Postauricular lymphadenopathy.
    G. Eczema or other dermatologic condition.
    H. Malignant otitis externa.

VII. Treatment

    A. Clean debris from canal: insert small gauze wick or absorbent sponge into external canal to carry antibiotic corticosteroid solution into canal if needed (severe swelling).
    B. Ciprofloxacin hydrochloride/hydrocortisone otic suspension (Cipro HC Otic Suspension) has broad spectrum for covering resistant organisms or combination eardrops of antibiotics, hydrocortisone, propylene glycol.
        1. Not recommended for children <1 year of age.
        2. Advise parents to warm bottle in hands for 1–2 minutes before use and then place 3 drops in affected ear(s) 2 times a day for 7 days.
    C. Ofloxacin solution 0.3% otic drops (Floxin) every 12 hours.
        1. Highly effective if *Pseudomonas aeruginosa* and *Staphylococcus aureus* are causes in patients 1 year of age and older.
        2. Age 1–12 years: 5 drops in affected ear(s) 2 times daily for 10 days.
        3. >12 Years of age: 10 drops in affected ear(s) twice daily for 10 days.
    D. Analgesics for pain.
    E. Oral antibiotics only if signs of invasive infection.
        1. Cellulitis of auricle.
        2. Fever.
        3. Tender postauricular lymph nodes.
    F. Topical treatment is always also needed to treat otitis externa.
    G. Keep ear dry.
    H. Do not use cotton swabs.

VIII. Follow-up

    A. Mild cases: none.
    B. Immediate recheck: pain worsens or sensitivity to eardrops.
    C. Return visit in 2–3 days if marked cellulitis or tympanic membrane was not visualized.
    D. Return visit if symptoms worsen, do not improve in 48 hours, or recur.

  E. Telephone if severe pain.

  F. Recheck in 10 days and continue treatment, if not completely resolved.

IX. Complications

Cellulitis of surrounding tissue, **380.10**	Stenosis of auditory canal, **380.50**
Irritated furunculosis, **680.0**	Transient conductive hearing loss, **388.02**
Malignant otitis externa, **172.3**	

  A. Cellulitis of surrounding tissue.

  B. Irritated furunculosis.

  C. Malignant otitis externa (uncommon) seen in chronically ill or immunosuppressed children.

  D. Stenosis of auditory canal.

  E. Transient conductive hearing loss.

X. Education

  A. Explain cause and treatment plan.

  1. Keep ear dry: no swimming during acute phase, can use cotton coated with petroleum jelly or lamb's wool when showering or shampooing to occlude canal; remove immediately when finished.

  2. Side effects of eardrops: local stinging or burning sensation and rash where drops have come in contact with skin.

  3. Avoid earplugs and use of cotton swabs.

  4. Acute pain should subside within 48 hours.

  B. Keep foreign objects out of ears.

  C. Prevention of recurrence (common): instill 2–3 drops of isopropyl alcohol in ear canals after swimming, showering, or during hot humid weather; shake excess water out of ears.

ACUTE OTITIS MEDIA (AOM)

Enlarged tonsils (pharyngitis), **462.**	Otitis media, chronic, **381.01**
Fever, **780.6**	Perforation of tympanic membrane, **384.20**
Influenza virus (types A and B), **487.1**	Respiratory syncytial virus (RSV), **079.6**
Otitis media, **382.9**	Upper respiratory infection, **465.9**
Otitis media, acute, **392.9**	

I. Etiology

  A. *Streptococcus pneumoniae* (most common causative organism).

  B. Nontypeable *Haemophilus influenzae* causes about 27% of the bacterial otitis.

  C. Less frequent pathogens include *Moraxella (Branhamella) catarrhalis* and Group A beta-hemolytic streptococci.

  D. *Staphylococcus aureus* and *Pseudomonas aeruginosa:* common in chronic serous otitis media, especially if perforation of tympanic membrane present.

  1. Group A beta-hemolytic streptococci, *Escherichia coli, S. aureus:* more common in neonates.

E. Viruses, particularly respiratory syncytial virus (RSV), influenza virus (types A and B), and adenovirus, increase the risk, possibly by impairing eustachian tube function. Infants have increased susceptibility to OM, possibly due to short horizontal position of eustachian tube.

F. Viruses may be involved in about 40% of cases of AOM.

G. Bacterial resistance is increasing problem: certain strains of *H. influenzae* and most strains of *M. catarrhalis* are resistant to amoxicillin because of beta-lactamase production. Another concern is drug-resistant *S. pneumoniae* (DRSP).

H. The groups most at risk for DRSP are:
1. Children <24 months of age.
2. Those who have recently received beta-lactam drugs, were recently treated with antibiotics, and/or had a recent ear infection.
3. Children exposed to large numbers of other children (e.g., day care attendance in children 2 months to <5 years of age, or household crowding >2 years of age).
4. Those with immune deficiencies (e.g., sickle cell disease, HIV, malignancy). The proportion of penicillin-resistant *S. pneumoniae* strains may be 40–50% and half of these may be highly resistant.

II. Occurrence

A. After upper respiratory infection (URI), OM most common disease of childhood; peak prevalence from 6 to 36 months of age. Incidence declines at about 6 years of age.

B. Incidence has dramatically increased during the past 25 years; greatest in children <2 years of age.

C. By 3 years of age, most have had at least 1 acute infection; $\frac{1}{3}$ have had 3.

D. Those with first episode early in life: increased risk for developing chronic ear disease.

E. More common in boys than in girls.

F. Caucasians, Native Alaskans, Native Americans have higher incidence than African Americans.

G. More frequent in low-income and large families and those children in group day care settings.

H. Those immunocompromised, including those with AIDS, have higher incidence.

I. Smoking in household increases incidence.

J. Bottle-fed infants have higher incidence than breastfed infants.

K. Incidence, prevalence of otorrhea: tympanostomy tubes in place longer.

III. Clinical manifestations

Diagnosis of AOM requires:
- History of acute onset of signs and symptoms.
- Presence of middle ear effusion.
- Signs and symptoms of middle ear inflammation.
- Distinct erythema of TM or distinct otalgia (discomfort clearly related to the ear(s) that causes sleep disturbances and/or interferes with normal activity).

A. Most common <2 years of age.

B. Acute onset of ear pain and fever; pulling, tugging, rubbing at infected ear.

    C. Occasionally asymptomatic.

    D. Fever in 50% of cases.

    E. Other associated symptoms: irritability, disturbed sleep, restlessness, rhinorrhea or URI, cough, malaise, sore throat, stiff neck, refusal of bottle, change in eating habits, vomiting, diarrhea.

    F. May report recent URI, previous ear infections, allergies, taking bottle to bed, infant supine when feeding bottle, attending day care, other siblings sick.

    G. Hearing loss.

IV. Physical findings

    A. Fever is common.

    B. Signs of URI or allergies.

    C. Possible red, enlarged tonsils (pharyngitis).

    D. Cervical nodes often enlarged.

    E. Otoscopic findings: middle ear effusion must be present as evidenced by any of the following: bulging TM, decreased or absent mobility of the TM as noted with pneumatic otoscopy, air fluid level behind the TM, otorrhea reflectometry.

V. Diagnostic tests

    A. Pneumatic otoscopy to assess mobility of TM.

    B. Tympanometry: to supplement but not replace pneumatic otoscopy, for children >6 months of age.

    C. Acoustic reflectometry.

    D. Tympanocentesis with culture and sensitivity testing is diagnostic of organism.

VI. Differential diagnosis

Dental abscess, **522.5**	Mastoiditis, **389.3**
Eustachian tube dysfunction, **381.81**	Otitis externa, **380.10**
Foreign body, ear, **931.**	Otitis media, acute with effusion, **381.00**
Furuncle, **680.0**	Sinusitis, **473.9**
Immune deficiency, **279.3**	Temporomandibular joint (TMJ)
Impacted teeth, **520.6**	dysfunction **524.60**
Lymphadenitis, **289.3**	Tonsillitis, **463.**

    A. Otitis externa, otitis media with effusion (OME), sinusitis.

    B. Mastoiditis, furuncle.

    C. Foreign body, trauma.

    D. Eustachian tube dysfunction.

    E. Lymphadenitis.

    F. Dental abscess, tonsillitis, impacted teeth.

    G. Temporomandibular joint (TMJ) dysfunction.

    H. Immune deficiency.

VII. Treatment (Table 22-1)

    A. Pain management, especially during the first 24 hours, is a priority regardless if antimicrobial agents are prescribed. Acetaminophen and ibuprofen are the mainstays. Adequate dosage is important.

TABLE 22-1 ● Recommended antibacterial agents for patients who are being treated initially with antibacterial agents or have failed 48 to 72 hours of observation or initial management with antibacterial agents

Temperature ≥39°C and/or severe otalgia	At diagnosis for patients being treated initially with antibacterial agents		Clinically defined treatment failure at 48–72 hours after initial management with observation option		Clinically defined treatment failure at 48–72 hours after initial management with antibacterial agents	
	Recommended	Alternative for penicillin allergy	Recommended	Alternative for penicillin allergy	Recommended	Alternative for penicillin allergy
No	Amoxicillin, 80–90 mg/kg per day	Non-type I: cefdinir, cefuroxime, cefpodoxime; type I: azithromycin, clarithromycin	Amoxicillin, 80–90 mg/kg per day	Non-type I: cefdinir, cefuroxime, cefpodoxime; type I: azithromycin, clarithromycin	Amoxicillin-clavulanate, 90 mg/kg per day of amoxicillin component, with 6.4 mg/kg per day of clavulanate	Non-type I: ceftriaxone, 3 days: type I: clindamycin
Yes	Amoxicillin-clavulanate, 90 mg/kg per day of amoxicillin, with 6.4 mg/kg per day of clavulanate	Ceftriaxone, 1 or 3 days	Amoxicillin, clavulanate, 90 mg/kg per day of amoxicillin, with 6.4 mg/kg per day of clavulanate	Ceftriaxone, 1 or 3 days	Ceftriaxone, 3 days	Tympanocentesis, clindamycin

From American Academy of Pediatrics/American Academy of Family Physicians Subcommittee on Management of Acute Otitis Media, *Pediatrics* 113(5) 1451–1465, 2004. http://aappolicy.aappublications.org/cgi/content/full/pediatrics:1135/14512fulltext-otitis&search

B. Observation involves deferring treatment for 48 to 72 hours in otherwise healthy children 6 months to 2 years of age with nonsevere illness at presentation *AND* uncertain diagnosis and in children ages 2 years and older who present without severe symptoms *OR* an uncertain diagnosis. There should also be a reliable parent or caregiver able to obtain medication if needed and adequate facilities for follow up and reevaluation.

C. Prescribe antibiotics with caution. Over 80% of cases resolve spontaneously.

D. Begin antimicrobial therapy (Box 22-1) if no improvement or condition has worsened within 24 to 72 hours.

E. Antibiotic therapy is indicated for symptomatic AOM particularly in children <2 years of age.

F. Prescribe amoxicillin (drug of choice) or ampicillin if causative organism unknown (most cases).

BOX 22-1 • **Antibiotics Labeled for the Treatment of Acute Otitis Media**

Penicillins
Amoxicillin
Amoxicillin-clavulanate (Augmentin)

Sulfa-based combinations
Erythromycin-sulfisoxazole (Pediazole)
Trimethoprim-sulfamethoxazole (Bactrim, Septra)

Macrolide/azalide
Azithromycin (Zithromax)
Clarithromycin (Biaxin)

Second-generation cephalosporins
Cefaclor (Ceclor)
Cefprozil (Cefzil)
Cefuroxime axetil (Ceftin)
Loracarbef (Lorabid)

Third-generation cephalosporins
Cefdinir (Omnicef)
Cefixime (Suprax)
Cefpodoxime proxetil (Vantin)
Ceftibuten (Cedax)
Ceftriaxone (Rocephin)

Topical antimicrobial agents (approved for use with tympanostomy tubes or nonintact tympanic membrane
Ciprofloxacin/dexamethasone (Ciprodex Otic Suspension)
Otloxacin (Floxin Otic Solution)

From Pichichero, ME: Acute otitis media: Part II. Treatment in an era of increasing antibiotic resistance, *Am Fam Phys* 61:2410-6, 2000. Website: www.aafp.org/afp/20000415/2410.html; and Rosenfeld, RM: Antibiotic use for otitis media: Oral, topical, or none? *Pediatr Ann* 33:837, 2004.

G. Initially prescribe amoxicillin 40–45 mg/kg per day for 5–7 days in uncomplicated cases in children >2 years of age who do not attend day care, have not taken antibiotics within the past 3 months, except in areas of high resistance. This dose may fail to eradicate drug-resistant *S. pneumoniae* (DRSP).

H. If child attends day care, has taken antibiotics recently, or has history of recent AOM, prescribe amoxicillin 80–90 mg/kg per day in 2 divided doses for 10 days.

I. Prescribe adequate dose for initial treatment of symptomatic children. If allergic to penicillin, treat with azithromycin (for children allergic to beta-lactam).

J. Not recommended in children <6 months of age: 30 mg/kg (max 500 mg) once daily for 3 days; or 10 mg/kg (max 500 mg) once, then 5 mg/kg (max 250 mg) once daily for 4 days. Can also prescribe oral cephalosporins, macrolides, or trimethoprim-sulfamethoxazole (TMP-SMX) (rates of resistance to pneumococci are high). Treat for 10 days.

K. Begin second-line therapy in cases of documented amoxicillin failure (e.g., persistent fever, ear pain, irritability, TM findings after 3 days of treatment of redness, bulging, or otorrhea). Drug must be active against beta-lactamase-producing strains of *H. influenzae* or *M. catarrhalis*, DRSP (e.g., oral amoxicillin-clavulanate [Augmentin]); give in higher doses of 80–90 mg/kg per day of amoxicillin component, clavulanate dose remains at 10 mg/kg per day or ceftriaxone (Rocephin) 50 mg/kg (max 1 g) IM once for severe infections and/or if compliance is concern.

L. If recurrence of acute symptoms after full course of amoxicillin, retreat with second-line antibiotic. First drug of choice is amoxicillin-clavulanate. Oral cephalosporins (except cefuroxime axetil) and macrolides do not provide adequate coverage against resistant strains of *S. pneumoniae*.

M. Pain control (see above): warm compresses, an analgesic with antipyretic effects (e.g., acetaminophen or ibuprofen), and eardrops with benzocaine and antipyrine (Auralgan).

N. Children with frequent AOM: evaluate for anemia. If iron deficiency is diagnosed (hemoglobin <10 g/dL), begin iron supplementation to achieve at least a hemoglobin level of 11 g/dL.

O. Persistent AOM likely caused by different pathogen than initial infection: treat with antibiotic (e.g., cefaclor, TMP-SMX, erythromycin-sulfisoxazole, amoxicillin-clavulanate potassium, cefixime).

P. Recurrent AOM: American Academy of Pediatrics and the CDC suggest placement of tympanostomy tubes rather than antibiotic prophylaxis. If must prescribe antibiotics: sulfisoxazole most effective at preventing recurrences.

Q. Pneumococcal vaccine (PCV 7, Prevnar) in children during first year of life, as well as high risk children >1 year of age.

R. Influenza vaccine in high-risk children.

    S. Surgical intervention: tympanostomy tubes (performed by an ENT surgeon) possible in children with chronic middle ear fluid (3 months or 4 persistent episodes) who fail to respond to antimicrobial therapy; children with recurrent AOM; suppurative complications; those with eustachian tube dysfunction.

    T. Adenoidectomy in children >4 years of age with recurrent AOM may be performed as substitute for, or in conjunction with, insertion of tympanostomy tubes.

    U. Tympanocentesis (performed by an ENT specialist) and culture of exudate: if diagnosis is uncertain, child is seriously ill or toxic, response to antibiotic therapy is unsatisfactory, suppurative complications develop, otitis media in newborn or in immunologically deficient patients, or AOM develops despite receiving antibiotic therapy.

    V. Refer for audiologic testing if fail hearing screen.

    W. Consult/refer to physician: infant <2 months of age, signs of meningitis.

    X. ENT referral: hearing loss or delayed speech, 3 infections in 6 months or 4 in 12 months

VIII. Follow-up

    A. <3 Months of age: revisit 1 to 2 days (higher incidence of treatment failure).

    B. Children 3 months of age and older: revisit in 48–72 hours if no improvement or condition worsens (need to change antibiotics).

    C. Return visit 4–8 weeks to evaluate for OME and reinforce teaching.

    D. Persistent AOM: prescribe second-line antibiotic (e.g., amoxicillin-clavulanate, cefuroxime, or ceftriaxone IM); recheck every 2 to 4 weeks until resolved.

    E. Return visit if signs or symptoms of ear infection, trouble hearing, fever with/without ear pain.

IX. Complications

Cerebral thrombophlebitis, 325.	Meningitis, 322.9
Cholesteatoma, 385.30	Ossicle necrosis, 385.24
Facial nerve paralysis, 767.5	Otitis media, acute, 382.9
Hearing loss, 389.9	Otitis media, acute with effusion, 381.00
Labyrinthitis, 386.30	Perforation of tympanic membrane, 384.20
Language delay, 315.39	Pseudotumor cerebri, 348.2
Mastoiditis, 389.3	Tympanosclerosis, 385.09

    A. Perforation of TM.

    B. Hearing loss, language delay.

    C. Persistent AOM, persistent OME.

    D. Mastoiditis, cholesteatoma.

    E. Meningitis.

    F. Facial nerve paralysis.

G. Labyrinthitis.

H. Tympanosclerosis.

I. Ossicle necrosis.

J. Pseudotumor cerebri.

K. Cerebral thrombophlebitis.

X. Education

A. Causes of ear infections.

B. Risk factors/modification: passive smoke, bottle propping, allergies, sinusitis, use of pacifier after age 6 months, breastfeeding (may protect), immunizations.

C. Treatment plan: if antibiotics prescribed, call if symptoms worsen or do not improve in 48 hours; give exactly as prescribed.

D. Pain relief measures.

E. Importance of follow-up.

OTITIS MEDIA WITH EFFUSION (OME)

Allergies, 477.9	Otitis media, 382.9
Cervical lymphadenopathy, 785.6	Otitis media, acute, 382.9
Enlarged tonsils, 474.11	Otitis media with effusion, chronic, 380.23
Eustachian tube dysfunction (ETD), 381.81	Perforated tympanitic membrane, 384.2
Hearing loss, 389.9	Sleep disturbances, 780.50
Irritability, 799.2	Speech and language disorder, 315.39

I. Etiology

A. Multifactorial: eustachian tube dysfunction (ETD), infection, allergies.

B. Bacteria are same as for AOM, except frequency of *H. influenzae* is greater in OME.

C. If TM perforated in chronic OME: *S. aureus* and *P. aeruginosa* most likely causative organisms.

II. Occurrence

A. See AOM above.

B. Usually follows episode of AOM.

C. Children who are diagnosed with AOM during the first year of life are much more likely to develop chronic OME.

D. $^2/_3$ of children with AOM have middle ear effusion or high negative middle ear pressure 2 weeks after diagnosis; $^1/_3$ have middle ear effusion 1 month after diagnosis, regardless of antibiotic therapy.

E. OME most common cause of hearing loss in children.

III. Clinical manifestations

A. May be asymptomatic.

B. Complaint of hearing loss (older children).

C. Possible language delay.

D. Feeling of fullness in affected ear, clogged/crackling sensation in ear, "talking in tunnel."

    E. Irritability.

    F. Sleep disturbances.

    G. Poor school performance.

    H. Allergies.

    I. Frequent episodes of otitis media.

IV. Physical findings

    A. Possible indicators of allergies.

    B. Possible enlarged tonsils.

    C. Possible cervical lymphadenopathy.

    D. External canal may have discharge.

    E. TM: often retracted or convex, opaque; diffuse light reflex; may be translucent with air-fluid level or air bubbles present or amber with blue gray fluid noted, no visible landmarks.

    F. Pneumatic otoscopy: decreased or irregular mobility to both negative and positive pressure.

    G. Weber test: lateralization to involved ear.

    H. Rinne test: BC > AC (abnormal).

    I. Hearing impairment.

    J. Tympanometry: fluid present.

V. Diagnostic tests

    A. Pneumatic otoscope for primary diagnosis, confirmed by tympanometry.

    B. Tympanometry: tympanogram is flat with an effusion.

    C. Audiometry.

    D. Acoustic reflectometry.

    E. Otoacoustic emissions.

    F. Tympanocentesis.

VI. Differential diagnosis

Anatomic abnormalities, 759.9	Nasopharyngeal carcinoma, 147.9
Hearing loss, 389.9	Otitis media, acute, 382.9

    A. All possible causes of hearing loss.

    B. Anatomic abnormalities.

    C. AOM.

    D. Nasopharyngeal carcinoma (if unilateral OME).

VII. Treatment

    A. Most cases of OME resolve spontaneously within 3 months.

    B. Document at each visit: laterality, duration of effusion, and presence and severity of associated symptoms.

    C. Distinguish the child who is at risk for speech, language, or learning problems from other children with OME and more quickly evaluate hearing, speech, and language and need for intervention in children at risk.

    D. Refer for hearing evaluation when OME persists for 3 months or longer or at any time there is a language delay, learning problems, or a significant hearing loss is suspected in a child with OME.

E. Not recommended for treatment of OME in an otherwise healthy child 2 months through 12 years. Antihistamines and decongestants are ineffective for OME and should not be used for treatment. Antimicrobials and corticosteroids do not have long-term efficacy and should not be used for routine management.

F. Observation or antibiotic therapy treatment options for children with effusion less than 4–6 months and any time in children without a 20-dB hearing threshold level or worse in the better hearing ear.

G. Antibiotics: consider beginning with a beta-lactamase-resistant antibiotic (e.g., amoxicillin-clavulanate potassium) for 2–3 weeks.

H. Myringotomy and tympanostomy tubes: *consider* if bilateral effusion for a total of 3 months and bilateral hearing deficiency (defined as a 20-dB hearing threshold level or worse in the better hearing car). *Recommended* after a total of 4–6 months of bilateral effusion with a bilateral hearing deficit.

VIII. Follow-up
 A. Return visit in 1 month, sooner if acute symptoms develop.

IX. Complications

Hearing loss, 389.9
Otitis media, acute, 382.9
Speech delay, 315.39

 A. Hearing loss, speech delay.
 B. Recurrent AOM.

X. Education
 A. Diagnosis; OME usually resolves spontaneously without treatment in 3 months.
 B. Treatment plan.
 C. Signs of hearing loss.
 D. Modify risk factors.
 E. Relationship between speech and language development and hearing.
 F. Importance of follow-up.

BIBLIOGRAPHY

American Academy of Family Physicians, American Academy of Otolaryngology-Head and Neck Surgery, and American Academy of Pediatrics Subcommittee on Otitis Media with Effusion: Clinical practice guideline: Otitis media with effusion, Published May 3, 2004 (http://www.aafp.org.otitis media.xml).

American Academy of Pediatrics and American Academy of Family Physicians Subcommittee on Management of Acute Otitis Media: Diagnosis and management of acute otitis media, *Pediatrics* 113(5):1451–1465, 2004.

Asch-Goodkin J: Acute otitis media: What the evidence says, *Contemp Pediatr* (Supplement), 4, March 2002.

Finkelstein J, et al: Reduction in antibiotic use among US children, 1996–2000, *Pediatrics* 112:620, 2003.

Fox J, Verst A : Eyes and ears. In Fox J, editor: *Primary health care of infants, children, & adolescents,* ed 2, St Louis, 2002, Mosby.

Garbutt J, Jeffe D, Shackelford P: Diagnosis and treatment of acute otitis media: An assessment, *Pediatrics* 112:143, 2003.

Hoberman A, et al: Treatment of acute otitis media consensus recommendations, *Clin Pediatr* 373:6, 2002.

Rosenfeld, RM: Antibiotic use for otitis media: Oral, topical, or none? *Pediatr Ann* 33:833–842, 2004.

Stool SE, et al: Managing otitis media with effusion in young children. In *Quick reference guide for clinicians.* AHCPR Publication 94-0623. Rockville, MD, July 1994, Agency for Health Care Policy and Research, Public Health Service, US Department of Health and Human Services.

Takata G, et al: Evidence assessment of management of acute otitis media: I. The role of antibiotics in treatment of uncomplicated acute otitis media, *Pediatrics* 108:239, 2003.

Takata G, et al: Evidence assessment of the accuracy of methods of diagnosing middle ear effusion in children with otitis media with effusion, *Pediatrics* 112:1379, 2003.

CHAPTER 23

Sinus, Mouth, Throat, and Neck Disorders

SUSAN G. RAINS

ALLERGIC RHINITIS

Allergic conjunctivitis, 372.14	Nasal obstruction, 478.1
Allergic rhinitis due to other allergens, 477.8	Noisy breathing/snoring, 786.09
Allergic rhinitis due to pollen (seasonal rhinitis), 477.9	Sneezing, 784.9
	Stuffy nose, 478.1
Cough, 786.2	Rhinorrhea, 478.1
Halitosis, 784.9	Wheezing, 786.07

I. Etiology

A. Atopic predilection.
   1. Very common atopic disease of childhood, second only to asthma.
   2. Often same mediators that produce asthma.
   3. Genetic factors: increased IgE production in response to allergens.
B. Environmental factors.
   1. Common allergens.
      a. Seasonal (rare in children <3 years of age).
         • Nonflowering, wind-pollinated plants.
         • Tree pollens: early spring.
         • Grasses: late spring and early summer.
         • Weeds: fall.
      b. Perennial: animal dander, dust (mites), molds (spores), mildew, feathers, cockroaches.

II. Occurrence

A. Affects about 20% of children and 30% of adolescents.
B. If one parent affected, child has 30% chance of developing allergies; both parents, 70% chance.
C. The incidence in males is slightly higher.

III. Clinical manifestations

A. Stuffy nose, sneezing, itching, runny nose, noisy breathing/snoring, cough, halitosis, frequent clearing of throat, plugged ears, wheezing.

    B. Possibly associated signs of allergic conjunctivitis: itchy, injected conjunctiva, puffy lids, tearing or clear mucous drainage in eye.

IV. Physical findings

    A. Nasal mucosa is usually pale, edematous, boggy.

    B. Thin, watery rhinorrhea.

    C. Allergic salute may cause external, transverse crease near end of nose.

    D. Nasal obstruction may cause mouth breathing.

    E. Allergic shiners (dark circles under eyes), due to venous pooling.

V. Diagnostic tests

    A. Nasal smear for presence of eosinophils: >10% is positive (intranasal steroids may decrease percentage).

    B. Skin testing.

VI. Differential diagnosis

Choanal atresia, 748.0	Rhinitis, drug or food induced, 477.1
Cystic fibrosis, 277.00	Rhinitis medicamentosus, 372.05
Dermatoid cyst, 706.2	Rhinorrhea, 478.1
Deviated septum, 470.	Sinusitis, 473.9
Headache, 784.0	Sinusitis, chronic, 473.9
Nasal foreign body, 932.	Upper respiratory infection, 465.9
Nasal glioma, 748.1	Vasomotor rhinitis, 477.9
Nasal polyp, 471.9	Viral URI, 465.9

    A. Infection.

        1. Viral upper respiratory infection (URI): red and swollen turbinates, thicker, more purulent rhinorrhea; duration 10–14 days, clustered fall–spring.

        2. Sinusitis: possibly symptoms of URI, in addition headache, facial pressure; duration longer than viral URI but more limited than solely allergic rhinitis.

    B. Nasal foreign body: unilateral purulent nasal discharge, foul odor.

    C. Nasal polyp, dermatoid cyst, nasal glioma.

    D. Cystic fibrosis (patients often have nasal polyps and chronic sinusitis).

    E. Choanal atresia, deviated septum.

    F. Vasomotor rhinitis: sudden appearance and disappearance of symptoms in response to irritants.

    G. Rhinitis medicamentosus: abuse of nasal spray/drops.

    H. Drug- or food-induced rhinitis.

VII. Treatment

    A. Avoidance.

        1. Minimize exposure to dust mites, especially in child's bedroom: remove wall-to-wall carpets, curtains, bed ruffles, stuffed animals; wash cotton bedding in hot water frequently, use nonallergic bedding covers.

        2. Minimize exposure to animal dander.

        3. Minimize exposure to pollens: close windows, use air conditioning, filters on air systems, keep humidity low in home, remove house plants.

    4. Avoid activities such as leaf raking, lawn mowing, furniture dusting.

    5. Avoid talcs, perfumes, cigarettes, wood smoke.

B. Pharmacotherapy.

    1. Antihistamines.

        a. First generation (sedating unless child has adverse hyperactive response):

          • Diphenhydramine (Benadryl), chlorpheniramine, combined products: 5 mg/kg/day, divided qid.

        b. Second generation:

          • Loratadine (Claritin, generic preparations now available OTC).

            • Age 2–5 years: 5 mg PO daily.

            • >6 Years: 10 mg.

          • Cetirizine (Zyrtec).

            • Age 2–5 years: 2.5–5 mg PO daily.

            • >6 Years: 10 mg.

          • Fexofenadine (Allegra).

            • >12 Years: 60 mg tab bid or 180 mg daily.

    2. Intranasal steroids, e.g., fluticasone propionate (Flonase 0.05%), mometasone furoate (Nasonex):

        a. 4–12 Years of age: 1 spray each nostril daily.

        b. >12 Years of age: 2 sprays/nostril.

    3. Topical cromolyn (NasalCrom): 1 spray tid-qid, 2–4 weeks for effect.

    4. Nasal decongestants.

        a. Oral often combined with antihistamines.

        b. Topical not recommended due to rebound and abuse potential.

C. Immunotherapy (hyposensitization): "allergy shots" especially recommended for children who suffer perennially and do not respond to medications.

VIII. Follow-up

A. 2–4 Weeks after initial treatment, sooner if needed, then 3–6 months.

IX. Complications

Dental malocclusion, 524.5	Loss of smell, 781.1
Hearing loss, **389.9**	Otitis media, **382.9**
Hoarseness, **784.49**	Sinusitis, chronic, **473.9**

A. Chronic sinusitis.

B. Recurrent otitis media.

C. Hoarseness.

D. Loss of smell or hearing.

E. High-arched palate, dental malocclusion from chronic mouth breathing.

X. Education

A. Chronicity of problem.

B. Avoidance of allergens (recent evidence that exposure to cats, dogs in first year of life decreases development of allergies later in childhood).

C. Medication administration and side effects.

APHTHOUS STOMATITIS

Aphthous stomatitis, 528.2	Fever, 780.6
Deficiencies of B_{12}, 266.2	Lymphadenopathy, 785.6
Deficiencies of folic acid, 266.2	Malabsorption syndromes, 579.9
Deficiencies of iron, 280.9	Painful sores in mouth, 528.9

I. Etiology
A. Commonly known as canker sores, aphthous stomatitis is recurrence of painful, discrete, shallow ulcers on unattached mucous membranes of mouth.
B. Considered to be immune-mediated destruction of epithelium, cause is multifactorial, but *not* herpes simplex.
C. Associated risk factors.
  1. Genetic: positive family history.
  2. Deficiencies of iron, vitamin B_{12}, folic acid.
  3. Childhood: higher incidence (peak 10–19 years).

II. Occurrence
A. Incidence: up to 20% of population.
B. Precipitating factors.
  1. Stress/trauma: emotional, physical, hormonal.
  2. Foods: chocolate, nuts, tomatoes.
  3. Malabsorption syndromes.

III. Clinical manifestations
A. Patient complains of single or multiple painful sores in mouth.
B. Tingling or burning may precede appearance of lesions.
C. Smaller lesions may heal in a week, larger 10–30 days.

IV. Physical findings
A. Ulcerative lesions on mucosa.
B. 1–5 Ulcerative oval or circular ulcers with an erythematous periphery and pale white/gray or yellow center.
C. Size: 2–10 mm.
D. Absence of systemic symptoms (i.e., fever, lymphadenopathy).

V. Diagnostic tests
A. None.

VI. Differential diagnosis

Fever, 780.6	Herpes simplex, 054.9
Herpangina-ulcerative pharyngitis, 074.0	Lymphadenopathy, 785.6

A. Herpes simplex:
  1. Small, irregular vesicles that rupture and leave ulcers.
  2. Red at periphery with gray center.
  3. Patient often febrile with significant lymphadenopathy.
  4. Recurrent herpes infections remain localized to lips, rarely cross mucocutaneous junction. Primary infections sometimes involve oral mucosa.
B. Herpangina-ulcerative pharyngitis (not stomatitis); fever, lymphadenopathy.

VII. Treatment
A. Supportive.
1. Oral analgesics such as acetaminophen or ibuprofen.
2. Topical anesthetics: especially prior to eating/drinking.
   a. Viscous Xylocaine dabbed on lesions with cotton swab.
   b. Mouthwashes.
   - Diphenhydramine elixir: antacid suspension (aluminum and magnesium hydroxide combination): mix 1:1 (parent can do this).
   - Pharmacist may add lidocaine for older child to swish and spit.
   c. 0.1% Triamcinolone (Kenalog) in Orabase: dab on lesions qid.
3. Avoid acidic, salty foods and drinks.
4. Good oral hygiene.
   a. Rinse mouth frequently with clear water.
   b. Offer water to young children frequently, especially after eating or drinking other fluids.

VIII. Follow-up
A. None if healed.

IX. Complications
A. Generally none. Young child may refuse to drink.
B. Referral if persists >3 weeks or no urine output for 12 hours.

X. Education
A. Avoidance of triggers/precipitating factors.

CAT-SCRATCH DISEASE

Cat-scratch disease, 078.3	Nonpruritic vesicle or papule(s), 216.3
Conjunctivitis, nonsuppurative, 372.30	Ocular granuloma, 376.11
Fever, 780.6	Skin lesion, 709.9
Lymphadenopathy, 785.6	

I. Etiology
A. Bacteria *Bartonella henselae* infects human through scratch or possibly other methods of entry into body.
B. 87–99% of patients have had contact with kitten <6 months; 50% have history of scratch.

II. Occurrence
A. More common in children, esp. boys.
B. 20,000 Cases/year in US, primarily September–March.

III. Clinical manifestations
A. Primary skin lesion appears 3–10 days following inoculation.
B. Up to 10% of children have primary lesion present as nonsuppurative conjunctivitis or ocular granuloma.
C. Lymphadenopathy develops in about 2 weeks, persists sometimes for months.
D. Fever, mild systemic symptoms occur in $1/3$ of patients.
E. 30% of nodes may suppurate spontaneously.

IV. Physical findings
   A. Nonpruritic vesicle or papule(s) over site of inoculation.
   B. Lymphadenopathy of area that drains site of inoculation. Most commonly axillary, cervical, epitrochlear, or inguinal nodes.
   C. Skin over affected nodes is warm, taut, tender, indurated.
V. Diagnostic tests
   A. Direct fluorescence antibody testing (for detection of antibodies specific to *B. henselae*). Reliable only through CDC.
   B. Enzyme immunoassay for detection of IgG antibodies to *B. henselae*.
   C. Analysis of tissue specimens or nodal aspirate may be helpful.
   D. Blood cultures if bacteremia suspected.
   E. Skin test not recommended.
VI. Differential diagnosis

Cytomegalovirus, 078.5	Lymphadenopathy, 785.6
Epstein-Barr virus, 075.	Mycobacterium, 031.9
Group A streptococcus, 041.01	Neck masses, 784.2
Group B streptococcus, 041.02	Staphylococci, 041.10
HIV, V08.	Toxoplasmosis, 130.9
Infectious mononucleosis, 075.	

   A. Other causes of lymphadenopathy.
      1. Common viral and bacterial infections such as Group A beta-hemolytic streptococci (GABHS), staphylococci, cytomegalovirus (CMV), Epstein-Barr virus (EBV; infectious mono), HIV.
   B. Subacute and chronic lymphadenopathy more likely associated with mycobacterium and toxoplasmosis.
   C. Neck masses from other sources.
VII. Treatment
   A. Symptomatic.
      1. Antipyretics and analgesics.
      2. Moist wraps/compresses.
      3. Aspiration of painful nodes (avoid I&D).
      4. Antimicrobial treatment for severely ill patients or those with other chronic condition.
      5. Trimethoprim-sulfamethoxazole (Bactrim).
         a. Child: 8 mg/kg daily divided bid.
         b. Adult: 160 mg daily bid.
      6. Azithromycin (Zithromax).
         a. 500 mg day 1; 250 mg days 2–5.
         b. Younger children 10 mg/kg day 1; 5 mg/kg days 2–5.
      7. Ciprofloxacin (Cipro): Adult 500–750 mg bid.
VIII. Follow-up
   A. Every week until resolution of symptoms, dependent on severity of symptoms.

IX. Complications

Aseptic meningitis, 047.9	Osteomyelitis, 730.28
Encephalitis, 323.9	Parinaud oculoglandular syndrome, 378.81
Erythema nodosum, 695.2	Pneumonia, 486.
Hepatosplenomegaly, 571.8	Submandibular lymphadenopathy, 785.6
Neuroretinitis, 363.05	Thrombocytopenia purpura, 287.3

A. Parinaud oculoglandular syndrome: inoculation of conjunctiva results in ipsilateral preauricular or submandibular lymphadenopathy.
B. Less commonly: encephalitis, aseptic meningitis, neuroretinitis, thrombocytopenia purpura, erythema nodosum, pneumonia, hepatosplenomegaly, osteomyelitis, none of which have caused severe sequelae.

X. Education

A. Avoid scratches by decreasing rough play with kittens.
B. Immediately cleanse wounds from cats.

CERVICAL LYMPHADENITIS

Adenopathy, 785.6	Hepatosplenomegaly, 571.8
Arthralgias, 719.4	Infectious mononucleosis, 075.
Cat-scratch disease, 078.3	Lymphoma, 202.8
Cervical lymphadenitis, 289.3	Malnutrition, 263.9
Cervical lymphadenitis, acute, 683.	Mycobacterial infections, 031.9
Cervical lymphadenopathy, 785.6	Night sweats, 780.8
Collagen vascular disease, 459.9	Pharyngitis, 462.
Cough, 786.2	Rubella, 056.9
Enlargement of lymph glands, 785.6	Sore throat, 462.
Epstein-Barr virus, 075.	Staphylococci, 041.10
Fatigue, 780.79	*Staphylococcus aureus*, 041.11
Fever, 780.6	Toxoplasmosis, 130.9
Group A streptococcus, 041.01	Upper respiratory infections, 465.9
Group B streptococcus, 041.02	Weight loss, 783.21

I. Etiology

A. Enlargement of lymph glands of neck generally due to:
1. Infection: which causes proliferation and invasion of inflammatory cells.
   a. Viruses:
      • Upper respiratory: respiratory syncytial virus (RSV), adenoviruses, influenza, parainfluenza, rhinoviruses.
      • EBV.
      • CMV.
      • Rubella, rubeola, roseola.
      • Varicella zoster.
      • HSV.
      • Coxsackie.
      • HIV.

  b. Bacteria:
  - *Staphylococcus aureus* and GABS: 40–80% of cases.
  - Anaerobes.
  - *Corynebacterium diphtheriae.*
  - *Bartonella henselae* (cat-scratch disease).
  - Gram-negative rods: *Haemophilus influenzae*, pseudomonas, salmonellae, shigellae, *Francisella tularensis* (tularemia).
  c. Mycobacterium.
  - *Mycobacterium tuberculosis.*
  - Nontuberculous mycobacteria (NTM).
  d. Spirochetes.
  e. Rickettsiae.
  f. Fungi: including *Histoplasma capsulatum* (histoplasmosis).
  g. Protozoa: including *Toxoplasma gondii* (toxoplasmosis).
 2. Other causes.
  a. Neoplasms that cause infiltration of neoplastic cells.
  b. Histiocytosis.
  c. Collagen vascular diseases: juvenile rheumatoid arthritis (JRA), lupus.
  d. Sarcoidosis.
  e. Kawasaki disease.
  f. Postvaccination: DTaP, polio, typhoid.

II. Occurrence
A. About 40% of all children have palpable cervical lymph nodes.
B. Most cases of cervical lymphadenitis resulting from common bacterial and viral infections occur in toddler and preschool age groups.
C. Etiologic and age-related occurrence.
 1. Neonate.
  a. Acute unilateral cervical lymphadenitis: *S. aureus.*
  b. "Cellulitis-adenitis" syndrome: late-onset Group B streptococcus.
 2. <5 Years of age.
  a. Acute pyogenic cervical lymphadenitis: *S. aureus* and GABHS.
  b. NTM lymph node infection.
  c. Kawasaki disease (also usually unilateral).
 3. School-aged and adolescents: more likely chronic cervical lymphadenitis than acute pyogenic disease.

III. Clinical manifestations
A. Acute bilateral cervical lymphadenopathy generally caused by URI or strep pharyngitis. Generalized associated with EBV (infectious mononucleosis).
B. Acute unilateral cervical lymphadenitis variably associated with fever and suppuration, most often caused by staph and Group A streptococcus.
C. Subacute and chronic lymphadenitis is found in cat-scratch disease, toxoplasmosis, and mycobacterial infections. Nodes become fluctuant and are generally nontender.

    D. Painless, possibly matted nodes and especially those in supraclavicular area are more likely malignant.

    E. Associated symptoms.

        1. With URI: fever, sore throat, cough.

        2. Lymphoma, TB: fever, nights sweats, weight loss.

        3. Collagen vascular disease or serum sickness: fever, fatigue, arthralgias.

IV. Physical findings

    A. General.

        1. Signs of malnutrition including poor growth: suggestive of chronic disease.

        2. Generalized adenopathy and hepatosplenomegaly: suggestive of malignancy or other noninfectious illnesses and some infectious diseases such as EBV, HIV, TB, histoplasmosis.

    B. Enlargement of the lymph nodes: >1 cm.

        1. Node-bearing areas: occipital, cervicofacial, axillary, epitrochlear, inguinal, popliteal.

        2. Nodes may be warm, mobile, fixed, fluctuant, solid, smooth.

    C. Presentation, distribution, associated diseases.

        1. Acute posterior cervical lymphadenopathy: rubella, infectious mononucleosis.

        2. Supraclavicular or posterior cervical lymphadenopathy: risk for malignancy.

        3. Cervical lymphadenopathy, associated generalized lymphadenopathy: viral infection.

        4. Generalized lymphadenopathy: associated with leukemia, lymphoma, collagen vascular disease.

        5. Nodes bilateral and soft (not fixed): viral infection.

        6. Tender nodes, possibly fluctuant, not fixed: bacteria.

        7. Redness and warmth: acute pyogenic process.

        8. With fluctuance: abscess formation.

        9. Matted or fluctuant nodes, skin overlying red but not warm: TB.

      10. Nodes hard and fixed, without signs of acute inflammation: associated malignancy.

    D. Associated physical signs.

        1. Markedly red pharynx, possibly exudates, soft palate petechiae: GABHS.

        2. Swelling, redness, tenderness of gums: periodontal disease.

        3. Edema of the soft tissues of the neck: diphtheria.

        4. Sinus tract formation: TB.

        5. Gingivostomatitis: HSV.

        6. Herpangina: coxsackievirus.

        7. Rash: infectious mono, scarlet fever.

        8. Pallor, petechiae, bruises, sternal tenderness.

        9. Hepatosplenomegaly: leukemia.

V. Diagnostic tests

    A. Appropriate for suspicion of specific entity.

B. Throat culture.

C. PPD.

D. CBC.

E. Erythrocyte sedimentation rate (ESR).

F. Blood cultures.

G. Liver enzymes.

H. Serology for specific microorganisms.

I. Chest x-ray.

J. Ultrasound of nodes.

K. Echocardiogram, ECG.

L. Fine-needle aspiration for Gram stain and culture.

M. Biopsy: if malignancy suspected.

VI. Differential diagnosis

Neck masses, 784.2

A. Neck masses.
  1. Congenital lesions are generally painless and most likely identified in infancy.
  - Thyroglossal duct cyst: midline between thyroid bone and suprasternal notch, moves upward.
  - Branchial cleft cyst: smooth, fluctuant, proximal, anterior border of sternocleidomastoid muscle.
  - Sternocleidomastoid tumor: mass in belly of the muscle caused by perinatal injury; associated torticollis.
  - Cervical ribs: bony anomaly.
  - Cystic hygroma: fluid filled, easily transilluminated.
  - Hemangioma.
  - Laryngocele: cystic mass extending through the thyrohyoid membrane.
  - Dermoid cyst: midline cyst, also contains solid components.

B. Parotitis: swelling crosses angle of jaw; mumps.

VII. Treatment

A. Acute cervical lymphadenitis.
  1. Staphylococcus or Group B streptococcus.
    a. Patient nontoxic, no abscesses or cellulitis.
    - Cephalexin.
      - Child: 40 mg/kg/day divided into 4 doses.
      - Adult: 250–500 mg qid.
    - Oxacillin.
      - Child: 50–100 mg/kg/day qid.
      - Adult: 2–6 g/day qid.
    - Clindamycin.
      - Child >1 month of age: 8–25 mg/kg/day in divided doses q6–8h.
      - Adult: 150–450 mg q6h, max: 1.8 g/day.

      b. Patient toxic or immunocompromised.
- IV cefazolin, nafcillin, or clindamycin.

  2. Anaerobes: seen with periodontal/dental disease.
- Penicillin or clindamycin.

  3. Oral analgesia, warm compresses.

  4. Incision and drainage for suppurative, fluctuant nodes.

 B. Biopsy if significant lymphadenopathy persists >4–6 weeks and serious etiology is suspected.

VIII. Follow-up
 A. Call if node enlarges, becomes markedly tender, erythematous, indurated.

 B. Call if child appears toxic, has difficulty breathing or swallowing.

 C. If being treated for bacterial infection, call if not better in 48 hours (fever down, tenderness decreased, size of node stable).

 D. Recheck at end of treatment.

 E. Recheck if node(s) persist longer than several weeks.

IX. Complications
 A. Bacterial: suppuration, bacteremia.

 B. Undiagnosed infectious process or malignancy.

X. Education
 A. Address family's fears: primarily those of malignancy.

 B. Compliance with medications.

 C. Observation: when to call, return to clinic.

 D. Hydration.

EPISTAXIS

Allergies, unspecified, 477.9	Lymphadenopathy, 785.6
Epistaxis, 784.7	Nosebleeds, 784.7
Hepatomegaly, 789.1	Pale skin, 709.9
Hypertension, 401.9	Petechial rashes, 782.1
Hypovolemia, 276.5	Upper respiratory infections, 465.9

I. Etiology
 A. Bleeding from the nose can be anteriorly from nares (commonly Kiesselbach plexus) or posteriorly into nasopharynx. The nasal mucosa has rich, yet relatively unprotected blood supply. The mucosa is thin, especially in children.

 B. Causative factors.

  1. Inflammation.

    a. Infectious processes.

    b. Allergies.

  2. Neoplasms, polyps.

  3. Trauma.

    a. External injury.

    b. Nose picking.

      c. Foreign bodies.

      d. Chemical or caustic agents (including drugs).

C. Rarely.

  1. Systemic illnesses.

      a. Hematologic diseases.

      b. Hypertension.

II. Occurrence

A. Very common in children.

B. Highest incidence 2–10 years of age.

C. Often familial history.

III. Clinical manifestations

A. Complaints of persistent, recurrent nosebleeds.

B. May have history of:

  1. Recent or current URI.

  2. Allergies (especially nasal).

  3. Tarry stools.

  4. Medication or drug use.

  5. Persistent bleeding or bruising.

  6. Family history of epistaxis or bleeding disorders.

  7. Trauma: nose picking or foreign body insertion.

IV. Physical findings

A. Vital signs may reflect hypovolemia or underlying cause such as hypertension.

B. Inspection of nose, nasopharynx, and oropharynx may reveal:

  1. Bleeding most commonly from medial anterior nares.

  2. Dry, crusted mucosa.

  3. Excoriation of mucosa, site of bleeding.

C. General exam may find lymphadenopathy, hepatomegaly, petechial rashes, or pale skin, mucosa, nail beds.

V. Diagnostic tests

A. Vital signs, including blood pressure.

B. Hematocrit or CBC with platelets.

C. If severe and persistent:

  1. CBC with platelets.

  2. Prothrombin and partial thromboplastic bleeding time.

VI. Differential diagnosis

Bleeding disorders, 289.9	Polyps, 471.9
Foreign body, nose, 932.	Renal disease, 593.9
Hypertension, 401.9	Vascular abnormalities, 785.9

A. Bleeding disorder: if severe and recurrent, child <2 years, positive family history.

B. Polyps, vascular abnormalities.

C. Foreign body.

D. Hypertension, renal disease.

VII. Treatment
   A. Elevate head and lean forward.
   B. Pinch nares together for at least 10 minutes.
   C. Ice to nasal dorsum may be added.
   D. Packing (preferably absorbable), topical vasoconstrictive drugs may be needed.
   E. Referral to ENT if unmanageable or prolonged or abnormalities of nose.
VIII. Follow-up
   A. Hct, 6–12 hours after bleed if concern for anemia.
   B. Return if unmanageable and/or persistent.
 IX. Complications
   A. Possibly mild anemia.
   B. Rare: airway obstruction, aspiration, vomiting.
  X. Education
   A. Prevention.
      1. Humidification of air in home, esp. bedroom.
      2. Nasal saline sprays, drops.
      3. Petroleum jelly applied sparingly to anterior nares.
      4. Protective athletic gear.
      5. Discouragement of nose-picking behaviors and vigorous blowing.
   B. Reassurance: amount of blood always looks greater than it is.

FOREIGN BODY

Choking, 784.9	Foreign body, nosc, 932.
Cough, 786.2	Vomiting, 787.03
Dysphagia, 787.2	

  I. Etiology
   A. Small objects are often inserted into nose by children, causing full or partial obstruction of nares.
 II. Occurrence
   A. Frequent, especially in young children age 3–6 years.
III. Clinical manifestations
   A. Child may have been observed.
   B. Initially, local symptoms of obstruction: swelling, sneezing, mild discomfort.
   C. Subsequently, persistent, purulent, *unilateral* discharge; may be bloody or foul smelling.
 IV. Physical findings
   A. Dependent on length of time obstruction has been present: see above symptoms. Obstruction is almost always unilateral.
   B. Examiner may be able to visualize object with nasal speculum or otoscope.
  V. Diagnostic tests
   A. None.

VI. Differential diagnosis

Adenoiditis, 474.01
Nasal tumors, 471.9
Rhinosinusitis, 473.9

    A. Infection.
        1. Rhinosinusitis.
        2. Adenoiditis.
    B. Polyps.
    C. Nasal tumors.

VII. Treatment

    A. Purulent discharge may need to be suctioned in order to visualize object.
    B. An older child may be told to occlude one side of nares and blow vigorously.
    C. Removal requires:
        1. Good lighting.
        2. Topical anesthesia.
        3. Vasoconstrictor drugs.
        4. Alligator forceps, cerumen spoon.
        5. Narrow tip suction.

VIII. Follow-up

    A. None, if successful removal and signs of infection clear within 1–2 days.
    B. Referral to ENT if unable or unlikely to remove easily.
    C. Consider behavioral/emotional assessment if is recurrent problem or developmentally inappropriate behavior.

IX. Complications

    A. Chronic infection if undetected and/or not removed.
    B. Trauma to nares from removal procedure.

X. Education

    A. Close observation of children by caregivers.
    B. Limit access by small children to small objects.
        Note: If child *swallows* foreign body, especially coin, radiographic survey must be done to ensure object is in stomach. Child must be observed closely for dysphagia, drooling, gagging, vomiting, coughing, choking, airway compromise.

INFECTIOUS MONONUCLEOSIS

Abdominal pain, 789.00
Fatigue, 780.79
Fever, 780.6
Group A streptococcus, 041.01
Group B streptococcus, 041.02
Hemolytic anemia, 283.9
Infectious mononucleosis, 075.
Lymphadenopathy, 785.6
Lymphocytosis, 288.8
Malaise, 780.79

Mild hepatitis, 573.3
Myalgia, 729.1
Myocarditis, 429.01
Palatal petechiae, 782.7
Pharyngitis, 462.
Rash, 782.1
Splenomegaly, 789.2
Thrombocytopenia, 287.5
Tonsillitis, 463.

I. Etiology
   A. Epstein-Barr virus: 90% of cases.
   B. Clinical symptoms result from proliferation of *b*-lymphocyte cells in tonsils, lymph nodes, spleen.
   C. Latent, lifelong infection occurs and may be reactivated during immunosuppression.

II. Occurrence
   A. Humans.
      1. Endemic worldwide in younger children, especially Third World countries.
      2. $1/3$ of cases in adolescents in more affluent populations of developed countries.
      3. Almost all adults in US are seropositive for EBV.

III. Clinical manifestations
   A. Primary EBV infection.
      1. Incubation is 30–50 days.
      2. Primary EBV infection in adolescents presents in >50% of cases with:
         a. Fatigue, malaise, myalgia.
         b. Generalized lymphadenopathy.
         c. Pharyngitis.
         d. Possibly fever or prodrome of malaise and fever.
      3. Younger children may experience mild febrile episode, rash, abdominal pain.

IV. Physical findings
   A. Tonsillitis, pharyngitis: possibly exudative.
   B. Palatal petechiae.
   C. Lymphadenopathy.
      1. Anterior and posterior cervical nodes.
      2. Large, mildly tender.
      3. Epitrochlear nodes highly indicative.
   D. Splenomegaly.
      1. Frequent false negatives, if done too early in 50% of cases.
      2. 2–3 cm below costal margin.
      3. Persists for 2–4 weeks past resolution of other symptoms.

V. Diagnostic tests
   A. "Monospot" (mononucleosis rapid slide agglutination test for heterophil antibodies disease process and in children <6 years of age).
   B. CBC with differential.
      1. Lymphocytosis with up to 20,000 WBCs.
      2. Up to 40% atypical lymphocytes.
      3. Mild thrombocytopenia >50% of cases.
      4. Positive monocytes on differential (give specific range).
   C. Liver enzymes.
      1. Mild hepatitis common.
      2. Usually asymptomatic.
   D. EBV serology: indicated in acutely ill patient.
      1. If monospot negative and strong suspicion.
      2. Acute or postinfection differentiated.

    E. Throat culture.
       1. Rule out other causes.
       2. 5–25% Cases have concurrent GABHS infection.

VI. Differential diagnosis

Adenovirus, **079.0**	Leukemias, **208.9**
Cytomegalovirus, **078.5**	Pharyngitis, **462.**
Group A streptococcus, **041.01**	Rubella, **056.9**
Group B streptococcus, **041.02**	Tonsillitis, **463.**
HIV, **V08.**	*Toxoplasmosis gondii,* 130.9
Human herpes virus, **054.9**	

    A. Other causes of infectious mononucleosis syndrome:
       1. Adenovirus.
       2. Cytomegalovirus.
       3. *Toxoplasmosis gondii.*
       4. Human herpesvirus.
       5. HIV.
       6. Rubella.
    B. Pharyngitis/tonsillitis.
       1. GABHS.
       2. Other bacterial causes.
       3. Viruses other than EBV.
    C. Leukemias.

VII. Treatment

    A. Supportive.
       1. Analgesics and antipyretics.
       2. Hydration support if needed.
       3. Corticosteroids may be indicated if:
          a. Impending airway obstruction or dehydration secondary to severe tonsillopharyngitis.
          b. Massive splenomegaly.
          c. Myocarditis.
          d. Hemolytic anemia.
          e. Hemophagocytic syndrome.

VIII. Follow-up

    A. Fatigue may persist months after recovery. Patient should be allowed to resume school and activities as energy level permits.
    B. Splenomegaly.
       1. Recheck at weekly intervals.
       2. Avoid contact sports until fully recovered and spleen no longer palpable.

IX. Complications

Airway obstruction, **519.8**	Dehydration, **276.5**
Antibiotic-induced rash, **693.0**	Splenic rupture, **289.59**

A. Complications are rare, but include:
1. Dehydration.
2. Antibiotic-induced rash (most commonly with ampicillin or amoxicillin).
3. Splenic rupture: $\frac{1}{2}$ spontaneously, $\frac{1}{2}$ with blunt trauma.
4. Airway obstruction.

X. Education
A. Close personal contact is required for transmission.
B. Recovery often biphasic, with worsening of symptoms after period of improvement.
C. Full recovery may take months.
D. Patient should not donate blood.

PHARYNGITIS

Adenovirus, 079.0	*Neisseria gonorrhoeae*, 032.9
Coxsackievirus, 079.2	Peritonsillar abscess, 475.
Epstein-Barr virus, 075.	Pharyngitis, 462.
Group A streptococcus, 041.01	Rheumatic fever, 390.
Group B streptococcus, 041.02	Rhinovirus, 079.3

I. Etiology
A. Inflammation of mucous membranes and underlying structures of pharynx and tonsils, usually caused by infection.
B. Causative agents.
1. Respiratory viruses, including rhinovirus, adenovirus, coxsackievirus, Epstein-Barr virus.
2. GABHS.
3. Group C beta-hemolytic strep (not a cause of rheumatic fever), *Neisseria gonorrhoeae* rarely.
4. *Mycoplasma pneumoniae*: possibly 10% in adolescents.
5. *Corynebacterium diphtheriae*.

II. Occurrence
A. Peak incidence late fall through early spring.
B. Younger children more commonly present in winter months and with viral pharyngitis.
C. GABHS has proclivity for 5- to 15-year age group, also peaking in winter.

III. Clinical manifestations
A. Viral pharyngitis.
1. Gradual onset.
2. Prominent nasal symptoms: rhinorrhea, mild cough.
B. Coxsackievirus (see Physical Findings next).
C. Streptococcal.
1. Rapid onset.
2. See Physical Findings next.

IV. Physical findings

A. Viral pharyngitis.
   1. Sore throat, dysphagia.
   2. Low-grade fever.
   3. Possibly diarrhea.
B. Coxsackievirus.
   1. Fever, headache.
   2. GI complaints.
   3. Possibly papular rash of hand-foot-mouth disease.
C. Streptococcal GABHS.
   1. Moderate to high fever, headache.
   2. Red pharynx: beefy red swollen uvula and tonsils.
   3. Yellow, blood: tinged exudates.
   4. Petechiae on soft palate, strawberry (coated) tongue.
   5. Tender cervical lymphadenopathy.
   6. Multiple GI complaints.
   7. Accompanying scarlatiniform rash: red, sandpaper-like, clustered in body's "hot spots" (axillae, neck, inguinal, flexor surface of arms, behind knees).

V. Diagnostic tests

A. Throat swab for rapid antigen detection test for GABHS. Negative should also have follow-up throat culture (can also identify carrier state).
B. Heterophil antibody test for EBV.
C. CBC.

VI. Differential diagnosis

Allergic rhinitis, generalized, 477.9	Group G streptococcus, 041.05
Group C streptococcus, 041.03	Infectious mononucleosis, 075.

A. Viral vs. bacterial entity.
   1. Infectious mononucleosis.
   2. Group C or G streptococcus.
B. Allergic rhinitis.

VII. Treatment

A. Nonpharmacologic.
   1. Encourage fluids: may prefer hot or cold for pain relief.
B. Pharmacologic.
   1. Topical and oral analgesics and antipyretics.
   2. Antimicrobials: penicillin V recommended.
      a. Children <27 kg: 250 mg bid or tid for 10 days.
      b. Children >27 kg: 500 mg bid or tid for 10 days.
      c. IM benzathine penicillin G: if compliance, vomiting issues.
         • Children <27 kg: 600,000 units.
         • Children >27 kg: 1.2 million units.
      d. Amoxicillin: substituted for taste issues (may benefit 40% of children with adenotonsillar disease, who yield beta-lactamase-producing bacteria).

- Preliminary data also suggest once daily dosing of amoxicillin for 10 days is effective.
  - **e.** Penicillin allergic options.
    - Erythromycin estolate or ethylsuccinate: 40 mg/kg/day in 2–4 divided doses.
    - Clarithromycin.
      - Child: 15 mg/kg/day, max: 1000 mg divided q12h for 10 days.
      - Adult: 500 mg q12h for 10 days.
    - Azithromycin: 12 mg/kg/day for 5 days.
    - First-generation cephalosporin such as cephalexin: also appropriate if retreatment necessary.
  - **f.** If illness recurs shortly after treatment:
    - May be retreated with same drug.
    - IM penicillin if compliance an issue.
    - Narrow-spectrum cephalosporin (cephalexin).
    - Amoxicillin-clavulanate potassium.

VIII. Follow-up

- **A.** Routine reculturing is not necessary.
- **B.** Encourage patients to call if:
  1. Unable to complete course of medication or retain medication.
  2. Siblings complain of sore throat within 2–5 days: amoxicillin-clavulanate 90 mg/6.4 mg per kg/day. If allergic: 6 months to 12 years of age, cefdinir 7 mg/kg bid or 14 mg/kg daily; >13 years, 300 mg bid 10 days.
  3. No improvement in patient in 48 hours.
  4. Signs and symptoms of renal complications.
  5. Drug reaction.
- **C.** Possible assessment of carrier state and treatment if indicated.
  1. Clindamycin most effective treatment.
  2. ENT referral for possible surgical candidates:
  3. Multiple bouts of tonsillectomy in 1 year despite adequate treatment.
  4. Significant upper airway obstruction.
  5. Peritonsillar abscess.

IX. Complications

Cervical lymphadenitis, **683.**	Poststreptococcal glomerulonephritis, **580.0**
Mastoiditis, **383.0**	Rheumatic heart disease, acute, **391.9**
Peritonsillar abscess, **475.**	Streptococcal pharyngitis, **034.0**

- **A.** Streptococcal pharyngitis.
  1. Suppurative.
     - **a.** Peritonsillar abscess.
     - **b.** Cervical lymphadenitis.
     - **c.** Mastoiditis.
  2. Acute rheumatic fever.
  3. Post-strep glomerulonephritis.

X. Education
A. Transmission is person to person via respiratory tract secretions.
B. Medication compliance is essential.
C. May return to school/day care 24 hours after beginning antibiotic therapy.

RHINOSINUSITIS

Allergic rhinitis, 477.9	Immunodeficiency, 279.2
Ciliary dyskinesia, 781.3	Nasal obstruction, 478.1
Cough, 786.2	Nasal speech, 784.5
Cystic fibrosis, 277.00	Postnasal secretions, 473.9
Dental pain, 529.6	Proptosis, 376.30
Ear pressure, 388.70	Rhinorrhea, 478.1
Fatigue, 780.79	Rhinosinusitis, bacterial, 473.9
Frontal sinusitis, 473.1	Rhinosinusitis, viral, 472.0
Gastroesophageal reflux, 530.81	Smoke exposure, 987.9
Halitosis, 784.9	Snoring, 786.09
Headache, 784.0	Upper respiratory infection, 465.9

I. Etiology
A. Each case of viral rhinitis is also rhinosinusitis, because mucous membranes of nasal passages, sinus cavities are identical.
B. Sinusitis is inflammation of mucous membranes lining paranasal sinuses, commonly used to describe bacterial rhinosinusitis.
C. Factors that increase risk of sinusitis are:
  1. Smoke exposure.
  2. Cold and dry inspired air.
  3. Preceding or concurrent URI.
  4. Allergic rhinitis.
  5. Swimming.
  6. Gastroesophageal reflux.
  7. Cystic fibrosis.
  8. Immunodeficiency.
  9. Ciliary dyskinesia.
  10. Factors associated with nasal obstruction.
D. Stagnation of secretions occurs within sinus cavities, becoming culture medium for bacteria.
E. Common pathogens:
  1. *Streptococcus pneumoniae.*
  2. *Haemophilus influenzae.*
  3. *Moraxella catarrhalis* (becoming most common in children).

II. Occurrence
A. Complication of 5–10% of viral upper respiratory illnesses in children.
B. In young children, occurs primarily in maxillary sinuses, ethmoids secondly.
C. Frontal sinusitis is rare prior to age 10 years.

III. Clinical manifestations

A. Acute and persistent nasal and sinus symptoms for 10–30 days.
   1. Subacute: clinical symptoms for 4–12 weeks.
   2. Chronic: symptoms lasting at least 12 weeks.
   3. Recurrent: 4+ incidents/year with complete resolution in interim.
   4. Mild: 10 days of persistent anterior and posterior rhinorrhea and fatigue.
   5. Moderate: 10 days of nasal congestion, fever, increased maxillary or frontal tenderness/pressure.
B. May complain of cough (worsening at night), rhinorrhea, postnasal secretions, halitosis, dental pain, headache, fatigue, ear pressure, snoring, nasal speech.

IV. Physical findings

A. Fever.
B. Nasal speech.
C. Halitosis.
D. Purulent drainage in posterior pharynx and/or nose.
E. Nasal mucosa may be erythematous and swollen.
F. Face over paranasal sinuses may be tender to palpation.
G. Headache, especially when bending over.
H. Sinuses opaque, especially in older children.
I. Puffiness around eyes.
J. Proptosis, impaired extraocular movements: associated with orbital infection.

V. Diagnostic tests

A. X-rays.
   1. Not helpful in chronic sinusitis.
   2. May be helpful in acute sinusitis, but does not differentiate viral from bacterial. Positive signs include air fluid levels, opacification and mucosal thickening in sinuses.
B. CT scan of paranasal sinuses: indicated in complicated and severe cases.

VI. Differential diagnosis

Adenoidal hypertrophy, 474.12	Foreign body, nose, 932.
Allergic rhinitis, 477.9	Septal deviation, 470.
Choanal atresia, 748.0	Viral URI, 465.9

A. Viral URI.
B. Allergic rhinitis.
C. Drug induced (rhinitis medicamentosa).
D. Tumors: polyps, neoplasms, adenoidal hypertrophy.
E. Foreign body.
F. Septal deviation, choanal atresia.

VII. Treatment

A. Acute bacterial rhinosinusitis (ABRS) in children.
   1. Mild symptomatology and no antibiotics within past 4–6 weeks.

    a. Amoxicillin (90 mg/kg/day).
    b. High-dose amoxicillin-clavulanate (90 mg/6.4 mg per kg/day).
    c. Cefpodoxime proxetil, cefuroxime axetil, cefdinir.
  2. Mild disease and HAVE received antibiotics within previous 4–6 weeks or in moderate disease.
    a. High-dose amoxicillin-clavulanate (same dose).
    b. Cefdinir if allergic.
    c. Azithromycin or clarithromycin if severely allergic.
  3. Consider switch in medications if no response in 72 hours.
B. Chronic sinusitis: may need to treat for 4 weeks.
C. Normal saline nasal sprays: assists drainage and ventilation.
D. Topical nasal steroids: may decrease swelling of turbinates and aid ostia to drain.
E. Mucolytics: may help mucous clearance.
F. Antihistamines: helpful if allergic component.
G. Decongestants: controversial benefit.
H. Humidified air.
I. Encourage fluids.

VIII. Follow-up
A. Patient to call if no response to medications in 72 hours.
B. Recheck in 2 weeks.
C. Referral to ENT or allergist if indicated or refractory.

IX. Complications

Brain abscess, 324.0	Orbital cellulites, 376.01
Cavernous sinus thrombosis, 325.	Osteomyelitis of maxilla or frontal
Exacerbation of asthma, 493.92	bone, 730.28
Optic neuritis, 377.30	Subdural empyema, 324.9

A. Orbital cellulites.
B. Intracranial complications such as cavernous sinus thrombosis, subdural empyema, brain abscess.
C. Exacerbation of asthma.
D. Optic neuritis.
E. Osteomyelitis of maxilla or frontal bone.

X. Education
A. Prevention: avoid allergens and treat allergies when appropriate.
B. Encourage humidified air on home unless it exacerbates mildew, mold allergies.
C. Emphasize that most rhinitis and sinusitis are viral in etiology and antibiotics are not indicated.
D. Encourage compliance with prescribed antimicrobial agents.
E. Advise patient against diving (including scuba).

BIBLIOGRAPHY

American Academy of Pediatrics Subcommittee on Management of Sinusitis and Committee on Quality Improvement: *Pediatrics* 108:798-808, 2001.

American Academy of Pediatrics: *2003 Red book: report of the Committee on Infectious Diseases*, ed 26, Elk Grove Village, IL, 2003, American Academy of Pediatrics.

Behrman RE, et al: *Nelson textbook of pediatrics*, ed 17, Philadelphia, 2000, WB Saunders.

Feder HM: Periodic fever, aphthous stomatitis, pharyngitis, adenitis: a clinical review of a new syndrome, *Clin Opin Pediatr* 12:233-236, 2000.

Hayden G, Hendley J: An up-to-date approach to pharyngitis in children, *Resp Dis Pediatr J* 3:125-131, 2001.

Kelley PE: Foreign bodies in the nose and pharynx. In Burg FD, et al, editors: *Gellis and Kagan's current pediatric therapy*, ed 16, Philadelphia, 1999, WB Saunders.

Leung A, Pinto-Rojas A: Infectious mononucleosis, *Consultant* 40:134-136, 2000.

Leung A, Robson L: Childhood cervical lymphadenopathy, *J Ped Health Care* 18:3-7, 2004.

Nimmagadda S, Evans R: Allergy: Etiology and epidemiology, *Pediatr Rev* 20:111-115, 1999.

Ownby DR, et al: Exposure to dogs and cats in the first year of life and risk of allergic sensitization at 6 to 7 years of age, *JAMA* 288:963-972, 2002.

Platts-Mills TAE: Allergen avoidance in the treatment of asthma and rhinitis, *N Engl J Med* 349:207-208, 2003.

Schutze GE: Diagnosis and treatment of *Bartonella henselae* infections, *Pediatr Infect Dis J* 19:185-7, 2000.

Sinus and Allergy Health Partnership: Antimicrobial treatment guidelines for acute bacterial rhinosinusitis, *Otolaryngol Head Neck Surgery J* 130(suppl):1-44, 2003.

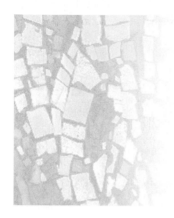

CHAPTER 24

Respiratory Disorders

MARTI MICHEL

CROUP

Airway obstruction, severe, 519.8
Anxiety, 300.00
Change in level of consciousness, 780.09
Croup, 464.4
Croup, spasmodic, 478.78
Cyanosis, 782.5
Edema of larynx, 478.6
Edema of nasal mucosa, 478.25
Fatigue, 780.79
Harsh, barking cough, 786.2
Hoarseness, 784.49
Hypoxemia, 799.0
Increased retractions, 786.00
Inspiratory stridor, 786.1
Laryngotracheitis, 464.20
Laryngotracheobronchitis, 490.
Laryngotracheobronchopneumonia, 485.
Mild erythema, 695.9
Mild fever, 780.6
Progressive restlessness, 799.2
Respiratory distress, 786.09
Restlessness, 799.2
Rhinorrhea, 478.1
Sore throat, 462.
Suprasternal, 738.3
Tachycardia, 785.0
Tachypnea, 786.06
Upper airway obstruction, acute, 519.8
Wheezing, 786.07

I. Etiology

A. Acute upper airway obstruction in children, most often caused by viral infection.
   1. Most common form of viral croup is laryngotracheitis resulting from inflammation and edema of larynx, subglottic area.
      a. Causative agents include parainfluenza 1, 2, 3 (parainfluenza 1 and 3 most common), influenza A and B, respiratory syncytial virus (RSV), adenovirus, measles.
   2. Spasmodic croup is similar to viral croup but is not associated with fever and symptoms, lasts only hours, not days.
      a. Onset typically occurs during night in a child who has been well.
      b. May represent allergic reaction to viral antigen.

    3. Laryngotracheobronchitis (LTB) and laryngotracheobronchopneumonia (LTBP) involve upper airway; also affect lower airway, specifically bronchi.

      a. Same viral agents are common to LTB and LTBP.

      b. Bacterial superinfection occurs more commonly in this croup variant; includes *Staphylococcus aureus, Streptococcus pyogenes, S. pneumoniae, Haemophilus influenzae, Corynebacterium diphtheria.*

        • Agents are infrequent causes but tend to cause more severe illness.

II. Occurrence

  A. Viral croup occurs at 6 months to 5 years of age, with peak in second year of life.

  B. Boys > girls.

  C. Occurs in late fall, early winter.

  D. Symptoms typically last 3–7 days.

III. Clinical manifestations

  A. Gradual onset with rhinorrhea, sore throat, mild fever.

  B. Disease has wide spectrum from very mild illness to severe illness.

  C. Harsh, barking cough.

  D. Hoarseness.

  E. Inspiratory stridor.

  F. Increasing obstruction.

    1. Tachycardia, tachypnea.

    2. Suprasternal and intercostal retractions.

    3. Paradoxical abdominal and chest wall movement.

    4. Progressive restlessness and anxiety correlates with hypoxemia.

IV. Physical findings

  A. Normal or mildly elevated temperature.

  B. Mild erythema and edema of nasal mucosa.

  C. Inspiratory stridor.

  D. Hoarseness.

  E. Harsh, barky cough.

  F. Nontoxic appearing.

  G. On auscultation, normal breath sounds except transmission of stridor.

  H. With increased obstruction: wheezing, prolonged expiration, decreased breath sounds.

V. Diagnostic tests

  A. Diagnosis made on basis of history and clinical exam.

  B. Anteroposterior neck x-rays.

    1. Classic "steeple sign": narrowed air column consistent with narrowing of subglottic space.

    2. Lateral view is useful in ruling out epiglottitis, retropharyngeal abscess, or radiopaque foreign body.

  C. If indicated, WBC normal or low with polymorphonucleotides (PMNs).

  D. Clinical croup score can classify severity of illness.

VI. Differential diagnosis

Diphtheria 032.9   Peritonsillar abscess, 475.
Epiglottitis, 464.30   Retropharyngeal abscess, 478.24
Foreign obstruction, 933.1

  A. Epiglottitis: toxic appearing, drooling, high fever.
  B. Laryngeal foreign body: history, age, sudden onset, unilateral physical findings.
  C. Diphtheria: characteristic thin, gray membrane extends from tonsil to associated soft/hard palate.
  D. Retropharyngeal or peritonsillar abscess: severe throat pain, refusal to swallow or speak, fever to 105°F (40.6°C).

VII. Treatment

  A. Most children have mild airway obstruction resolve without specific treatment.
  B. Symptomatic treatment at home includes taking child into bathroom with hot shower running, to provide warm mist or taking child outside in cool night air.
  C. Cool mist vaporizer may be used.
  D. Corticosteroids.
    1. Controversial use in mild croup.
    2. Decrease edema of laryngeal mucosa.
    3. Single dose 0.15 mg dexamethasone given orally or IM.
    4. Use cautiously with patients who have lower respiratory tract involvement (increased likelihood of bacterial infection).
    5. Consider use of single nebulized budesonide 2 mg.
  E. Criteria for hospitalization:
    1. Signs of moderate to severe airway obstruction.
    2. Increased work of breathing and respiratory distress.
    3. Hypoxemia.
    4. Restlessness, anxiety, or fatigue.
    5. Change in level of consciousness.

VIII. Follow-up

  A. Call health provider immediately if signs of respiratory distress increase.
  B. Increased respiratory rate.
  C. Stridor at rest.
  D. Increased retractions.
  E. Change in level of consciousness, restlessness, or anxiety.
  F. Cyanosis.

IX. Complications

  A. Acute deterioration in respiratory status requires hospitalization/intubation.

X. Education

  A. Croup usually lasts 3–7 days; typically worse at night.
  B. Give guidelines about oral intake (fluids) and urine output.

C. Use of bathroom mist, cool night air, cool mist vaporizer to relieve symptoms.
D. Signs of increasing respiratory distress and hypoxemia.
E. Good hand washing, containment of coughs/sneezes prevents spread of illness.
F. Maintain calm, reassuring manner. Avoid situations that provoke stress or crying, which can worsen respiratory distress.
G. Children may have repeated episodes of croup.
H. Antibiotics are not indicated for viral croup.
I. Avoid secondhand smoke exposure.

BRONCHIOLITIS

Apnea, 770.81	Poor appetite, 783.0
Atelectasis, 518.0	Poor feeding, 783.3
Bronchiolitis, 466.19	Respiratory syncytial virus, 079.6
Cough, 786.2	Rhinorrhea, 478.1
Dyspnea, 786.09	Sneezing, 784.9
Hypoxemia, 799.0	Subsegmental consolidation, 481.
Irritability, 799.2	Tachypnea, 786.06
Lethargy, 780.79	Upper respiratory tract infection, 465.9
Low-grade fever, 780.6	Vomiting, 787.03
Nasal congestion, 478.1	Wheezing, 786.07

I. **Etiology**
   A. Bronchiolitis is common viral illness.
      1. RSV, bronchiolitis is most common cause of acute lower respiratory infection (LRI) in first 2 years of life.
      2. Bronchiolitis is also caused by parainfluenza 1 and 3, adenovirus, rhinoviruses, influenza.
   B. Transmission.
      1. Highly contagious.
         a. Virus shed 5–12 days and up to 30 days with underlying disease.
         b. Virus spreads by large droplet aerosols generated by coughing, sneezing.
         c. Transmitted by direct contact with nasopharyngeal secretions from infected person.
            • Virus survives on skin approximately 20 minutes.
            • Virus survives on gowns/tissues approximately 30–60 minutes.
            • Virus survives on hard, nonporous surfaces approximately 6 hours.
         d. High-risk groups at risk for more severe disease: prematurity, chronic lung disease, congenital heart disease, immunosuppression.
      2. Reinfection occurs throughout life.
II. **Occurrence**
   A. Seasonal prevalence.
      1. Yearly epidemics in early winter/spring.

2. In temperate climates, typically start in November and persist through April.
3. Strains A and B circulated concurrently during outbreaks; strain A more dominant.
4. By age 3, most children have been infected with RSV.
5. Only 1–5% require hospitalization.
6. Adolescents, adults with RSV have symptoms of upper respiratory tract infection.

III. Clinical manifestations

A. Initial presentation.
1. Mild upper respiratory infection (URI) with rhinorrhea and nasal congestion.
2. Low-grade fever for 2–3 days.
3. Poor appetite.
4. Hoarse cough progresses to deep, wet cough.
   a. Often paroxysmal.
   b. Often associated with post-tussive vomiting.
   c. Associated with wheezing.
B. Clinical progression.
1. LRT involvement evident by:
   a. Tachypnea: 60–80 breaths/minute.
   b. Dyspnea.
   c. Coughing, wheezing.
2. Neonatal presentation.
   a. Lethargy, irritability.
   b. Poor feeding.
   c. URI symptoms.
   d. Apnea: occurrence is inversely proportional to age.

IV. Physical findings

A. Increased work of breathing.
1. Nasal congestion with thick purulent secretions.
2. Respirations rapid, shallow with accessory muscle use, retractions.
3. Nasal flaring, grunting, head bobbing.
4. Paroxysmal cough, wheezing, crackles.
5. Prolonged expiratory phase, chest hyperexpansion and hyperresonance.
6. Liver and spleen may be palpable secondary to chest hyperexpansion.
7. Hypoxemia correlates with severity of tachypnea.
8. Paradoxical abdominal and chest wall movement.

V. Diagnostic tests

A. Diagnosis often made on basis of clinical presentation, physical findings, epidemiology.
1. Definitive diagnosis may not be necessary in infants with mild disease.
B. Chest x-ray (CXR).
1. Hyperinflation may be only abnormality: flattened diaphragms, increased lucency.

2. Peribronchial thickening and increased interstitial markings.
3. Subsegmental consolidation in upper and middle lobes: patchy atelectasis or consolidation due to atelectasis.
C. Oximetry: to determine oxygenation status.
D. Laboratory tests.
   1. Identification of virus or viral antigen in respiratory secretions.
      a. Specimen obtained by nasal wash.
      b. Rapid diagnostic tests detect antigen using immunofluorescence techniques or enzyme-linked immunoassays.
      c. Viral culture.

VI. Differential diagnosis

Aspiration, 934.8	Hypoxemia, 799.0
Asthma, 493.90	Immunodeficiency, 279.3
Bacterial pneumonia, 482.9	*Mycoplasma pneumoniae,* 483.0
Cervical lymphadenopathy, 785.6	Nasal congestion, 478.1
Chlamydial infection, 079.98	Pneumonia, 486.
Congenital heart disease, 746.9	Poor feeding, 783.3
Congestive heart failure, 428.0	Poor growth, 764.9
Cough, 786.2	Respiratory distress, 786.09
Cystic fibrosis, 277.02	Respiratory failure, 518.81
Fever, 780.6	Rhinitis, 477.9
Foreign body, 934.8	Tachypnea, 786.06
Heart murmur, 785.2	Upper respiratory infection, 465.9

A. Cystic fibrosis: sweat test is gold standard for diagnosis.
B. Pneumonia: viral URI symptoms and coryza with low-grade fever; bacterial pneumonia; abrupt onset with high fever; *Mycobacterium pneumoniae* (insidious onset and nontoxic appearance).
C. Asthma: pattern of symptoms, absence of fever, inspiratory wheezing, prolonged expiratory phase.
D. Foreign body aspiration: typically in toddler; may be detected on x-ray or by bronchoscopy.
E. Aspiration: swallowing study to determine silent or free aspiration.
F. Chlamydial infection: manifests from 3 to 19 weeks of age, afebrile, repetitive, staccato cough with tachypnea; wheezing is rare; cervical lymphadenopathy.
G. Immunodeficiency: systemic illness following vaccination with live virus; severe, life-threatening illness with viral infection.
H. Congenital heart disease: accompanied by heart murmur, signs of CHF, poor feeding, poor growth.

VII. Treatment

A. Treatment is supportive, maintaining adequate hydration, oxygenation; monitor closely for increasing respiratory distress.
   1. Management of nasal congestion and rhinitis.
   2. Use of antipyretics.

    3. Guidelines for feeding and urine output.

    4. Recognition of signs of increasing respiratory distress.

  B. Criteria for hospitalization.

    1. Age (younger more likely).

    2. Tachypnea/hypoxemia.

    3. Hydration management.

VIII. Follow-up

  A. Most infants improve within 3–5 days.

    1. Guidelines for parents to call health care provider: increased respiratory distress, poor fluid intake, or low urine output.

    2. Close outpatient follow-up by telephone or visit may be indicated.

IX. Complications

Lung disease, chronic, 518.89	Respiratory syncytial virus, 079.6
Pneumothorax, spontaneous, 512.8	Wheezing, 786.07
Respiratory failure, 518.81	

  A. Acute complications.

    1. Respiratory failure, apnea: rarely secondary bacterial infection.

    2. Spontaneous pneumothorax due to air trapping, airway narrowing.

    3. Worsening of chronic lung disease.

    4. Mortality 1–5% with higher rates in high-risk groups.

  B. Long-term complications.

    1. Recurrent episodes of wheezing.

    2. Infants have airway hyperreactivity and impaired pulmonary function for up to 10 years after RSV infection.

X. Education

  A. Avoid secondhand smoke exposure.

  B. Prevention.

    1. For high-risk populations passive immunity (monoclonal antibody technology) through monthly administration of palivizumab (Synagis) from October through April.

    2. Good hand washing, avoidance of ill contacts during bronchiolitis season.

  C. Post-illness.

    1. Reinfection common; having RSV offers no immunity to subsequent infections.

    2. May have period of prolonged wheezing after infection.

    3. Recurrent wheezing is common, especially with URIs.

INFLUENZA

Abdominal pain, 789.00	Increased retractions, 786.9
Anxiety, 300.00	Influenza, 487.1
Atelectasis, 518.0	Irritability, 799.2
Change in level of consciousness, 780.09	Myalgia, 729.1

Change in mental status, 780.99	Nausea, 787.02
Chills, 780.99	Pharyngitis, 462.
Conjunctivitis, 372.30	Pneumonia, 486.
Cough, 786.2	Respiratory distress, 786.09
Croup, 464.4	Respiratory rate, increased, 786.01
Cyanosis, 782.5	Restlessness, 799.2
Diffuse myalgia, 729.1	Shortness of breath, 786.05
Dyspnea, 786.09	Tachycardia, 785.0
Extreme fatigue, 780.79	Tachypnea, 786.06
Fever, 780.6	Upper respiratory infection, 465.9
Generalized malaise, 780.79	Vomiting, 787.03
Headache, 784.0	Wheezing, 786.07

I. Etiology

A. Influenza is highly contagious respiratory illness caused by influenza viruses.
  1. Influenza viruses are orthomyxoviruses.
  2. Type A and B are primary pathogens, responsible for community outbreaks.

B. Influenza is spread by respiratory droplet.
  1. Close contact with person with influenza.
  2. Direct contact with articles contaminated with nasopharyngeal secretions.
  3. Virus is shed 1 day prior to developing symptoms; children, immunocompromised persons may be contagious for >1 week.
  4. Incubation period is 1–4 days with average of 2 days after exposure.

II. Occurrence

A. Peak of flu season can occur from December through March.

B. About 1% of children require hospitalization annually.

C. Influenza can cause URI, croup, bronchiolitis, pneumonia.

III. Clinical manifestations

A. Abrupt onset of fever with rigors, chills.

B. Conjunctivitis.

C. Pharyngitis.

D. Cough.

E. Diffuse myalgia.

F. Extreme fatigue, headache, and generalized malaise.

G. Gastrointestinal symptoms: abdominal pain, nausea, vomiting.

H. With severe disease: irritability, change in mental status.

I. Symptoms progressively worsen over 12–24 hours.

J. May present with nonspecific signs of febrile illness, limited respiratory symptoms.

IV. Physical findings

A. High fever.

B. Tachycardia, tachypnea.

C. Nonproductive cough.

D. If lower respiratory tract infected, physical findings consistent with pneumonia or bronchiolitis.

V. Diagnostic tests
   A. Identification of virus or viral antigen in nasopharyngeal secretions.
      1. Specimens should be obtained within 72 hours of illness, due to decrease in viral shedding after that time.
      2. Specimen obtained by swab, nasal aspirate, or wash.
      3. Viral culture.
      4. Rapid diagnostic tests via fluorescent antibody staining, enzyme-linked immunoassay, or optical immunoassay.
         a. Rapid tests are more sensitive on pediatric specimens than adult specimens.
         b. Some tests detect both influenza A and B; some detect only one strain.
   B. Diagnosis of specific flu-related complications.
   C. Chest x-ray normal or areas of atelectasis.
VI. Differential diagnosis

Bronchiolitis, **466.19**
Laryngotracheobronchitis, **490.**
Pneumonia, **486.**

   A. Other lower respiratory illness (e.g., bronchiolitis, laryngotracheobronchitis, pneumonia).
VII. Treatment
   A. Encourage fluids.
   B. Antipyretics for fever (never use salicylates in children or adolescents).
   C. Monitor for complications of influenza.
   D. Antiviral therapy.
      1. Must be administered within 48 hours of onset of illness.
      2. Amantadine: administered orally to children ≥1 year of age for treatment, prophylaxis of influenza A.
      3. Rimantadine: administered orally for treatment of influenza A for those ≥13 years of age and for prophylaxis of influenza A in those ≥1 year of age.
      4. Zanamivir: administered by inhalation for treatment of influenza A and B for children ≥7 years of age.
      5. Oseltamivir: administered orally for treatment of influenza A and B for children and adults ≥1 year of age; prophylaxis of influenza A and B for those ≥13 years of age.
VIII. Follow-up
   A. Call health provider immediately if signs of respiratory distress increase.
      1. Increased respiratory rate, shortness of breath.
      2. Increased retractions.
      3. Change in level of consciousness, restlessness, or anxiety.
      4. Cyanosis.
   B. Close telephone follow-up for those at high risk for flu-related complications.

IX. Complications

Asthma, **493.90**	Dehydration, **276.5**
Bacterial pneumonia, **482.9**	Diabetes, **250.00**
Chronic heart failure, **428.0**	Viral pneumonia, **480.9**

    A. Viral and bacterial pneumonia.

    B. Severe illness requiring hospitalization.

    C. Dehydration.

    D. Worsening of chronic illness, including CHF, asthma, or diabetes.

    E. Death.

X. Education

    A. Prevention.

        1. Annual intranasal vaccine is an option for healthy children and adults 5–49 years of age.

        2. Yearly influenza vaccine in fall for all children 6–24 months of age and targeted high-risk children and adolescents with specific chronic medical conditions.

        3. Children <9 years of age require 2 doses of vaccine administered 1 month apart to produce sufficient antibody response.

        4. Good hand washing, avoidance of ill contacts during influenza outbreaks.

    B. Post-illness.

        1. Treat with antiviral agents within 72 hours after onset of symptoms to reduce duration of illness.

        2. Recognize signs of severe illness requiring medical intervention including shortness of breath, dyspnea, cyanosis, change in level of consciousness.

        3. Encourage fluids to maintain adequate hydration and urine output.

        4. Acetaminophen for treatment of myalgia, headache, fever.

        5. Recurrent wheezing is common, especially with URIs.

        6. Avoid secondhand smoke exposure.

BRONCHITIS

Bacterial infection, **041.9**	Mycoplasmal infection, **041.81**
Bronchitis, **490.**	Pharyngitis, **462.**
Bronchitis, acute, **466.**	Pulmonary disease, chronic, **518.89**
Bronchitis, chronic, **491.9**	Respiratory syncytial virus, **079.6**
Chest pain, **786.50**	Rhinitis, **472.00**
Cough, **786.2**	Upper respiratory infection, **465.9**
Fever, **780.6**	Vomiting, **787.03**
Fungal infection, **117.9**	Wheezing, **786.07**

I. Etiology

    A. Bronchitis is common respiratory problem of childhood characterized by cough.

    B. Most commonly occurs after viral infection.

        1. Rhinovirus, RSV, influenza, parainfluenza, adenovirus, coxsackievirus, paramyxoviruses can be etiologic agent.

    C. May occur with bacterial, mycoplasmal, or fungal infection.

    D. May occur as result of inflammation caused by frequent viral infection, secondhand smoke exposure, and air pollution.

    E. Chronic bronchitis is poorly defined in children.

II. Occurrence

    A. Peak months in young children are related to high RSV activity.

    B. Peak incidence is in winter months.

    C. Chronic/recurrent bronchitis: cough lasting >1 month or 4 episodes within 1 year.

III. Clinical manifestations

    A. Mild URI symptoms including rhinitis and pharyngitis.

    B. Dry hacking cough begins 3–4 days after onset of rhinitis.

    C. Cough often becomes productive after a few days.

    D. Older patients may complain of chest pain, worse with coughing.

    E. As cough progressively worsens, the child has more signs of generalized illness.

    F. Younger children may have post-tussive vomiting.

    G. Normal temperature or mild elevation.

IV. Physical findings

    A. Physical findings vary with phase of illness.

    B. Initially clear or mucopurulent nasal secretions.

    C. Auscultation initially may be normal.

    D. Cough is dry hacking in nature.

    E. Normal or slightly elevated temperature.

    F. Over next week, cough becomes productive as condition progresses to include lower respiratory symptoms.

        1. Coarse crackles with variable wheezing may be present.

        2. Moderate to severe productive cough, chest pain.

        3. Post-tussive vomiting, thick yellow mucopurulent sputum.

    G. Elevated temperature is likely during this time.

V. Diagnostic tests

    A. Diagnosis is often diagnosis of exclusion (see differential diagnosis).

    B. Assessment of general health status including height, weight, signs of chronic pulmonary disease.

    C. Elevated neutrophil count or C-reactive protein is suggestive of bacterial etiology.

    D. CXR is usually normal, but may show peribronchial thickening.

    E. RSV wash for rapid testing.

VI. Differential diagnosis

Anorexia, 783.0	Headache, 784.0
Asthma, 493.90	Heart murmur, 785.2
Bronchiectasis, 494.0	Immunodeficiency, 279.3
Bronchopulmonary dysplasia, 770.7	Irritability, 799.2
Chronic pulmonary disorders, other, 518.89	Poor feeding, 783.0

Congenital heart disease, 746.9
Congestive heart failure, 428.0
Digital clubbing, 781.5
Foreign body aspiration, 934.8
Gastroesophageal reflux, 530.81

Poor growth, 764.9
Purulent rhinitis, 472.0
Sinusitis, 473.9
Wheezing, 786.07

A. Asthma: pattern of symptoms, absence of fever, expiratory wheezing, prolonged expiratory phase.
B. Bronchiectasis: recurrent pulmonary infections, anorexia, irritability, poor growth, digital clubbing, rule out other chronic pulmonary disorders.
C. Bronchopulmonary dysplasia: history of prematurity, treatment with oxygen therapy and or mechanical ventilation during neonatal period.
D. Immunodeficiency: systemic illness following vaccination with live virus; severe life-threatening illness with viral infection.
E. Gastroesophageal reflux: barium swallow demonstrates reflux of barium into esophagus; esophageal pH monitoring.
F. Congenital heart disease: accompanied by heart murmur, signs of CHF, poor feeding, poor growth.
G. Sinusitis: purulent rhinitis lasting >2 weeks, facial/dental pain, headache, pressure over affected area.
H. Foreign body aspiration: typically in toddler, x-ray or by bronchoscopy.

VII. Treatment
A. Treatment is supportive.
B. Cough suppressants should be avoided in children with productive cough.
C. Rest as needed.
D. Avoidance of environmental irritants.
E. Empiric trial of bronchodilator therapy.
F. Acetaminophen for chest pain, fever.
G. Antibiotic therapy may be considered if bacterial infection is strongly suspected (prolonged symptoms, patient's age, high fever).
H. Humidification of air promotes comfort.
I. Chest physiotherapy may be indicated if productive cough, coarse crackles on exam.

VIII. Follow-up
A. If cough for >2 weeks or worsens, fever, or signs of respiratory distress: contact health care provider.

IX. Complications

Otitis media, chronic, 382.9
Pneumonia, 486.
Sinusitis, 473.9

A. In healthy children not serious illness.
B. In chronically ill children, may develop concurrent otitis, sinusitis, pneumonia.

X. Education
A. Avoid large day care settings for young children to minimize frequency of viral infection.

B. Avoid secondhand smoke exposure.

C. Bronchitis is usually caused by viral infection; antibiotics are not effective.

D. Acute bronchitis is benign, self-limited illness usually lasting 2 weeks.

E. Should consult with health care providers before administering cough suppressants.

F. If child has signs of respiratory distress, contact health care provider.

G. If cough does not resolve within 2 weeks or worsens or fever recurs, contact health care provider.

PERTUSSIS

Apnea, 770.81	Lymphocytosis, 288.8
Atelectasis, 518.0	Pertussis, 033.9
Choking, 784.9	Petechiae, 782.7
Cough, 786.2	Pneumonia, 486.
Cough, paroxysmal, 780.2	Rhinorrhea, 478.1
Cyanosis, 782.5	Sneezing, 784.9
Exhaustion, 780.79	Subconjunctival hemorrhages, 372.72
Fever, 780.6	Upper respiratory infection, 065.9
Lacrimation, 375.20	Vomiting, 787.03
Leukocytosis, 288.8	Whooping cough, 033.9

I. Etiology

    A. Pertussis: highly contagious, vaccine-preventable bacterial infection caused by *Bordetella pertussis*, less commonly by *B. parapertussis* (gram-negative coccobacillus).

    B. Transmission: airborne, occurs by contact with respiratory droplets of infected person or by indirect contact with contaminated surfaces.

II. Occurrence

    A. Pertussis causes disease in every age group.

        1. Significantly impacts nonimmunized or partially immunized young children; can cause severe disease. Highest mortality in infants <6 months of age.

    B. Incubation period is 7–21 days.

    C. Persons with pertussis are considered infectious from 7 days after exposure to 3 weeks after person enters paroxysmal stage.

        1. Pertussis is most contagious from catarrhal stage until 2 weeks after onset of cough without appropriate therapy.

III. Clinical manifestations

    A. Pertussis is lengthy disease, divided into 3 stages:

        1. Catarrhal stage lasts 1–2 weeks, may not be recognized in infants <3 months.

            a. Characterized by URI symptoms such as rhinorrhea, sneezing, mild cough, low-grade fever.

        2. The paroxysmal stage last 2–4 weeks or longer.

            a. Characterized by paroxysmal cough/bouts of rapid cough, sudden coughing.

      b. Have color change, bulging eyes, tearing, tongue protrusion.

      c. May be triggered by feeding, crying, excitement, activity.

      d. May have multiple episodes each hour during peak but appear well between episodes.

      e. May have characteristic whoop during forceful inspiration.

      f. Post-tussive vomiting, exhaustion are common following episode.

      g. Infants <3 months of age have apnea, choking, gasping.

    3. Convalescent stage lasts 1–2 weeks, but cough can persist for several months. During this stage, cough and post-tussive vomiting decrease.

IV. Physical findings

  A. Cough.

    1. Catarrhal stage: mild.

    2. Paroxysmal cough: associated with cyanosis, lacrimation, exhaustion, post-tussive vomiting.

    3. Subconjunctival hemorrhages and petechiae on head and neck.

  B. Breath sounds are normal, unless significant atelectasis or pneumonia.

V. Diagnostic tests

  A. Consider in cases of prolonged cough with history of post-tussive vomiting, whoop, paroxysmal cough.

  B. Viral culture.

    1. Most likely to be positive during catarrhal stage to peak of paroxysmal stage.

    2. Use calcium alginate or Dacron swab of posterior nasopharynx for 15–30 seconds or by nasal wash and plate on specialized media, incubate for 7 days.

  C. Rapid testing by nasal wash for direct fluorescent antibody (DFA) or polymerase chain reaction (PCR).

  D. Serology.

    1. Enzyme immunoassay detects antibody to B pertussis in acute and convalescent samples: not helpful during acute illness and difficult to interpret in immunized persons.

  E. CBC: leukocytosis with lymphocytosis in catarrhal and early paroxysmal stages.

VI. Differential diagnosis

Adenoviral infection, 079.	Chlamydial infection, unspecified, 079.98
Bordetella parapertussis infection, 033.1	Cytomegalovirus, 078.5

  A. Adenoviral infection: presence of fever distinguishes from pertussis.

  B. *Mycoplasma* infection: causes prolonged cough but fever, systemic symptoms, crackles on auscultation help differentiate from pertussis.

  C. *B. parapertussis* infection: less severe illness.

  D. In infancy, consider chlamydia, cytomegalovirus (CMV).

VII. Treatment

  A. Most children beyond infancy can be managed at home.

  B. Treatment of choice: erythromycin 40–50 mg/kg/day divided every 6 hours for 14 days.

1. Do not use in young infants because of association with infant hypertrophic pyloric stenosis.
C. Alternatively use trimethoprim-sulfamethoxazole (TMP-SMX), 8–40 mg/kg/day divided every 12 hours for 14 days, if unable to take erythromycin or culture resistant to erythromycin. The newer macrolides clarithromycin and azithromycin are alternatives for those who cannot tolerate erythromycin.
D. Those with pertussis should be considered contagious until treatment with erythromycin for 5 days.
E. Treat all household and close contacts including day care and school regardless of age, immunization status, symptoms.
F. In addition to chemoprophylaxis, for children <7 years of age who are not immunized or partially immunized, follow schedule for accelerated vaccination.
G. Reportable disease to local and state health departments.

VIII. Follow-up
A. Guidelines for parents to call health care provider for poor fluid intake, low urine output, change in level of consciousness, cyanosis, or respiratory distress.
B. Close outpatient follow-up by telephone to monitor and reassure family.

IX. Complications

Apnea, 770.81	Fluid and electrolyte imbalances, 276.9
Bacterial pneumonia, 482.9	Otitis media, 382.9
Conjunctival hemorrhage, 372.72	Petechiae, 782.7
Encephalopathy, 348.30	Seizures, 780.39
Epistaxis, 784.7	Viral pneumonia, 480.9

A. Infants <6 months of age have increased morbidity and mortality.
B. Children with history of prematurity or underlying chronic heart, pulmonary, or neurologic disease are at high risk for severe disease.
C. Apnea.
D. Secondary infection causing viral or bacterial pneumonia or otitis media.
E. Neurologic complications include encephalopathy and seizures.
F. Sequelae of violent coughing including conjunctival hemorrhage, CNS hemorrhage, epistaxis, petechiae.
G. Fluid and electrolyte imbalances.
H. Death. Infants <1 year of age are at highest risk.

X. Education
A. Very contagious and spread by direct or indirect contact with respiratory droplets.
B. Good hand washing, containment of coughs/sneezes prevents spread of illness.
C. Guidelines about adequate hydration and nutrition.
D. Children may continue to have cough for several months.
E. Provide adequate rest and avoid activity that triggers cough.
F. Need for antibiotic treatment of all household and close contacts.

G. Household and close contacts are considered contagious until completed 5 days of erythromycin therapy.
H. Need for accelerated immunization for contacts <7 years of age partially immunized/not immunized.
I. Avoid secondhand smoke exposure.

ASTHMA

Airflow obstruction, episodic, **519.8**	Family history of eczema, dermatitis, **V19.4**
Allergens, inhalant, **477.9**	Fatigue, **780.79**
Allergens, outdoor, **477.9**	Itching, **698.9**
Animal allergens, house-dust mites,	Mucosal swelling, **784.2**
cockroach allergens, molds, **477.8**	Nasal polyps, **471.9**
Asthma, **493.90**	Otitis, **382. 9**
Bronchiolitis, recurrent, **466.19**	Pneumonia, **486.**
Bronchitis, allergic, **493.90**	Rhinitis, **472.0**
Chest pain, **786.50**	Rhinorrhea, clear, **478.1**
Chest tightness, **786.59**	Shortness of breath, **786.05**
Conjunctivitis, **372.30**	Sinusitis, **473.9**
Cough, **786.2**	Sleep disturbances, **780.50**
Eczema, **691.8**	Sneezing, **784.9**
Family history of allergy, **V19.6**	Upper respiratory infection, **465.9**
Family history of asthma, **V17.5**	Wheezing, **786.07**

I. Etiology
  A. Asthma is chronic inflammatory disorder of airways in which many cells and cellular elements play a role.
   1. Mast cells, eosinophils, T-lymphocytes, neutrophils.
  B. May have genetic predisposition (with critical interaction with environment).
  C. The characteristics of asthma are:
   1. Symptoms of episodic airflow obstruction that is reversible.
   2. Airway inflammation.
   3. Increased airway responsiveness to variety of stimuli.
  D. Hyperresponsiveness.
   1. Chronically inflamed airways are hyperresponsive.
   2. When exposed to "triggers," there is bronchoconstriction and airflow limitation.
   3. Inflammation contributes to airway edema and increased mucous production.
   4. Cough and wheeze are characteristic of asthma but are also common nonspecific symptoms associated with many other clinical entities.
  E. Common triggers.
   1. Inhalant allergens: animal allergens, house-dust mites, cockroach allergens, molds, outdoor allergens.
   2. Irritants: active/passive tobacco smoke exposure, indoor and outdoor air pollution, strong odors, chemical cleaning products.

3. Viral illness.
   a. URI, sinusitis, rhinitis, otitis, lower respiratory infection.
   b. Viral illness is primary trigger for asthma in young children.
4. Weather: rapid change in weather, hot, humid weather, or cold air.
5. Exercise.
6. Emotions or stress.
7. Occupational exposures: farm and barn exposures, formaldehydes, paint fumes, smoke, strong odors.
8. Aspirin sensitivity (more common in adults): includes other NSAIDs.
9. Sulfite sensitivity: in many processed foods, dried fruit, salad bars, beer, wine.
10. Risk factors.
    a. Atopy: family history or eczema.
    b. Gender: preadolescent boys are at higher risk.
    c. Smoking: history of mother smoking perinatally.
    d. Respiratory viral disease.
11. Aggravating factors: smoking, gastroesophageal reflux, sinusitis.

II. Occurrence
A. Most common serious chronic illness among children.
B. Onset at any age from infancy to old age; 50–80% of children develop asthma symptoms before 5 years of age.

III. Clinical manifestations
A. Recurrent wheezing.
B. Dry persistent cough, nocturnal cough.
C. Recurrent chest tightness or shortness of breath, chest pain.
D. Sputum production.
E. Exercise-induced cough, wheezing, shortness of breath, or chest tightness.
F. In younger children, difficulty keeping up with their peers.
G. Atopic profile.
   1. Eczema.
   2. Seasonal or perennial allergy symptoms.
   3. Rhinitis, sneezing, itching and rubbing of nose, throat clearing.
   4. Conjunctivitis.
H. Fatigue secondary to sleep disturbance.
I. Poor school performance secondary to sleep disturbance.

IV. Physical findings
A. Upper respiratory tract.
   1. Allergic shiners, "allergic salute" (characteristic crease at bridge of nose due to chronic rhinitis).
   2. Conjunctivitis.
   3. Boggy, pale nasal mucosa, mucosal swelling, clear rhinorrhea, nasal polyps, nasal flaring.
   4. Grunting.
B. Chest exam.
   1. Normal chest examination does not rule out asthma.

    2. Bilateral wheezing, end-expiratory wheezing on forced expiration.

    3. Prolonged expiratory phase; rapid, shallow respirations.

    4. Hyperresonance to percussion.

    5. Hyperexpansion of chest, increased A-P diameter.

    6. Intercostal, suprasternal, and/or subcostal retractions.

    7. In infants, paradoxical breathing.

    8. In young children, pushing with abdominal musculature on expiration.

    9. Dry, tight sounding cough.

V. Diagnostic tests

    A. Detailed medical history.

        1. Family history of allergy, asthma, eczema, dermatitis.

        2. Identify symptoms consistent with asthma.

        3. Identify pattern of symptoms that occur or worsen in presence of triggers.

            a. Consider diagnosis after 3 episodes of cough and/or wheezing, once alternative diagnoses are excluded.

    B. Focused physical examination.

    C. Laboratory procedures.

        1. Spirometry.

            a. Age limited; difficult to accurately test children <5–7 years of age in most settings.

            b. Pre- and postbronchodilator to validate reversibility:

                • May be normal.

                • Essential for diagnosis.

                • Annually to establish baseline pulmonary function.

        2. Peak flow is monitoring tool, not diagnostic tool.

    D. Chest x-ray: important in newly diagnosed asthmatic, rules out alternative diagnoses.

    E. Special studies.

        1. Sinus x-rays or CT to evaluate sinusitis.

        2. pH probe or barium swallow to evaluate gastroesophageal reflux (GER).

        3. Allergy testing.

            a. Referral to board-certified allergist to administer skin tests and interpret.

            b. RAST testing: not as sensitive as skin testing, results not immediate.

            c. Allergic bronchitis, wheezy bronchitis.

            d. Recurrent bronchiolitis or pneumonia.

                • Even children with mild persistent asthma have significant airway inflammation.

                • Without adequate anti-inflammatory therapy, there may be airway remodeling or irreversible changes in asthma airway.

    F. Asthma classification: presence of any one feature prior to treatment is sufficient to place patient in category (see Appendix G for details).

        1. Intermittent asthma.

            a. Symptoms ≤2 times per week, nighttime symptoms ≤2 times a month.

    b. Asymptomatic and normal peak flow between exacerbations.

    c. Exacerbations brief; intensity may vary.

    d. May have severe or lethal episodes.

  2. Mild persistent asthma.

    a. Symptoms >2 times per week but less than daily. Nighttime symptoms >2 times a month.

    b. Exacerbations may affect activity.

    c. Nighttime symptoms >2 times per month.

  3. Moderate persistent asthma.

    a. Daily symptoms, daily use of inhaled quick-relief bronchodilators.

    b. Nighttime symptoms >1 time a week.

    c. Exacerbations affect activity, occur 2 times per week; may last days.

  4. Severe persistent.

    a. Continual symptoms; frequent exacerbations, nighttime symptoms.

    b. Limited physical activity.

VI. Differential diagnosis

Bronchiolitis, viral, **466.19**	Malabsorption, **579.9**
Bronchopulmonary dysplasia, **770.7**	Poor growth, **764.9**
Cystic fibrosis, **277.00**	Pulmonary infection, chronic, **518.89**
Foreign body aspiration, **934.8**	Tracheoesophageal fistula, **530.84**
Gastroesophageal reflux, **530.81**	

  A. Vocal cord dysfunction: paradoxical adduction of vocal cords during inspiration (often in adolescent girls). Symptoms of distress including inspiratory wheezing and are out of proportion to clinical exam, including normal oxygen saturations. Diagnosis established by direct visualization of vocal cords using flexible rhinolaryngoscopy or flexible laryngoscopy.

  B. Congenital pulmonary malformations: radiologic testing, bronchoscopy to rule out abnormality.

    1. Tracheoesophageal fistula.

    2. Vascular ring, sling, or extrinsic mass.

  C. Foreign body aspiration: focal findings on auscultation; medical history key.

  D. Bronchopulmonary dysplasia: history of prematurity, treatment with oxygen therapy, mechanical ventilation during neonatal period.

  E. Viral bronchiolitis: virus may be identified by antigen testing or culture; may be trigger for asthma. Asthma differentiated by pattern of symptoms over time.

  F. Gastroesophageal reflux: reflux of barium into esophagus by barium swallow or esophageal pH monitoring. Can be aggravating factor in asthma control.

  G. Cystic fibrosis: genetic disease characterized by excessive production of thick, tenacious respiratory secretions, chronic pulmonary infection, malabsorption, subsequent poor growth.

VII. Treatment

  A. Goals of treatment.

        1. No coughing, shortness of breath/rapid breathing, wheezing, chest tightness.

        2. No waking up at night because of asthma symptoms.

        3. Normal activities including play, sports, exercise.

        4. No absences from school or activities or work (for parent or caregiver).

        5. Normal lung function.

B. Key principles.

        1. Prevent airway inflammation by eliminating or avoiding triggers.

        2. Asthma can be controlled, not cured.

        3. Reverse and suppress inflammation.

C. Nonpharmacologic therapy.

        1. Patient education.

        2. Objective measures of lung function using peak flow monitoring and follow-up spirometry.

        3. Control or avoid aggravating factors.

D. Pharmacologic therapy.

        1. Simplify treatment plan whenever possible.

        2. Classification of severity guides choice and frequency of therapy.

        3. Persistent asthma is most effectively controlled with daily anti-inflammatory medications.

        4. National Asthma Education and Prevention guidelines support aggressive therapy to achieve rapid control of symptoms and then step down to lowest level of therapy to maintain control.

        5. Goals in treatment of acute episode are:

           a. Rapid reversal of acute airway obstruction.

           b. Identify causes of asthma episode.

           c. Adjust chronic maintenance to prevent recurrence of asthma flare.

        6. Inhaled beta$_2$-agonist is quick-relief medication for all levels of severity and treatment of choice for prevention of exercise-induced asthma.

        7. Short "burst" of oral glucocorticoids is used to reduce inflammation during acute episode.

E. Build child/family and health care provider partnership.

        1. Understand and address reasons for adherence problems in asthma.

        2. Explore patient/family misconceptions about asthma.

        3. Agree on goals and expectations of treatment.

        4. Jointly develop treatment plan.

VIII. Follow-up

A. Before increasing medications, investigate reasons for poor asthma control.

        1. Improper inhaler technique.

        2. Adherence issues, knowledge deficit.

        3. Environmental exposures.

        4. Exacerbation of aggravating conditions (i.e., GER, sinusitis).

B. Many children have multiple caretakers.

        1. Each caretaker must have access to medications, appropriate devices, asthma action plan.

2. Provide information to all caregivers including day care providers, teachers, coaches, school nurses.
3. Ensure reliable, immediate access to medications in all settings including school.

C. Regular use of quick-relief medicine indicates deterioration in control of asthma and need to assess maintenance therapy.
D. Regular follow-up visits are encouraged to achieve and maintain control with appropriate intensity of therapy.
E. Monitor child for side effects of medications.
F. Refer to asthma specialist for difficult-to-control asthma in children >5 years of age: consider at step 3; refer at step 4.
G. For children <5 years of age: consider referral at step 2; refer at step 3 and 4.
H. Peak flow monitoring to establish personal best: more specific than predicted value.
I. At each encounter, reassess concerns and correct misconceptions.
J. Monitor quality of life on regular basis.
K. Recognize and address barriers to asthma self-management.
L. Assess source of social support for child and family.
M. Assess child and family satisfaction with asthma care.
N. Yearly influenza vaccine for child and household contacts.

IX. Complications

Pneumonia, 486.
Pneumothorax, 512.8

A. Pneumothorax, pneumonia.
B. Acute exacerbation requiring hospitalization, intubation, mechanical ventilation.
C. Death.

X. Education

A. Asthma education should begin at diagnosis and continue at every encounter: include child as developmentally appropriate and all caregivers.
B. Key components.
   1. Basic asthma facts to enable child and family to understand rationale for treatment decisions and asthma self-management.
   2. Roles of medications in treating acute symptoms and achieving/ maintaining asthma control.
   3. Environmental avoidance and control measures.
   4. Teach relevant skills: how to use devices such as spacers, other medication delivery devices, peak flow meter; have child demonstrate relevant skills at each encounter.
   5. Provide asthma action plan: daily maintenance therapy including avoidance of triggers, plan for recognizing and treating worsening asthma, and when to seek medical attention.
C. Establish goals of therapy jointly and monitor child and family's perception of progress toward reaching goals.

PNEUMONIA

Abdominal distention, 787.3
Anorexia, 783.0
Arthritic symptoms, transient, 716.4
Arthropathy, 716.9
Cervical lymphadenopathy, 785.6
Conjunctivitis, unilateral, 372.30
Coryza, 460.
Cough, 786.2
Cyanosis, 782.5
Dehydration, 276.5
Diarrhea, 787.9
Drowsiness, 780.09
Dyspnea, 786.09
Ear pain, 388.70
Empyema, 510.9
Fever, 780.6
Headache, 784.0
Hoarseness, 784.49
Hypoxemia, 799.0
Lethargy, 780.79
Leukocytosis, 288.8
Malaise, 780.79
Meningismus, 781.6
Mycoplasma pneumoniae, 483.0
Nasal congestion, 478.1
Nausea, 787.02
Nuchal rigidity, 781.6
Otitis media, 382.9
Parainfluenza infection, 480.2

Pleural effusion, 511.9
Pleuritic pain, 786.52
Pneumonia, 486.
Pneumonia, bacterial, 482.9
Pneumonia, bronchopneumonia, 485.
Pneumonia, interstitial, 516.8
Pneumonia, lobar, 481.0
Pneumonia, mycoplasma, 483.00
Pneumonia, *Staphylococcus aureus*, 482.41
Pneumonia, viral, 480.9
Respiratory distress, 786.09
Respiratory syncytial virus, 079.6
Restlessness, 799.2
Retractions, substernal, 738.3
Retractions, suprasternal, 738.8
Rhinitis, 472.0
Rigors, 780.99
Seizure, 780.39
Sneezes, 7884.9
Sore throat, 462.
Staphylococcus pneumoniae, 482.30
Tachycardia, 785.0
Tachypnea, 786.06
Tactile fremitus, 785.3
Upper respiratory infection, 465.9
Urticaria, 708.9
Vomiting, 787.03
Wheezing, 786.07

I. Etiology

A. Pneumonia is inflammation and infection of lung parenchyma due to infectious pathogens.

B. It represents wide spectrum of signs/symptoms and disease severity.

C. Pathogens vary depending on age of patient.

D. Classification.

1. By pathogen (bacterial, including mycoplasma or viral).

2. By anatomic location: lobar, interstitial, bronchopneumonia.

E. Common viral pathogens.

1. RSV; adenovirus; parainfluenza 1, 2, 3; influenza A and B; rhinovirus.

2. Transmission: highly contagious.

a. Transmitted by direct contact with nasopharyngeal secretions from infected person.

  b. Pneumonia results from spread of infection along airways.
  - Causes direct injury to respiratory epithelium, resulting in airway obstruction, abnormal secretion and necrotic debris in airway lumen and lymphocytic infiltrations of interstitium and lung parenchyma.
  - Small airways are obstructed, resulting in poor oxygenation and air trapping, which leads to ventilation and perfusion mismatch.
- **F.** Common bacterial pathogens.
  1. *Streptococcus pneumoniae, Mycoplasma pneumoniae, Streptococcus* (group A) *pyogenes, Staphylococcus aureus.*
  2. Transmission: contagious.
     a. Bacterial pathogens may be aspirated or inhaled, rarely by hematogenous spread.
     b. Transmitted via person-to-person contact by large droplet aerosolization during coughing/sneezing.
     c. Viral infection damages hosts normal airway defense mechanisms facilitating secondary bacterial infection.
  3. *S. pneumoniae.*
     a. Many have *S. pneumoniae* colonization in upper respiratory tract.
     b. Gram + encapsulated diplococci produce local edema.
     - Organism is distributed into adjacent areas of lung, resulting in typical focal lobar consolidation.
     - >90 Serotypes exist.
  4. *S. aureus.*
     a. Gram-positive organism; beta-lactamase producer.
     b. Produces exoproducts, enzymes, toxins, which contribute to virulence of this organism.
     c. Causes confluent bronchopneumonia; often unilateral with areas of hemorrhagic necrosis, cavitation of lung parenchyma, resulting in formation of pneumatocele, empyema, or bronchopulmonary fistula.
  5. *M. pneumoniae.*
     a. Smallest self-replicating bacterium; lacks cell wall, dependent on host.
     b. Binds to ciliated respiratory epithelium and inhibits ciliary action.
     c. Airways and areas surrounding are filled with infiltrates.
     d. Causes cellular destruction and inflammatory response.

II. Occurrence
- **A.** Acute childhood respiratory infections results in 4.5 million deaths/year.
  1. 70% are pneumonia-related deaths.
  2. Bacterial pneumonia less common than viral pneumonia, but has highest mortality.
- **B.** Viral pneumonia.
  1. Peak attack rate between 2–3 years of life.
  2. More common in fall and winter.
     a. Fall: parainfluenza infection causing croup.
     b. Winter: RSV and influenza.
     c. Viral pneumonia can be complicated by secondary bacterial infection.

C. Bacterial pneumonia.
  1. More common in children >5 years of age.
  2. Occurs in winter to early spring.
  3. Organisms vary according to age of child.
     a. *S. pneumoniae.*
        • Children <4 years of age at highest risk.
        • Risks factors: male > female, day care attendance, frequent otitis media (>3 in 6 months), frequent URIs (3 in 6 months), prematurity, and previous hospitalization for respiratory disease.
        • Incubation period varies by serotype but generally short: 1–3 days.
     b. *M. pneumoniae.*
        • Leading cause of pneumonia in school-age children, adolescents.
        • Occurs year-round. Incubation period: 2–3 weeks (range: 1–4 weeks).
        • Rarely severe enough to warrant hospitalization.
     c. *S. aureus:* children <2 years of age at highest risk.

III. Clinical manifestations
  A. Viral pneumonia: symptoms variable depending on age.
     1. Onset may be acute or gradual but typically progresses more slowly than bacterial infection.
     2. Nasal congestion and coryza.
     3. Lower respiratory symptoms develop insidiously.
     4. Temperature variable depending on causative agent.
     5. Nontoxic appearing.
     6. History of URI symptoms, rhinitis, cough.
     7. Hoarseness, wheezing, rapid/shallow respirations.
  B. Bacterial pneumonia.
     1. *S. pneumoniae.*
        a. Infants initially.
           • Mild URI symptoms, unilateral conjunctivitis or OM.
           • Abrupt onset of fever to 104°F. May have seizure due to abrupt spike in temperature.
           • Mild cough; may have diarrhea, vomiting.
        b. Infants progress.
           • Restlessness, apprehension.
           • Nasal flaring, rapid shallow respiration, grunting.
           • Abdominal distention.
           • Cough may be absent.
           • Circumoral cyanosis.
        c. Older children and adolescents.
           • Onset abrupt with rigors followed by temperature 102–104°F.
           • Appears ill.
           • Headache.
           • Anorexia, nausea, vomiting, diarrhea, abdominal pain.
           • Dyspnea, pleuritic pain, and cough; cough may be productive.
           • Alternating restlessness and drowsiness.

C. *M. pneumoniae.*
1. Slow onset.
2. Malaise, transient arthritic symptoms.
3. Persistent dry, hacking cough; sore throat often followed by hoarseness.
4. Low-grade temperature and chills.
5. May have ear pain.

IV. Physical findings
A. Viral pneumonia: symptoms dependent on causative agent and age of child.
1. Nontoxic appearing.
2. Tachypnea, cough, diffuse bilateral wheezing, decreased breath sounds throughout lung fields.
3. Suprasternal, intercostal, substernal retractions.
4. Cyanosis.
B. Bacterial pneumonia.
1. *S. pneumoniae.*
   a. Infants.
      • Tachypnea; nasal flaring, grunting, retractions; diminished breath sounds; crackles, wheezing.
      • Fever.
      • Tachycardia.
      • Palpable liver or spleen secondary to abdominal distention.
      • Air hunger and cyanosis.
   b. Older children and adolescents.
      • Diminished breath sounds over affected area of lung.
      • Dullness to percussion over area of consolidation.
      • Increased tactile fremitus over area of consolidation.
      • Cough productive of bloody or rust-tinged sputum.
      • Crackles, wheezing, splinting of respirations on affected side.
      • Fever.
      • Nuchal rigidity and other signs of meningeus may be present if upper lobes are involved.
      • Drowsiness, restlessness.
      • Respiratory distress and hypoxemia are variable or mild without widespread disease or pleural effusion.
C. *M. pneumoniae.*
1. Fever.
2. Diminished breath sounds; coarse, harsh breath sounds.
3. May have macular rash, erythematous macular rash, urticaria.
4. Cervical lymphadenopathy.
5. Conjunctivitis, otitis media.
6. Arthropathy.

V. Diagnostic tests
A. Viral pneumonia.
1. Definitive diagnosis: viral isolation/viral antigens in respiratory tract infection.

    2. CXR: typically shows bilateral, diffuse infiltrates.

    3. WBC: normal or leukocytosis (not usually >20,000) with lymphocytosis.

B. Bacterial pneumonia.

    1. No "gold standard" definitive test.

    2. Blood cultures are positive for the causative agent only about 10% of the time.

    3. WBC: leukocytosis (15,000–40,000) with granulocytosis.

    4. CXR.

        a. *S. pneumoniae:* lobar consolidation; typically single focus but may be multiple foci; "spherical" infiltrate or round pneumonia; right lobes are preferentially affected.

        b. *S. aureus:* bronchopneumonia (multiple, central segmental infiltrates become confluent and diffuse); these infiltrates lead to necrosis, cavitation, pneumatoceles, and abscess formation.

C. *M. pneumoniae.*

    1. Clinical manifestation and physical exam are essential to diagnosis.

        a. Insidious onset, nontoxic.

        b. Child >5 years of age.

        c. Low-grade fever.

    2. *M. pneumoniae* detected by polymerase chain reaction (PCR) technology.

    3. Cold agglutinins (during acute phase) with titer 1:64 or greater are predictive of *M. pneumoniae.*

    4. WBC: normal.

VI. Differential diagnosis

Aspirations, **934.8**	Foreign body aspiration, **934.8**
Asthma, **493.90**	*Mycoplasma pneumoniae,* **483.0**
Bronchiolitis, **466.49**	Pneumonia, viral, **480.9**
Coryza, **460.**	Tracheoesophageal fistula, **530.84**
Cystic fibrosis, **277.00**	Upper respiratory infection, **465.9**
Fever, **780.6**	

A. Viral pneumonia: URI symptoms and coryza with low-grade fever; bacterial pneumonia: abrupt onset with high fever; *M. pneumoniae:* insidious onset and nontoxic appearance.

B. Foreign body aspiration: may be detected on x-ray or by bronchoscopy.

C. Cystic fibrosis: sweat test is definitive diagnostic test.

D. Asthma: pattern of symptoms, absence of fever; inspiratory wheezing; prolonged expiratory phase.

E. Aspiration: swallowing study to determine silent or free aspiration.

F. Tracheoesophageal fistula: gas-filled bowel on x-ray in an infant with respiratory problems and drooling at birth.

G. Bronchiolitis: rapid testing for viral antigen.

H. Right lower lobe pneumonia can present as GI process; x-ray can differentiate.

I. Right upper lobe pneumonia can present as meningitis, severity of illness, lumbar puncture.

VII. Treatment
A. Viral pneumonia.
   1. Supportive care; typically mild illness and can manage at home; young infant at risk for respiratory fatigue and more severe symptoms.
B. Bacterial pneumonia.
   1. Dependent on bacteria; dependent on condition of child (oxygenation, hydration status, age: infants <4–6 months are usually hospitalized).
   2. Acetaminophen for fever and chest pain.
   3. Antibiotic treatment is generally 7–10 days.
   4. Amoxicillin is outpatient drug of choice; alternative choices are clarithromycin for children 6 weeks to 4 years of age; erythromycin for children >4 years of age.
   5. With high level of penicillin-resistant pneumococci present in community, consider cefuroxime, Augmentin, or azithromycin.
C. *M. pneumoniae.*
   1. Usually mild disease that can be managed at home.
   2. Erythromycin is drug of choice.
   3. Antibiotic treatment is generally 7–10 days.
   4. Acetaminophen for fever.

VIII. Follow-up
A. Follow-up x-ray not needed in most cases of community-acquired pneumonia.
   1. Exceptions include severe illness requiring hospitalization, complications such as abscess, empyema, pleural effusion.
   2. May take up to 6 weeks for significant improvement.
B. Daily contact with health care provider may be indicated with more serious illness, in children with underlying conditions, and in very young children.
C. Recheck child if no improvement after 48 hours of treatment or if worsening occurs.
D. Follow-up visit at 10–14 days; occasional relapse may occur.

IX. Complications

Empyema, 510.9	Pleural effusion, 511.9
Encephalopathy, 248.30	Pulmonary abscess, 513.0
Guillain-Barré syndrome, 357.0	*Staphylococcus aureus,* 041.11
Meningoencephalitis, 323.9	Stevens-Johnson syndrome, 695.1
Mycoplasma pneumoniae, 483.0	Toxic shock syndrome, 040.82
Pericarditis, 423.9	Transverse myelitis, 323.9

A. Severe disease requiring hospitalization and ventilatory support.
B. Empyema, pulmonary abscess, pleural effusion, pericarditis.
C. *S. aureus:* toxic shock syndrome.
D. *M. pneumoniae:* Stevens-Johnson syndrome, transverse myelitis, meningoencephalitis, encephalopathy, Guillain-Barré syndrome.

X. Education
A. Immunizations are essential to decrease individual morbidity and mortality associated with pneumonia but also to reduce incidence in community.
B. Understand symptoms that warrant immediate attention (lethargy, seizure, severe respiratory distress) and symptoms that require follow-up (no improvement 48 hours after starting antibiotics, worsening of respiratory symptoms, signs of dehydration).
C. Need to give antibiotic as prescribed for full course.
D. Careful hand washing, containment of coughs/sneezes reduces spread of disease.
E. *M. pneumoniae:* common for close household contacts to develop illness.

BIBLIOGRAPHY

Behrman R, Kliegman R, Jenson H: *Nelson textbook of pediatrics,* ed 17, Philadelphia, 2004, WB Saunders.

CDC Fact Sheet: Influenza technical information, Atlanta, GA, December 2003, Centers for Disease Control and Prevention.

CDC Fact Sheet: Pertussis Technical Information, Atlanta, GA, December 2003, Centers for Disease Control and Prevention.

Klassen T, et al: Nebulized budesonide and oral dexamethasone for treatment of croup: a randomized controlled trial, *J Am Med Assoc* 279(20): 1635, 1998.

Long S, Pickering L, Prober C: *Principles and practice of pediatric infectious diseases,* ed 2, Philadelphia, 2003, Churchill Livingstone.

Michael M: Scope and impact of pediatric asthma, *Nurse Pract* 27(S):7, 2002.

National Heart, Lung, and Blood Institute, Global Initiative for Asthma: *Global burden of asthma,* NIH Publication No 02-3659: 3, Bethesda, MD, 2003, National Institutes of Health.

National Heart, Lung, and Blood Institute, National Asthma Education and Prevention Program: *NAEPP expert panel report guidelines for the diagnosis and management of asthma, Update on selected topics 2002,* NIH Publication No 02-5075, Bethesda, MD, 2002, National Institutes of Health.

National Heart, Lung, and Blood Institute, National Asthma Education and Prevention Program: *Practical guide for the diagnosis and management of asthma,* NIH Publication No 97-4053, Bethesda, MD, 1997, National Institutes of Health.

Pickering L: Influenza diagnosis and treatment in children: A review of studies on clinically useful test and antiviral treatment for influenza, *Pediatr Infect Dis J* 22(2):170.2003.

Pickering L: *Red book,* ed 26, Elk Grove Village, IL, 2003, American Academy of Pediatrics, p 383.

Storch G: Rapid diagnostic tests for influenza, *Curr Opin Pediatr* 15:79, 2003.

Taussig M, Landau L: *Pediatric respiratory medicine,* St. Louis, 1999, Mosby, p 565.

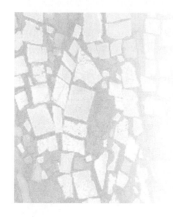

Cardiovascular Disorders

KAREN M. CORLETT

CHEST PAIN

Asthma, 493.81	Musculoskeletal, 786.59
Asthma, exercise-induced, 493.90	Myocarditis, 429.0
Cardiac murmur, 782.2	Obesity, 278.00
Cardiomegaly, 429.3	Palpitations, 785.1
Cardiomyopathy, 425.4	Pericarditis, 423.9
Chest pain, 786.50	Pneumonia, 486.
Chest pain, noncardiac, 786.59	Pneumothorax, 512.8
Congenital heart disease, 746.9	Presyncope, 780.2
Congestive heart failure, 428.0	Pulmonary, 786.52
Coronary artery anomalies, 746.9	Pulmonary embolus, 415.19
Coronary artery disease, 414.9	Rheumatic fever, 391.9
Dizziness, 780.4	Supraventricular tachycardia, 427.89
Dysrhythmias, 427.9	Syncope, 780.2
Enlarged liver, 789.1	Tachycardia, 785.0
Gastroesophageal reflux, 530.81	Tachypnea, 786.06
Heart disease, acquired, 429.9	Turner's syndrome, 758.6
Heart murmur, 785.2	Valvular defects, 424.0
Kawasaki disease 446.1	Ventricular tachycardias, 427.1
Marfan syndrome, 759.82	Weak peripheral pulses, 785.9

I. Etiology
   A. Classes of chest pain.
      1. Severe, acute, unremitting chest pain: refer immediately to pediatrician or urgent/emergent care facility. Rare and most often due to cardiac, pulmonary, or gastrointestinal causes.
      2. Chronic or recurrent chest pain: more likely.
         a. Typically patient has had several episodes of chest pain before medical attention is sought.

      b. Many times, physical exam may be normal.

      c. Patient history is crucial in elucidating etiology of chest pain although large percentage of chest pain in children will never have etiology determined.

      d. Chest pain is distressing to patients, families: chest pain in adult friends, relatives typically signifies cardiac event, most chest pain in childhood is noncardiac in origin.

      e. Thorough history and physical can rule out serious causes for chest pain.

  B. Chest pain, cardiac in origin.

    1. Coronary artery disease.

    2. Congenital heart disease.

    3. Typically have murmur.

    4. Acquired heart disease.

    5. Infectious etiologies.

    6. Cardiomyopathy pericarditis, Kawasaki disease, rheumatic fever.

    7. Myocardial issues, myocarditis.

    8. Cardiomyopathies.

    9. Dysrhythmias.

    10. Supraventricular or ventricular tachycardias.

  C. Chest pain, noncardiac in origin: most common.

    1. Musculoskeletal.

    2. Pulmonary.

    3. Gastrointestinal.

    4. Psychogenic.

II. Occurrence

  A. Few studies of overall incidence of chest pain in pediatric population due to wide range of specialists to whom these patients are referred.

  B. Incidence, particularly in adolescents, is significant.

III. Clinical manifestations

  A. Chronic or recurrent intermittent chest pain.

  B. Most often occurs in adolescent population.

  C. May or may not limit activities.

  D. Usually chest pain has been long standing before treatment is sought.

  E. Important to elucidate inciting factors and relieving factors.

  F. Relationship of pain to activity varies.

  G. Associated symptoms.

  H. Syncope, presyncope, dizziness, palpitations.

  I. Congenital heart disease or previous cardiac surgery is important factor in determining cardiac origin of chest pain; also increases likelihood of dysrhythmia as origin for chest pain.

IV. Physical findings

  A. Most commonly patients will have no significant physical exam findings. Physical exam findings may be clues to origin of chest pain.

  B. Stigmata of certain syndromes: Marfan, Turner's.

C. Cardiac murmur.

D. Evidence of congestive heart failure.

E. Obesity: increased incidence of gastroesophageal reflux (GER).

F. Reproducible pain with palpation.

G. Signs of trauma to chest wall.

H. Decreased breath sounds.

I. Tachypnea, increased work of breathing, retractions, flaring, tachycardia, weak peripheral pulses, cool extremities, delayed capillary refill, rales, enlarged liver, easily fatigued, edema.

V. Diagnostic tests

A. Refer to pediatrician/specialist if chest pain of cardiac origin is suspected; may conduct following tests as part of evaluation.

B. Chest x-ray (CXR).

   1. Evaluate for cardiomegaly. May also reveal rib fractures or pneumonia.

C. Electrocardiogram.

   1. Clue to cardiac origins: hypertrophied cardiac muscle, long QT syndrome.

D. Echocardiography.

   1. Structural abnormalities.

   2. Coronary artery anatomy.

   3. Cardiac function.

E. Exercise testing.

   1. ST segment response to exercise.

   2. May provoke dysrhythmias.

   3. May provoke exercise-induced asthma.

F. May reassure patient and parents.

VI. Differential diagnosis

Acute pancreatitis, 577.0	Peptic ulcer disease, 533.9
Asthma, 493.90	Pleural pain, 786.52
Asthma, exercise-induced, 493.81	Pleuritis, 511.0
Biliary colic, 574.2	Pneumonia, 486
Costochondritis, 733.6	Pneumothorax, 512.8
Esophagitis, 530.10	Precordial catch, 786.51
Gastroesophageal reflux, 530.81	Pulmonary embolus, 415.19
Muscular pain, 729.1	Slipping rib syndrome, 733.99

A. Musculoskeletal.

   1. Costochondritis.

     a. Most often at 2nd to 5th costal cartilages.

     b. Often reproducible pain with pressure at costochondral junctions.

     c. Treated with nonsteroidal anti-inflammatory drugs.

   2. Slipping rib syndrome.

     a. Pain at lower costal margin, often associated with click.

     b. Reproducible at times with anterior motion of lower rib.

     c. Treated with avoidance of inciting movements.

      3. Trauma (nonaccidental or accidental).
         a. Point tenderness at site of trauma.
         b. Pain is worse with movement of chest, self-limited.
      4. Muscular pain.
         a. History of new physical activity, pain is worse if affected muscles are used.
      5. Precordial catch.
         a. Sharp pain in anterior chest, often when child is bent over.
         b. Short, intermittent pain, relieved by shallow respirations.
      6. Pleural pain.
         a. Infection affecting intercostal and upper abdominal muscles, intensified with coughing.
         b. Tender muscles lasting 3–7 days.
         c. Intense pain separated by pain-free intervals.
  B. Pulmonary.
      1. Asthma, particularly exercise-induced asthma.
      2. Pneumonia.
      3. Foreign body aspiration.
      4. Pleuritis: often is remote occurrence to viral infection.
      5. Diaphragmatic irritation.
      6. Pulmonary embolus: associated with dyspnea, usually is acute episode.
      7. Pneumothorax: associated with dyspnea, usually is acute episode.
  C. Gastrointestinal: typically localized to substernal area.
      1. Gastroesophageal reflux.
      2. Related to mealtimes. Exacerbated by supine positioning.
      3. Esophagitis.
      4. Biliary colic.
      5. Acute pancreatitis: pain radiates to back.
      6. Peptic ulcer disease.
  D. Psychogenic causes: often have witnessed episodes of chest pain in family members.

VII. Treatment
  A. Musculoskeletal.
      1. Analgesics and anti-inflammatories.
      2. Avoidance of inciting movements, rest.
  B. Pulmonary.
      1. Asthma: trial of bronchodilators, particularly if exercise-induced symptoms.
      2. Immediate referral for concern of pulmonary embolus or pneumothorax.
  C. Gastrointestinal.
      1. GER: H_2 blockers, dietary modifications, weight loss if obesity contributing to symptoms.
      2. Referral to specialist if initial medical therapy does not relieve symptoms.

D. Psychogenic.
    1. Frank discussion with patient, family about nonorganic cause of chest pain.
        a. Changes in patient's life leading to stress or depression?
        b. Assess for secondary gain that pain yields patient.
        c. Counseling may be indicated.
    2. Refer to specialist.
E. Cardiac causes.
    1. Refer to specialist.
    2. Coronary artery anomalies, valvular defects: medical management, surgical repair.
    3. Infectious etiologies.
        a. Cardiomyopathy/myocarditis.
        b. Treatment of inciting infection if elucidated.
        c. Supportive care until recovery of function.
        d. Transplantation if function does not recover.
    4. Kawasaki disease (see later section).
    5. Myocardial issues.
        a. Obstructive cardiomyopathy.
        b. Activity restriction.
        c. Consideration of medical or surgical therapy.
    6. Dysrhythmias.
        a. Identification of dysrhythmia.
        b. Antidysrhythmic agents.
        c. Ablation of accessory pathways.

VIII. Follow-up
  A. Follow-up with pediatrician or specialist as indicated.
  B. Support for chronic pain.
  C. Assess for missed diagnosis if pain persists or worsens.
  D. No cause of chest pain may have been identified. Patient, family may require ongoing support, education, particularly if pain continues.

IX. Complications
  A. Misdiagnosis.
  B. Sudden cardiac death rare.

X. Education
  A. Most often require assurance and education as to noncardiac nature of chest pain and resumption of normal activities.
  B. If cause of chest pain found, education regarding cause and treatment plan.

HYPERTENSION

Adrenal disorders, 255.9	Papilledema, 377.00
Anorexia, 783.0	Papilledema with increased intracranial
Diabetes, 250.00	pressure, 377.01
Epistaxis, 784.7	Pheochromocytoma, 194.0

Headache, 784.0	Renal vascular diseases, 593.9
Hypertension, 401.9	Seizure, 780.39
Hypertension, family history of, V17.4	Stroke, 436
Hypertension, secondary, 405.99	Systemic lupus erythematosus, 710.0
Hyperthyroidism, 242.9	Tiredness, 780.79
Irritability, 799.2	Tuberous sclerosis, 759.5
Myocardial infarction, 410.	Turner's syndrome, 758.6
Nausea, 787.02	Vascular lesions, 459.9
Obesity, 278.00	Vomiting, 787.03

I. Etiology
   A. May be early onset of essential hypertension.
   B. Etiology of adult-onset essential hypertension is unclear and thought to be multifactorial with genetic, familial, environmental factors contributing to development of essential hypertension. Becoming more clear that elevations of blood pressure in childhood are beginnings of adult essential hypertension.
   C. May be a sign of underlying pathology (secondary hypertension).
   D. Renal, cardiac, endocrine diseases.

II. Occurrence
   A. By definition, 5% of children will have hypertension.

III. Clinical manifestations
   A. Definition is blood pressure consistently above 95th percentile for age, sex, height taken on 3 separate occasions.
   B. Secondary hypertension.
      1. Hypertension secondary to another cause.
      2. Severe elevation of blood pressure.
      3. Younger age.
      4. Severe elevation of blood pressure at any age should trigger an aggressive evaluation to look for an underlying cause.
   C. Essential hypertension.
      1. Typically milder elevation in blood pressure, but still >95th percentile.
      2. Often associated with obesity.
      3. Typically, family history of essential hypertension.
      4. Elevated heart rate is common.
      5. Variable blood pressure measurements on repeated evaluation.
      6. Often no additional findings on history or physical.
      7. For mild elevation of blood pressure in asymptomatic adolescent, minimal workup is indicated; it is more likely to be essential hypertension, particularly if positive family history.

IV. Physical findings
   A. Essential hypertension: may be few abnormal physical findings but patient history is important adjunct to determine whether hypertension is essential or secondary.

1. Family history of hypertension in 1st- or 2nd-degree relative, myocardial infarction, stroke, renal vascular diseases, diabetes, obesity.
   2. Obesity.
B. Secondary hypertension: may be physical findings or important clues in patient's history as to possible cause of secondary hypertension.
   1. Neonatal history of invasive umbilical lines.
   2. History of urinary tract infections.
   3. Medication history: OTC, prescribed, and illicit drugs.
      a. Tobacco, diet pills, anabolic steroids, oral contraceptive pills, pseudoephedrine, phenylpropanolamine.
   4. Headaches.
   5. Weight loss (pheochromocytoma, hyperthyroidism).
   6. Overall slowing of growth parameters may indicate underlying chronic disease.
   7. Webbed neck (Turner's syndrome associated with coarctation).
   8. Presence of skin lesions (tuberous sclerosis, systemic lupus erythematosus).
   9. Retinal exam: presence of vascular lesions due to chronic hypertension, papilledema with increased intracranial pressure.
   10. Dysmorphic features: William syndrome, Turner's syndrome.
   11. Adrenal disorders.
   12. Anorexia, nausea.
   13. Tiredness, irritability.
   14. Epistaxis.
   15. Neurologic symptoms.
      a. Headache, nausea, vomiting, anorexia, visual complaints, seizure, papilledema.

V. Diagnostic tests
A. Errors in blood pressure measurement are common: use correct technique, appropriately sized equipment for repeated measurement.
   1. All children ≥3 years of age: blood pressure measured at *every* pediatric visit.
   2. Appropriate cuff size essential for accurate measurement.
   3. Bladder width of cuff should be 40% of child's arm circumference, bladder should cover 80% or more of circumference of arm.
   4. At least 3 separate measurements.
   5. Measurement should occur after short period of rest.
   6. The younger the patient, the higher the blood pressure, the more concern for secondary hypertension. Refer to physician or specialist.
B. Any severe elevation in blood pressure: refer to physician or specialist.
C. Stepwise approach to evaluation.
   1. CBC.
   2. Urinalysis, urine culture.
   3. Serum blood urea nitrogen, creatinine, electrolytes, calcium.
   4. Lipid panel.

    5. Renal ultrasound.

    6. Echocardiography.

    7. Other, more invasive tests may be ordered by specialists.

VI. Differential diagnosis

Cushing's syndrome, 255.0	Systemic lupus erythematosus, 710.0
Hypertension, secondary, 405.99	Tuberous sclerosis 759.5
Hyperthyroidism, 244.9	Turner's syndrome, 758.6
Renal vascular disease, 593.9	

    A. Secondary hypertension.

    B. Renal vascular disease, renal parenchymal disease.

    C. About 60–80% of secondary hypertension in childhood is due to renal causes·

    D. Coarctation of aorta (Turner's syndrome).

    E. Endocrine and adrenal causes: hyperthyroidism, Cushing's syndrome.

    F. Systemic diseases: systemic lupus erythematosus, tuberous sclerosis.

    G. Pharmacologic effect: steroids, amphetamine or sympathomimetics, oral contraceptives, illicit drugs.

    H. CNS manifestations: increased intracranial pressure, intracranial mass.

VII. Treatment

    A. Treatment is targeted to cause if secondary hypertension.

        1. Treatment goal is to achieve blood pressure <95th percentile.

    B. Nonpharmacologic treatment.

        1. Weight loss if obese; prevention of obesity if normal weight.

        2. Dietary modification.

        3. Decreasing sodium intake if excessive. Salt restriction useful in patients with sensitivity to sodium.

        4. Exercise.

        5. Frequent blood pressure monitoring.

        6. Promotion of healthy lifestyle behaviors.

        7. Tobacco cessation; avoid drugs of abuse, particularly cocaine; healthy diet; regular exercise; moderate sodium intake.

    C. Pharmacologic treatment.

        1. Diuretics.

        2. Vasodilators.

        3. Beta blockers.

        4. Angiotensin-converting enzyme (ACE) inhibitors.

        5. Calcium antagonists.

VIII. Follow-up

    A. Continued monitoring of blood pressure.

    B. Encouragement and follow up of lifestyle changes.

    C. Refer back to pediatrician or specialist if treatment goals not achieved with lifestyle changes, current medication regime.

IX. Complications

    A. End-organ dysfunction.

B. No good long-term follow-up studies for essential hypertension in children, but seems to be precursor for adult essential hypertension.

C. Extrapolated to same morbidity/mortality of adult essential hypertension over time.

X. Education

A. Essential hypertension.

1. Chronicity of disease, likely long-term morbidity, end-organ damage if not controlled.
2. Potential improvements with dietary, lifestyle changes and medications if necessary.
3. Need for continuous follow-up.
4. Adherence to medication regime if prescribed.
5. Encourage patients to return to prescriber if side effects unacceptable because many classes of medications are available for blood pressure control.
6. Goals of therapy.

B. Suspected or known secondary hypertension.

1. Thorough evaluation of cause, may be extensive testing.
2. Follow up with specialists.
3. Adherence to treatment or medication regimen.

INNOCENT HEART MURMURS

Bruit, 785.9	Peripheral pulmonary arterial stenosis
Chromosomal abnormality, 758.89	murmur, 747.3
Clubbing of digits, 781.5	Pulmonary flow murmur, 424.3
Cyanosis, 782.5	Shock, 785.50
Diaphoresis, 780.8	Splenomegaly, 789.2
Easily fatigued, 780.79	Still's murmur, 782.2
Edema, 376.33	Tachycardia, 785.0
Hepatomegaly, 789.1	Tachypnea, 786.09
Hypotension, 458.9	Weak pulses, 785.9
Innocent heart murmurs, 785.2	

I. Etiology

A. Innocent murmur is abnormal heart sound caused by turbulent blood flow not associated with structural heart disease, also called functional or nonorganic murmur.

II. Occurrence

A. Cardiac murmurs are noted in 50–70% of children who are asymptomatic.

B. Vast majority of murmurs heard in infants and children are innocent in nature.

III. Clinical manifestations

A. Innocent murmur is typically found on routine physical exam.

B. Presence of other clinical manifestations: concern for congenital, acquired heart disease.

C. Any murmur, innocent or organic, is typically louder with fever, anemia, other high cardiac output states.

IV. Physical findings

A. Absence of physical findings other than murmur should be expected if innocent murmur is suspected. Innocent murmurs often more prominent during high cardiac output states such as fever, anemia, pregnancy.

B. Physical exam findings of congenital or acquired heart disease as below should specifically be evaluated.

1. Known or suspected syndrome or genetic or chromosomal abnormality.
2. Failure to grow.
3. Easily fatigued.
4. Tachypnea, increased work of breathing, retractions, flaring, grunting.
5. Diaphoresis particularly with exertion, feeding in the infant.
6. Cyanosis, central or peripheral.
7. Clubbing of digits.
8. Tachycardia.
9. Edema, particularly periorbital and facial in infant.
10. Active precordium.
11. Palpable thrill.
12. Weak pulses, delayed capillary refill, hypotension, or other signs of shock.
13. Differential between upper and lower extremity pulses or blood pressures.
14. Hepatomegaly or splenomegaly.
15. Murmur of grade IV (Box 25-1) or higher in intensity.
16. Diastolic murmur.

C. Careful consideration as to murmur description.

1. Location.
   a. Where murmur is heard best, described by location over cardiac structures or location on chest.
   b. Most common areas to auscultate innocent murmurs are left upper sternal border and left lower sternal border.
2. Radiation.
   a. Descriptor of where else murmur can be heard.
   b. Innocent murmurs rarely radiate to distant parts of chest.
3. Timing: where in the cardiac cycle the murmur is heard.
   a. Systole: between S_1 and S_2.

BOX 25-1 • Grading of Cardiac Murmurs

Grade I/VI: soft, difficult to hear unless room quiet and child cooperative.
Grade II/VI: soft but heard immediately.
Grade III/VI: easily heard, moderately loud, no thrill associated.
Grade IV/VI: loud, can palpate the thrill of turbulent flow on chest wall.
Grade V/VI: loud, has thrill, able to hear murmur with stethoscope barely off chest wall.
Grade VI/VI: loud, has thrill, able to hear murmur with stethoscope off chest wall.

---

   b. Diastole: between S_2 and S_1.
   c. Continuous: starts in systole, continues into diastole, does not need to continue throughout cardiac cycle, but has same sound for duration of murmur.
   d. Innocent murmurs are typically systolic, venous hum is continuous murmur. Solely diastolic murmur is never innocent and should be referred.
   e. Children with innocent murmurs typically have normal first and second heart sounds (S_1 and S_2) that are audible in addition to murmur. Rapid heart rates of infants, particularly febrile infants, may make it difficult to distinguish between systole and diastole.
4. Pitch: sound frequency of murmur. Innocent murmurs typically low to medium in pitch.
5. Quality: Musical or vibratory in quality.
6. Intensity: loudness of the murmur (Box 25-1).
   a. Innocent murmurs, typically Grade I–II/VI. Often change in intensity with change in position: sitting to lying, standing to sitting. May change in intensity from one visit to the next.
   b. No clicks or extra sounds if murmur is innocent.
D. Types of innocent murmurs.
   1. Still's murmur.
      a. Most common innocent murmur in children; occurs typically in 2- to 6-year-olds.
      b. Low to medium in pitch, buzzing or vibratory in nature.
      c. Short murmur occurring in early systole.
      d. Grade I–III/VI.
      e. Loudest in supine position, diminished by standing.
      f. Heard best at left lower sternal border.
   2. Pulmonary flow murmur.
      a. Heard in children/adolescents.
      b. Harsh murmur, blowing, nonmusical.
      c. Systolic ejection murmur.
      d. Grade II–III/VI.
      e. Loudest in supine position, loudest on exhalation.
      f. Heard best in 2nd to 3rd intercostal space at left sternal border.
   3. Peripheral pulmonary arterial stenosis murmur.
      a. Heard frequently in infants and newborns.
      b. Medium in pitch.
      c. Short systolic ejection murmur.
      d. Grade I–II/VI.
      e. Often heard best in axillae and over back.
      f. Turbulence is due to relative smallness of peripheral pulmonary arteries in newborn and angulation of takeoff of right and left branch pulmonary arteries from main pulmonary artery.

4. Supraclavicular or brachiocephalic systolic murmur or bruit.
   a. Heard in children, young adults.
   b. Low to medium in pitch, harsh.
   c. Is short, systolic murmur.
   d. Grade I–III/VI.
   e. Heard best above clavicles, radiates to neck.
   f. Heard best in supine, sitting positions; changes with change in neck position.
5. Venous hum.
   a. Also known as cervical venous hum.
   b. Continuous murmur.
   c. Heard over neck, immediately below clavicles.
   d. Intensity varies, loudness varies with position, activity; best heard in sitting position.
   e. May disappear when head is turned toward side of murmur.
   f. Murmur results from turbulence of flow as large veins converge.

V. Diagnostic tests
A. When murmur is detected, refer to pediatrician or cardiologist to determine significance.
B. Many innocent murmurs do not require further diagnostic tests after thorough history, physical, auscultatory exam.
C. CXR, electrocardiogram, cardiac echocardiography may determine whether murmur is truly innocent.
D. Murmurs associated with structural abnormalities (organic murmurs) may require additional diagnostic evaluation.

VI. Differential diagnosis

Cardiomyopathy, 425.4	Kawasaki disease, 446.1
Congenital heart disease, 746.9	Rheumatic heart disease, 398.90
Cyanotic or acyanotic disease, 782.5	

A. Congenital heart disease.
B. Cyanotic or acyanotic disease.
C. Acquired heart disease.
D. Cardiomyopathy.
E. Kawasaki disease.
F. Rheumatic heart disease.

VII. Treatment
A. Innocent heart murmurs have no organic cause, no structural abnormality, therefore, no treatment required.
B. Education of patient, family is most important treatment modality.

VIII. Follow-up
A. If innocent murmur confirmed, patients may return to usual health maintenance schedule for follow-up visits.
B. If innocent murmur suspected, should return for reevaluation to physician.

IX. Complications
A. None, since no abnormality is present.

X. Education
A. Crucial for patient, family.
B. Explain murmur as noise.
C. Noise is result of blood flow, not structural problem.
D. No heart disease or abnormality is present.
E. Murmur may change or disappear with time but if persists still no problem with heart.
F. No activity restrictions required.
G. No treatment required.

KAWASAKI DISEASE

Abdominal pain, 789.00	Increased liver enzymes, 794.8
Bilateral conjunctivitis, 372.30	Irritability, 799.2
Cardiomegaly, 429.3	Jaundice, 782.4
Cervical lymphadenopathy, 785.6	Joint pain, 719.40
Coronary artery aneurysms, 414.11	Kawasaki disease, 446.1
Cough, 786.2	Murmur, gallop, 427.89
Diarrhea, 787.91	Peripheral arterial aneurysms, 442.89
Distention of gallbladder, 575.8	Polymorphous exanthem, 782.1
ECG changes, 794.31	Proteinuria, 791.0
Elevated white blood cell count, 288.8	Reye's syndrome, 331.81
Erythema, unspecified, 695.9	Rhinorrhea, 478.1
Erythematous rash, 782.1	Seizure, 780.39
Fever, 780.6	Strawberry tongue, 529.3
Hypoalbuminemia, 273.8	Systemic vasculitis, acute, 447.6
Ileus, 560.1	Vomiting, 787.03

I. Etiology
A. Syndrome of acute systemic vasculitis of unknown origin.
B. Affects mostly small- to medium-sized arteries, particularly coronary arteries.
C. Likely of infectious origin or infection-triggered immune disorder.

II. Occurrence
A. Most prominent in Japan.
B. Children of Asian descent more susceptible than Caucasians.
C. 50% of cases in <2-year-olds, 80% of cases in <5-year-olds. Peak incidence at 1 year. Rare after 10 years of age.
D. Boys 1.5 times > girls.
E. 1–2% of siblings affected.
F. Recurrence rate: 1–3%.

III. Clinical manifestations
A. Vasculitis of small- to medium-sized arteries, especially coronary arteries. May progress to aneurysm formation in coronary arteries; can lead to thrombosis or scarring, increased risk for myocardial infarction.

IV. Physical findings
A. Fever.
B. Reddened, edematous, indurated palms/soles progressing to desquamation. May be unwilling to walk/use hands to grasp objects.
C. Erythematous rash. Most prominent on trunk, groin.
D. Bilateral conjunctival injection. Particularly bulbar conjunctiva.
E. Red or peeling lips, strawberry tongue, injected oral, pharyngeal mucosa.
F. Cervical lymphadenopathy.
G. Irritability: particularly in infants.
H. Evidence of vasculitis in other systems.
   1. Cardiovascular: murmur, gallop, ECG changes, cardiomegaly, peripheral arterial aneurysms.
   2. Gastrointestinal: diarrhea, vomiting, abdominal pain, ileus, jaundice, increased liver enzymes, distention of gallbladder.
   3. Hematologic: elevated WBC count, elevated platelet count.
   4. Renal: proteinuria, hypoalbuminemia.
   5. Respiratory: cough, rhinorrhea.
   6. Joint: pain, swelling.
   7. CNS: pleocytosis of cerebral spinal fluid (CSF), seizure.

V. Diagnostic tests
A. No specific laboratory test to confirm diagnosis.
B. Diagnostic criteria to establish diagnosis.
C. Fever of >5 days *and* 4 of the following 5 criteria:
   1. Erythematous, edematous, indurated palms/soles progressing to desquamation later in course.
   2. Polymorphous exanthem.
   3. Bilateral conjunctival injection.
   4. Red or peeling lips, strawberry tongue, injected oral, pharyngeal mucosa.
   5. Cervical lymphadenopathy.
   6. *OR* Fever of >5 days, 3 of the above 5 criteria, and coronary aneurysms documented by echocardiography or cardiac angiography.
D. Additional criteria for all of above is no other explanation for current illness.

VI. Differential diagnosis

Hypersensitivity reactions, 995.2	Stevens-Johnson pharyngitis, 695.1
Juvenile rheumatoid arthritis, 714.30	Streptococcal, 041.00
Measles, 055.9	Systemic lupus
Polyarteritis nodosa, 716.59	erythematosus, 710.0
Rheumatic fever, 390	Toxic shock syndrome, 040.82
Staphylococcus aureus, 041.11	Viral exanthems, 057.9

A. Infectious illnesses, particularly streptococcal and staphylococcal infections.
B. Drug reactions or hypersensitivity reactions.
C. Stevens-Johnson syndrome: erythema, swelling, peeling all advance beyond hands, feet.
D. Other vasculitic diseases.
E. Polyarteritis nodosa, systemic lupus erythematosus.
F. Juvenile rheumatoid arthritis: smaller joints, morning stiffness, fingers involved, joint deformities.
G. Rheumatic fever: positive antistreptococcal antibody.
H. Viral exanthems: do not meet all criteria for Kawasaki disease.
I. Measles: rash more prominent on face and neck.
J. Toxic shock syndrome: sandpaper rash, more toxic-appearing child, often hypotension with evidence of shock.

VII. Treatment
A. Referral to pediatrician and specialist.
B. Hospitalization.
C. Aspirin.
1. Used for antipyretic, antiinflammatory, and antiplatelet effects.
2. Duration is minimum of 6–8 weeks or until coronary artery abnormalities are resolved.
D. IV immunoglobulin.
1. Thought to be protective for development of coronary artery aneurysms.

VIII. Follow-up
A. Pediatric cardiology for echocardiographic evaluation of coronary artery aneurysms. Aneurysms may not develop until after acute stage of illness.

IX. Complications

Congestive heart failure, 428.0	Myocarditis, 429.0
Coronary artery aneurysms, 414.11	Pericardial effusion, 423.9
Coronary artery thrombosis, 410.9	Pericarditis, 423.9
Intrahepatic vasculitis, 447.6	Valvular heart disease, 424.0

A. Coronary artery aneurysms: develop in <20% of individuals, fewer if treated with immunoglobulin.
B. If coronary artery aneurysms develop, increased risk of coronary artery thrombosis, stenosis and resultant myocardial infarction.
C. May also develop valvular heart disease; mitral valve is affected more frequently than aortic valve.
D. Pericarditis, myocarditis, pericardial effusion, congestive heart failure may occur.
E. Can have development of vascular aneurysms elsewhere in body.
F. Can have liver dysfunction from intrahepatic vasculitis.

X. Education
A. Serious nature of illness.
B. Importance of specialty care and follow-up.

   C. Possibility of complications after initial phase of illness.

   D. Importance of adherence to prescribed medication: aspirin.

   E. Importance of not using aspirin to treat fever in other childhood illnesses: association with Reye's syndrome.

   F. Consider influenza vaccine due to association of Reye's syndrome with flulike illnesses and aspirin.

RHEUMATIC FEVER

Arthralgia, 719.4	Pericarditis, 423.9
Cardiomegaly, 429.3	Polyarthritis, 716.59
Carditis, 429.89	Pulmonary edema, 514.
Chorea, 333.5	Rash, 782.1
Congestive heart failure, 428.0	Rheumatic fever, 390.
Diffuse vasculitis, 447.6	Rheumatic heart disease, acute, 391.9
Erythema marginatum, 695.0	Streptococcal pharyngitis, 034.0
Erythrocyte sedimentation rate, 790.1	Subacute bacterial endocarditis, 421.0
Fever, 780.6	Subcutaneous nodules, 782.2
Group A streptococcal pharyngitis, 041.01	Tachycardia, 785.0
Migratory polyarthritis, 390.	Valvular disease, 424.9
Myocarditis, 429.0	White blood cell count, 288.9

  I. Etiology

   A. Complication of Group A beta-hemolytic streptococcal (GABHS) pharyngitis.

   B. Thought to be unique host factors that make certain individuals more susceptible to rheumatic fever after GABHS pharyngitis.

   C. Rheumatic fever is classified as collagen vascular disease or connective tissue disease resulting in diffuse vasculitis.

  II. Occurrence

   A. Most common in underdeveloped countries but resurgence in US.

   B. Occurs in 2–3% of patients with untreated GABHS.

   C. Rheumatic fever is rare in infants, toddlers. Most cases >5 years of age.

  III. Clinical manifestations

   A. Inflammation of joints and heart.

   B. Rarely, inflammation of brain and skin.

  IV. Physical findings

   A. Migratory polyarthritis.

     1. Occurs in 75% of initial episodes, 50% of recurrent episodes.

     2. Arthritis is typically of larger joints (knees, elbows, wrists, ankles).

     3. Each joint typically affected for <1 week, often overlap so that more than 1 joint is affected at a time.

     4. Joints are painful to touch, red, swollen; painful with movement.

   B. Carditis.

     1. Up to 50% of patients with rheumatic fever have evidence of carditis.

     2. May manifest as myocarditis with poor function, valvular disease with audible murmur, pericarditis with friction rub, or as general symptoms of tachycardia, cardiomegaly, pulmonary edema or symptoms of congestive heart failure.

C. Subcutaneous nodule.

    1. Small, hard nodules typically found on elbows, knees, wrists; also felt in occipital area, over vertebrae. Relatively rare finding in rheumatic fever.

D. Chorea.

    1. Finding of abnormal, involuntary writhing, purposeless movements that extinguish with sleep.

    2. Patients often have uncontrollable facial grimacing.

    3. Often preceding emotional lability thought to be from CNS involvement.

    4. Chorea is often late sign with latent period of 1–6 months.

E. Rash.

    1. Erythema marginatum: typical rash of rheumatic fever; painless, does not itch. Spreads peripherally while central clearing, most common on trunk, limbs; face is usually spared.

F. Low-grade fever.

G. Painful joints without obvious joint inflammation.

V. Diagnostic tests

A. Evidence of previous GABHS.

B. Modified Jones criteria to make diagnosis.

    1. Major criteria.

        a. Carditis.

        b. Polyarthritis.

        c. Chorea.

        d. Erythema marginatum.

        e. Subcutaneous nodules.

    2. Minor criteria.

        a. Arthralgia.

        b. Fever.

        c. Elevated acute-phase reactants (erythrocyte sedimentation rate, C-reactive protein, WBC count).

        d. Prolonged PR interval.

    3. Diagnosis requires 2 major criteria, or 1 major and 2 minor criteria, *and* evidence of previous GABHS infection.

    4. Electrocardiogram and echocardiogram for confirmed diagnoses.

VI. Differential diagnosis

Congenital heart disease, 746.9	Kawasaki disease, 446.1
Infective carditis, 429.89	Myocarditis, 429.0
Juvenile rheumatoid arthritis, 714.30	

A. Juvenile rheumatoid arthritis: small joints involved, swelling and deformities of joints, morning stiffness, no positive antistreptococcal antibody.

B. Kawasaki disease.

C. Congenital heart disease: murmur without associated symptoms of rheumatic fever.

D. Infective carditis or myocarditis: positive viral or bacterial cultures.

VII. Treatment

A. Prevention: appropriate diagnosis and treatment of streptococcal pharyngitis.

B. Referral to pediatrician or specialist if diagnosis suspected.

C. Antibiotics to eradicate streptococcal infection (primary prevention) (Table 25-1).

D. Bed rest until fever, symptoms resolve. With carditis, bed rest may be indicated for longer period of time.

E. Aspirin.
   1. If no relief in arthritis with initiation of aspirin therapy, question diagnosis.
   2. 80–100 mg/kg/day in 4 divided doses. Once fever resolves, decrease dose to 3–5 mg/kg/day in single dose, continue for 6–8 weeks or until acute-phase reactants return to baseline. With coronary artery aneurysms, continue therapy until coronary arteries return to normal.
   3. Check salicylate level and liver enzymes weekly while on high-dose therapy. Goal salicylate level is 20–30 mg/dL.
   4. Check liver enzymes weekly.
   5. Steroids may be considered if no response to aspirin therapy.

F. Secondary prevention (Table 25-1).
   1. To prevent recurrence of rheumatic fever in susceptible individuals.
   2. Antibiotics until 21 years of age and minimum of 5 years if no cardiac involvement.
   3. Antibiotics until 40 years of age and minimum of 10 years if cardiac involvement.
   4. Lifelong antibiotic prophylaxis if persistence of valve abnormalities.

VIII. Follow-up

A. With specialist.

B. Subacute bacterial endocarditis (SBE) prophylaxis if valve involvement.

IX. Complications

Valvular heart disease, 424.9

A. Cardiac involvement.
   1. Valvular heart disease.

B. Recurrence.
   1. Increased risk of recurrence in susceptible hosts.
   2. Cardiac damage is cumulative with each recurrence.

X. Education

A. Nature of disease.

B. Recurrence risk.

C. Prompt diagnosis and treatment of Group A streptococcal pharyngitis.

D. Cumulative nature of cardiac damage with repeat episodes.

TABLE 25-1 • Primary and secondary antibiotic prophylaxis for rheumatic heart disease

Antibiotic	Dose	Route	Duration
Primary Prevention			
Benzathine penicillin G	Infants, children: 25,000–50,000 units/kg Max dose: 1.2 million units/dose	IM	Once
Penicillin V	Children: 250 mg 2–3 times/day Adolescents, adults: 500 mg 2–3 times/day	Orally	10 days
Erythromycin (if penicillin allergy)	20–40 mg/kg/day in 2–4 divided doses	Orally	10 days
Secondary Prevention			
Benzathine penicillin G	Children: 25,000–50,000 units/kg every 3–4 weeks	IM	See text
Penicillin V	Children, adults: 250 mg twice a day	Orally	See text
Erythromycin (if penicillin allergy)	250 mg twice a day	Orally	See text

From Oritz EE: Acute rheumatic fever. In Anderson R, et al, editors: *Paediatric cardiology,* ed 2, New York, 2002, Churchill Livingstone; and Takemoto CK, Hodding JH, Kraus DM: *Pediatric dosage handbook,* ed 9, Hudson, OH, 2002, Lexi-Comp.

    E. Long-term antibiotic prophylaxis.
    F. Secondary prevention.
    G. Importance of continued pediatric subspecialty follow-up.
    H. SBE prophylaxis if indicated.

BIBLIOGRAPHY

Flynn, JT: Recognizing and managing the hypertensive child, *Contemp Pediatr* 20(8):38-60, August 2003.

Danford DA, McNamara DG: Innocent murmurs and heart sounds. In Garson A, et al, editors: *The science and practice of pediatric cardiology,* ed 2, Baltimore, 1998, Williams & Wilkins.

Kato, H: Kawasaki disease. In Moller JH, Hoffman JIE, editors: *Pediatric cardiovascular medicine,* New York, 2000, Churchill Livingstone.

Lam JC, Tobias JD: Follow-up survey of children and adolescents with chest pain, *South Med J* 94(9):921-4, September 2001.

National High Blood Pressure Education Program Working Group on Hypertension Control in Children and Adolescents: Update on the 1987 task force report on high blood pressure in children and adolescents: a working group report from the national high blood pressure education program, *Pediatrics* 98(4):649-658, October 1996.

Oritz EE: Acute rheumatic fever. In Anderson R, et al, editors: *Paediatric cardiology,* ed 2, New York, 2002, Churchill Livingstone.

Takemoto CK, Hodding JH, Kraus DM: *Pediatric dosage handbook,* ed 9, Hudson, OH, 2002, Lexi-Comp.

CHAPTER 26

Gastrointestinal Disorders

ROBIN SHANNON

ABDOMINAL PAIN, ACUTE

Abdominal pain, acute, 789.00	Mittelschmerz, 625.2
Appendicitis, 541.	Ovarian cyst, 620.2
Cholelithiasis, 574.2	Pancreatitis, 577.0
Colic, 789.0	Pharyngitis, 462.
Constipation, 564.00	Pelvic inflammatory disease (PID), 614.9
Dysmenorrhea, 625.3	Pneumonia, 486.
Ectopic pregnancy, 633.90	Testicular torsion, 608.2
Incarcerated hernia, 552.9	Urinary tract infection, 599.0
Intussusception, 560.0	Viral gastroenteritis, 008.8

Pain located in abdomen of <2 weeks' duration. Symptom can originate from within or outside gastrointestinal (GI) tract.

I. Etiology
   A. Pain from visceral (stomach, intestine), parietal (peritoneum), or referred areas.
   B. Frequently caused by viral gastroenteritis, urinary tract infection (UTI), constipation.
   C. Other possible causes vary by age:
      1. Infant: colic, intussusception, incarcerated hernia, testicular torsion.
      2. Preschool: appendicitis, intussusception, pneumonia, pharyngitis, trauma.
      3. School age: appendicitis, pneumonia, pharyngitis, pancreatitis, trauma.
      4. Adolescent: appendicitis, pancreatitis, cholelithiasis. Female: mittelschmerz, pelvic inflammatory disease (PID), dysmenorrhea, ectopic pregnancy, ovarian cyst.

II. Occurrence
   A. Gastroenteritis, appendicitis are most common causes.

III. Clinical manifestations
   A. Must take child's age, developmental level into consideration regarding location, duration of pain. Younger children often indicate periumbilical region.

    B. Associated symptoms: fever, vomiting, diarrhea, cough, anorexia depending on etiology.

    C. Important subjective data should include:

        1. Location, duration, frequency of pain.

        2. Stool frequency, consistency; history of hematochezia or melena.

        3. Vomiting: frequency, presence of bile or hematemesis.

        4. Symptoms outside GI tract (cough, congestion, dysuria, sore throat, fever).

        5. Medication and diet history.

        6. Sexual activity, vaginal discharge.

        7. Alleviating and aggravating factors.

IV. Physical findings

    A. Weight, temperature, vital signs.

    B. General appearance: assess degree of discomfort and hydration.

    C. Complete physical exam with attention to following:

        1. Abdominal exam: ask child to indicate location of pain. Observe for peristaltic waves, distention, guarding. Palpate for masses, stool, hepatosplenomegaly, tenderness. Percuss for rebound tenderness. Have child stand, jump to assess for signs of peritoneal irritation.

        2. Rectal exam: Assess for fissures, erythema.

V. Diagnostic tests

    A. May include CBC, comprehensive metabolic panel, amylase, lipase, and urinalysis. Consider pregnancy test in postmenarchal girls.

    B. Test stool for occult blood if history dictates.

    C. Chest x-ray (CXR) if pneumonia suspected.

    D. Abdominal x-ray if intestinal obstruction or perforation suspected. Useful to rule out fecal impaction.

    E. Abdominal ultrasound if appendicitis, ovarian cyst, ectopic pregnancy suspected.

VI. Differential diagnosis

Appendicitis, 541.
Cholelithiasis, 574.2
Pancreatitis, 577.0

    A. Appendicitis.

        1. Vague periumbilical pain, localized to right lower/middle quadrant.

        2. Often associated with fever, vomiting; may see elevated WBC count.

        3. Guarding, rebound, signs of peritoneal irritation on abdominal exam.

    B. Constipation, gastroenteritis, intussusception, incarcerated hernia, colic, peptic ulcer.

    C. Pancreatitis.

        1. Inflammation of pancreas from infection, medications, trauma, genetic defect, or structural abnormality.

        2. Epigastric pain often with nausea, vomiting.

        3. Elevated amylase, lipase.

   D. Cholelithiasis.
   1. Epigastric or right upper quadrant pain, often radiates to back.
   2. Ultrasound shows stones in gallbladder or bile duct.
VII. Treatment
   A. Appendicitis, cholelithiasis: surgical consult.
   B. Pancreatitis: possible hospital admission for IV hydration, pain control.
   C. Intussusception: admission for diagnosis and barium enema incarcerated hernia: admission for surgery.
VIII. Follow-up
   A. Telephone contact for any changes/increase in symptoms.
   B. Ensure follow-through with any consults that have been requested.
 IX. Complications
   A. School absence.
  X. Education
   A. Reassure if physical exam consistent with nonsurgical abdomen. Parents most often concerned about appendicitis.
   B. Review hydration/nutrition needs.
   C. Treat fever as needed.
   D. Monitor for any changes in symptoms or worrisome signs such as hematochezia, hematemesis, increased or newly localized pain.
   E. Education otherwise depends on final diagnosis.

ABDOMINAL PAIN, RECURRENT ABDOMINAL PAIN SYNDROME (RAP)

Recurrent abdominal pain syndrome (RAP), **789.0**

At least 12 weeks of continuous/intermittent abdominal pain in school-age child or adolescent with little/no occasional relationship of pain to physiologic events. Pain is not fabricated. Child otherwise well with normal growth and development. Commonly interrupts normal activities.
   I. Etiology
   A. Considered to be functional disorder: defined as absence of specific structural, infectious, inflammatory, or biochemical abnormalities as cause of pain.
   B. No longer thought to be caused by psychologic stressors. However, coping skills may be different in patients with RAP. Stress may effect pain experience, perpetuate symptoms.
   C. May be greater likelihood of anxiety, somatization in parents of children with RAP.
  II. Occurrence
   A. Equal incidence among males and females until age 10 years; then female-to-male ratio is 1.5:1.0.
 III. Clinical manifestations
   A. Periumbilical abdominal pain lasts from <1 hour to 3 hours.

    B. Occurs daily or intermittently over at least 12-week period.

    C. May be associated with nausea, fatigue, headache, pallor.

    D. Patient may assume fetal position, grimace/cry during episode.

    E. Pain does not wake child from sleep.

    F. Patient may have school absence, withdraw from social/extracurricular activities.

    G. No weight loss or growth delay.

    H. Not associated with fever, vomiting, melena, or hematochezia.

    I. Important subjective data to obtain:

        1. Description of normal elimination pattern; alleviating or aggravating factors.

        2. Dietary history, medications.

        3. Psychosocial stressors, parent/caregiver usual reaction to the pain.

IV. Physical findings

    A. Weight/height: plot on growth curve and compare with previous.

    B. Perform thorough physical exam at first visit with attention to following:

        1. Abdominal exam: ask patient to indicate location of pain. Assess for tenderness, masses, hepatosplenomegaly.

        2. Rectal exam: inspect for erythema, fissures, skin tags. Perform digital exam.

    C. Tanner staging.

V. Diagnostic tests

    A. No diagnostic test to make diagnosis of RAP.

    B. Screening laboratories to obtain:

        1. Urinalysis, urine culture.

        2. Complete blood count, erythrocyte sedimentation rate (ESR), comprehensive metabolic panel, amylase, lipase.

        3. Stool for occult blood, ova and parasite, giardia antigen.

        4. Consider lactose breath hydrogen test to rule out lactose intolerance.

VI. Differential diagnosis

Abdominal tenderness, 789.6	Lactose intolerance, 271.3
Constipation, 564.00	Melena hematochezia, 578.1
Crohn's disease, 555.9	Rectal skin tags, 455.9
Diarrhea, 787.31.	Ulcerative colitis, 556.9
Inflammatory bowel disease, 569.9	Upper respiratory infection, 465.9
Intestinal parasite, 129.	Weight loss, 783.21
Irritable bowel syndrome (IBS), 564.1	

    A. Irritable bowel syndrome (IBS).

    B. Infection: UTI, intestinal parasite.

    C. Lactose intolerance: positive lactose breath test or okay after no lactose in diet.

    D. Constipation.

    E. Inflammatory bowel disease (Crohn's disease, ulcerative colitis): associated with melena, hematochezia, and/or diarrhea. Possible weight loss, growth delay. Physical exam may reveal abdominal tenderness, multiple anal fissures/skin tags, possible joint symptoms. Refer to pediatric gastroenterologist.

VII. Treatment
A. Most valuable treatment is establishment of strong relationship with family and patient. Discuss possibility of RAP at first visit.
B. Can do trial of lactose-reduced diet. Eliminate caffeine.
C. Trial of fiber supplementation: may regulate intestinal motility. AAP recommends: child's age + 5 = grams of fiber/day.
D. Counseling: relaxation therapy, biofeedback.

VIII. Follow-up
A. Arrange for clinic visit about 1 month after diagnosis of RAP.
B. Telephone contact for any changes in symptoms.

IX. Complications
A. School absence or avoidance, decreased participation in extracurricular activities.
B. Interference with peer relationships.

X. Education
A. If physical exam normal, reassure family that is it unlikely any specific cause will be found.
B. Acknowledge pain is real, not fabricated.
C. Insist on return to normal, daily activities, school participation.
D. Educate family about reaction to the pain: may be altered reaction to pain or secondary gain if too much attention is given to symptom.
E. Discuss prognosis: pain may persist for months or years.

COLIC

Colic, 789.0

Often defined by "rule of 3": crying for >3 hours a day on >3 days a week for >3 weeks during first 3 months of life in otherwise healthy infant.

I. Etiology
A. Unknown, probably multifactorial.

II. Occurrence
A. Most studies estimate incidence rates of 10–20% of infants. Equal incidence among males and females, all socioeconomic levels, breastfed versus bottle-fed.

III. Clinical manifestations
A. Inconsolable crying for 3–6 hours per day, clustering in afternoon or evening.
B. Associated symptoms may include pain facies/grimacing, clenched fists, taut/distended abdomen, drawing legs up to abdomen, flatus.
C. Crying often described as intense.
D. Ask parents to describe quality, frequency, duration, timing of crying.
E. Ask about any other symptoms such as vomiting, regurgitation.
F. Detailed diet history, including mother if breastfeeding.
G. Frequency, consistency of stool, hematochezia.
H. Alleviating or aggravating factors.

    I. Medications given to baby or that breastfeeding mother is taking.

    J. Ask about coping skills of caregivers and opportunity for respite.

IV. Physical findings

    A. Weight/length/head circumference, temperature, vital signs.

    B. Complete physical exam.

    C. Abdominal exam may reveal mild distention.

    D. Check baby for evidence of incarcerated hernia, testicular torsion, hair tourniquet.

    E. Observe caregiver and infant: assess caregiver's anxiety, coping skills.

V. Diagnostic tests

    A. No test to diagnosis colic: made by history and physical exam.

VI. Differential diagnosis

Constipation, 564.00	Milk protein intolerance, 578.8
Gastroesophageal reflux, 530.81	Parental stress, 308.9
Inappropriate feeding, 783.3	Testicular torsion, 608.2
Incarcerated hernia, 552.9	

    A. Inappropriate feeding: assess infant's intake by history.

    B. Milk protein intolerance or allergy: usually associated with vomiting/diarrhea. May have history of hematochezia.

    C. Constipation: hard or dry stools regardless of frequency.

    D. Incarcerated hernia.

    E. Parental stress tension, poor coping.

    F. Testicular torsion: testis tender, cord thickened/shortened.

    G. Gastroesophageal reflux (GER).

VII. Treatment

    A. Consider 2-week trial of hypoallergenic formula.

    B. Encourage continued breastfeeding; eliminate caffeine from mother's diet.

    C. Swaddling of infant, rhythmic movement, gentle massage, warm baths.

    D. "White noise" such as soft music.

    E. Avoid overstimulation.

    F. Counsel parents: alleviate guilt about cause of colic, need for respite. Reassure them: infant is not in pain. Acknowledge importance of problem, discuss prognosis.

VIII. Follow-up

    A. Frequent clinic and/or telephone follow-up may be necessary to assess any formula changes, parental coping skills.

    B. Plan to see baby 2 weeks after initial diagnosis.

IX. Complications

    A. Poor parental coping skills.

    B. Disruption of maternal–infant relationship.

    C. Child abuse.

X. Education

    A. Discuss normal crying patterns. Infants cry more in first 3 months of life than at any other time. Crying increases at 2 weeks and usually peaks in

second month with gradual decline thereafter. Pattern of crying different in all babies.
- B. Explain that taut/distended abdomen and flatus are probably result of, not cause of, crying. Reassure them that infant not in pain.
- C. Alleviate parental guilt and discuss range of emotions may be experiencing.
- D. Stress need for respite: suggest parents leave baby with reliable caregiver for few hours. Infant may sense tension in parents if do not allow themselves break.
- E. Trial of hypoallergenic formula may be indicated, but multiple formula changes are not warranted and should be discouraged.

CONSTIPATION

Anal stenosis, 569.2	Hirschsprung's disease, 751.3
Anterior ectopic anus, 751.5	Hypercalcemia, 275.42
Change in diet, 269.9	Hypothyroidism, 244.9
Constipation, 564.00	Malnutrition, 263.9
Cow's milk protein intolerance, 579.8	Obesity, 278.00
Cystic fibrosis, 277.00	Sexual abuse, 995.53

Difficult defecation for >2 weeks; passage of hard and/or dry stools.
- **I. Etiology**
  - A. Functional: most common, no underlying pathology.
    1. Diet low in fiber/fluids; sudden change in diet (e.g., formula/breast to cow's milk).
    2. Lack of exercise, obesity.
    3. Stool withholding secondary to painful defecation ("pain-retention cycle").
    4. Family history.
  - B. Outlet dysfunction: Hirschsprung's disease, anterior ectopic anus, tethered spinal cord (secondary to occult spinal dysraphism), anal stenosis.
  - C. Metabolic: hypothyroidism, hypercalcemia.
  - D. Other: cystic fibrosis, malnutrition, sexual abuse, cow's milk protein intolerance (infants), medications (e.g., narcotics).
- **II. Occurrence**
  - A. Accounts for about 3% of visits to general pediatrics, 25% to pediatric gastroenterology.
- **III. Clinical manifestations**
  - A. Hard bowel movements (BMs), usually infrequent. May be dry, small (incomplete evacuation).
    1. Size, consistency, frequency of BMs: when did change in stool become apparent?
    2. Stool-withholding symptoms (hides for BM, crosses legs, dances around)?
    3. Blood associated with stool?
    4. Fecal soiling in underwear of previously toilet-trained child?
    5. Did child pass meconium within first 48 hours of life?
    6. What treatments have been instituted thus far?

    B. Associated symptoms: abdominal pain/distention, poor appetite, irritability.

    C. Other important questions: Diet history, any changes? Child on any medications? Child toilet trained? Any possibility of sexual abuse?

IV. Physical findings

    A. Height/weight: plot on growth curve.

    B. Complete physical exam with attention to:

        1. Abdomen: assess for fecal masses, particularly in lower quadrants. Assess for distention, tenderness.

        2. Anus: assess for placement, fissures, erythema. Digital exam to assess anal tone, quality of stool present. Observe for soiling at anal opening.

        3. Lower back: assess for tuft of hair over lumbar sacral area or deep sacral dimple above gluteal crease. Assess for deviated gluteal crease.

        4. Assess muscle tone throughout.

V. Diagnostic tests

    A. Testing not usually necessary.

    B. Abdominal flat-plate x-ray to assess fecal load if question diagnosis/to tailor disimpaction.

    D. X-ray of lumbar/sacral spine: assess for occult spinal dysraphism if abnormality on L/S spine area and/or history of lower extremity weakness. If abnormal: MRI.

    E. Labs only if red flags in history/physical exam: serum electrolytes, calcium, lead level, thyroid function (TSH, free T_4). Celiac screen and sweat test if poor growth.

    F. Unprepped barium enema: if history of delayed passage of meconium, to assess for transition zone associated with Hirschsprung's disease.

VI. Differential diagnosis

Anal stenosis, 569.2	Hirschsprung's disease, 751.3
Anterior ectopic anus, 751.5	Infant dyschezia, 564.00
Constipation, 564.00	Sexual abuse, 995.53
Cow's milk protein intolerance, 579.8	Side effect of narcotics, 564.09 ·
Encopresis, 787.6	

    A. Vast majority have functional constipation, diagnosis by history and physical exam.

    B. Infant dyschezia: at least 10 minutes of crying and straining before passage of soft stools in healthy infant <6 months of age. Reassure, self-limited.

    C. Encopresis: constipation with fecal soiling.

    D. Hirschsprung's disease: absence of ganglion nerve cells in colon to varying degrees. History usually delayed passage of meconium. May have thin caliber stools, abdominal distention, failure to thrive. No stool in rectal vault on digital exam.

    E. Structural: anterior ectopic anus, anal stenosis.

    F. Sexual abuse.

    G. Side effect of drugs such as narcotics.

H. Cow's milk protein intolerance: anal irritation/fissures, subsequent stool retention.

VII. Treatment

A. Stool softeners: most children will benefit from stool softener as first-line treatment.

1. Lactulose/sorbitol: 1 mL/kg/dose bid, maximum 30 mL bid. Must be ingested quickly. May mix in beverage.

2. MiraLax: for children >1 year of age and <5 years start with 2 teaspoons in 4 ounces of any noncarbonated beverage/day; ≥5 years can increase to 17 g (~1 heaping tablespoon) in 8 ounces beverage/day.

3. Mineral oil: never give to infants <1 year or patients at risk for aspiration (e.g., neurologically impaired). Difficult to regulate dose, start with 1–3 mL/kg/day.

4. Milk of magnesia: 1–3 mL/kg/day. Avoid in infants.

B. Laxatives/cathartics: used for disimpaction only, usually over period of 1–3 days.

1. Magnesium citrate: >1 year: 1–3 mL/kg/day.

2. Senna: 2–6 years: 2.5–7.5 mL/day; 6–12 years: 5–15 mL/day.

3. Bisacodyl: >2 years: 1–2 tablets/dose.

C. Enemas/suppositories: for disimpaction only, over 1–3 days.

1. Glycerin suppository: for children <2 years.

2. Bisacodyl suppository: >2 years: 1/2–1 suppository/day.

3. Pediatric Fleet enema: >2 years: 1–2 times/day for 1–3 days.

D. High-fiber diet.

E. Toilet training, not yet trained: delay until constipation resolved. Trained: encourage scheduled time on toilet bid following meal, for 5–10 minutes. Provide footstool.

F. Positive reinforcement for toilet sitting, successful passage of stool.

VIII. Follow-up

A. Close telephone contact after disimpaction, to monitor response to stool softeners.

B. Refer to pediatric surgery if Hirschsprung's disease/anal abnormalities concerns.

IX. Complications

Anal fissure, 565.0
Encopresis, 787.6

A. Encopresis.

B. Anal fissure (treat with stool softening agents, diet, topical cream, e.g., Anusol).

C. Delayed toilet training.

X. Education

A. Reassure family if history and physical consistent with functional constipation. Explain pain-retention cycle.

    B. Reassure that stool softeners are not habit forming and are necessary part of breaking pain-retention cycle.

    C. Parents may report child unable to have BM despite effort; explain that what appears to be straining may be child's attempt to withhold stool to avoid pain.

    D. Avoid chronic use of laxatives, enemas, suppositories.

    E. School-age children frequently avoid using bathroom at school for BM.

    F. Explain normal defecation patterns: not necessary to have BM every day; goal is passage of soft, comfortable stools in good quantities.

    G. Instruct family to call if soiling occurs or if child not responding to treatment.

DIARRHEA, ACUTE

Diarrhea, acute, 787.91

Noticeable or sudden increase in frequency, fluid content of stools; usually infectious, self-limited lasting for <2 weeks. Diarrhea is symptom, can result from disorders involving digestive, absorptive, secretory functions of intestine.

I. Etiology

    A. Infectious: intestinal.

        1. Viral: rotavirus, adenovirus, Norwalk.

        2. Bacterial: salmonella, shigella, *Clostridium difficile, Escherichia coli* 0157:H7.

        3. Parasite: giardia, cryptosporidium.

    B. Infectious: outside GI tract: may be concurrent symptom of systemic illness.

    C. Dietary, medications, toxic ingestion.

II. Occurrence

    A. Common symptom in children.

    B. Most commonly caused by infection in older infants/children.

    C. Dietary changes or indiscretions common in early infancy.

III. Clinical manifestations

    A. Increased frequency, fluid content of stools.

        1. Frequency, consistency of diarrhea?

        2. Hematochezia, melena, mucus or pus in stool?

        3. Any fecal incontinence in toilet-trained child?

        4. Anyone else in family/school or day care have diarrhea?

    B. Possible associated symptoms: abdominal pain or cramping, fever, vomiting.

    C. Systemic illness: are there signs of illness outside the GI tract?

    D. Medication history: recent antibiotics? OTC diarrhea remedies? others?

    E. Travel history.

    F. Toxic ingestions?

    G. Complete diet history: type, quantity of fluids; appetite; new/contaminated foods.

    H. Urine output.

IV. Physical findings

    A. Height, weight, temperature, vital signs.

   B. Complete physical exam with attention to following:
1. Abdomen: assess bowel sounds, tenderness, organomegaly, masses, distention.
2. Rectal: observe for stool around anus, erythema, fissures.

   C. Assess hydration: activity level, irritability; degree of thirst; degree of dehydration (Table 26-1) and signs/symptoms of dehydration (Table 26-2).

V. Diagnostic tests
   A. If patient appears nontoxic, mild/no dehydration: none; most episodes isonatremic.

   B. Moderate to severe dehydration: serum electrolytes.

   C. Test stool for occult blood (Table 26-3).

   D. When testing for *C. difficile,* ask for toxins A and B.

TABLE 26-1 • Assessment of degree of dehydration

	Mild	Moderate	Severe
Infant	5%	10%	15%
Adolescent	3%	6%	9%
Infant/young children	Thirsty, alert, possibly restless	Thirsty, restless, or lethargic	Drowsy, limp, cold, sweaty
Older child	Thirsty, alert, restless	Thirsty, usually alert	Usually apprehensive, cold, sweaty

TABLE 26-2 • Signs and symptoms of dehydration

	Mild	Moderate	Severe
Tachycardia	−	+	+
Palpable pulses	Normal	Weak	Decreased
Blood pressure	Normal	Orthostatic hypotension	Hypotension
Skin turgor	Normal	Slight decrease	Decreased
Mucous membranes	Moist	Dry	Dry
Fontanel	Normal	Normal to slightly depressed	Sunken
Urine output	Normal	Decreased	Oliguria, anuria
Tears	+	+/−	Absent

TABLE 26-3 • Diagnostic testing for diarrhea

Symptom	Stool C&S	Stool C. difficile	Stool O&P/giardia	Serum electrolytes	CBC w/diff
Well appearance	−	−	−	−	−
Toxic, 323.7	+	−	−	+	+
Blood in stool, 578.1	+	+	−	−	+
Blood in stool, history of antibiotics	+	+	−	−	+
Weight loss, 783.20	−	−	−	+	+

   E. Not usually necessary to check for parasites unless diarrhea becomes chronic.
   F. Test for rotavirus in stool if infant with moderate to severe symptoms.
   G. Stool for *E. coli* 0157:H7 is ordered separately.

VI. Differential diagnosis

Adenovirus, **008.62.**	Giardia, **007.1**
Allergic gastroenteritis, **558.3**	Norwalk, **008.63**
Antibiotic induced, **960.9**	Rotavirus, **008.61**
Bacterial, **008.5**	Salmonella, **003.9**
Clostridium difficile, **008.45**	Shigella, **004.9**
Cryptosporidium, **007.4**	Toxic ingestions, **558.2**
Diarrhea, **787.91**	Viral, **008.8**
Escherichia coli, **008.00**	

   A. Viral: most common GI infectious cause: rotavirus, adenovirus, Norwalk.
   B. Bacterial.
      1. Salmonella: food-borne. Most resolve in 5–7 days without treatment. Fever, diarrhea +/− blood, abdominal cramping for 4–7 days.
      2. Shigella: food-borne, usually during warmer months. Sudden high fever, abdominal cramps, nausea, vomiting, diarrhea with blood, mucus, pus. Usually self-limited. Dehydration common.
      3. *E. coli* 0157:H7: strain that produces toxin. Bloody diarrhea. Most common form of traveler's diarrhea, cause of most cases of hemolytic uremic syndrome (HUS).
      4. *C. difficile:* found frequently in stool of children with antibiotic-associated diarrhea and in healthy infants, role as etiologic agent in these cases controversial. In pathologic cases, diarrhea can occur within days or up to 8 weeks after antibiotic use or any drugs that alter GI flora. Watery diarrhea, +/− blood. Fecal–oral route. Common in hospitals.
   C. Parasitic.
      1. Giardia: waterborne, food-borne. Diarrhea, bloating, abdominal cramping, nausea. Temporary lactase deficiency. Often self-limited. Outbreaks can occur in day care and long-term care facilities.
      2. Cryptosporidium: mild diarrhea, usually self-limited.
   D. Dietary.
      1. Increase in fluids with high osmotic load: fruit juices, sports drinks, or any sugared beverages can cause temporary osmotic diarrhea in otherwise healthy infant/child.
      2. Introduction of new food: possible allergic response.
   E. Antibiotic induced.
   F. Toxic ingestions.
   G. Systemic illness: may have history of upper respiratory infection (URI) or other illness.

VII. Treatment
   A. Viral: self-limited, supportive care (see rehydration guidelines on p. 269).

B. Bacterial.

1. Salmonella: supportive.
2. Shigella: although can be self-limited, severity and duration of illness usually warrants antibiotic therapy: cefixime (8 mg/kg/day divided bid for 5 days) or ceftriaxone (50 mg/kg/day once a day for 5 days) oral.
3. *E. coli* 0157:H7: supportive.
4. *C. difficile:* metronidazole (30 mg/kg/day divided qid for 10 days) oral.

C. Parasite:

1. Giardia: metronidazole (15 mg/kg/day divided tid for 5 days) or nitazoxanide (Alinia) for children 1–11 years; 12–47 months: 5 mL bid for 3 days; 4–11years: 10 mL bid for 3 days, oral.
2. Cryptosporidium: supportive.

D. Rehydration.

1. Mild dehydration: oral replacement solution 50 mL/kg + replacement of stool losses (~10 mL/kg/stool) over 4 hours.
2. Moderate dehydration: oral replacement solution 100 mL/kg + replacement of stool losses over 4 hours, reassess hourly.
3. Severe dehydration: IV fluid: normal saline or lactated Ringer's beginning with bolus of 20 mL/kg over 1 hour. Transfer to tertiary care facility.
4. No dehydration: continue to feed age-appropriate diet including milk.

E. Dietary.

1. Remove possible offending/allergenic foods.
2. No fruit juice, sports drinks, other sugared beverages.
3. Feed full diet: restricting food deprives gut of nutrients needed for healing.
4. Continue to breast/formula feed, can alternate with oral replacement solution (ORS).
5. Eliminate dairy only if known *Giardia* infection or if symptoms severe.
6. With dehydrated patient: refeed age-appropriate diet as soon as rehydrated.

F. Antidiarrheal medication/bismuth: avoid; not advised for children.

VIII. Follow-up

A. Telephone: instruct parent to call and arrange for immediate clinic visit if not improving, new symptoms develop, signs of dehydration.

B. Return to clinic next day with mild-moderate dehydration.

C. Referral to MD or local ED for severe dehydration.

D. Repeat stool studies after treatment for *C. difficile,* giardia if symptoms persist.

IX. Complications

Dehydration, 276.5	Hemolytic uremic syndrome (HUS), **283.11**
Diarrhea, chronic, 787.91	Malnutrition, **263.9**
Escherichia coli, **008.00**	Shigella, **004.9**

    A. Dehydration, malnutrition.

    B. Chronic diarrhea may develop, especially if restricted diet/inappropriate fluids.

    C. Hemolytic uremic syndrome (*E. coli*), bacteremia (shigella).

X. Education

    A. Reassure: most cases viral, self-limited.

    B. Review proper hygiene, hand washing techniques, handling of soiled objects.

    C. Review dehydration signs/symptoms: instruct parent when to call.

    D. Review dietary instructions: explain restricting diet may prolong diarrhea. Appropriate beverage selection essential.

    E. Skin care: prevent diaper rash with effective barrier ointment.

ENCOPRESIS

Abdominal distention, 787.3	History of urinary tract infection, V13.00
Abdominal pain, 789.00	Poor appetite, 783.0
Encopresis, 787.6	Sexual abuse, 995.53
History of enuresis, V13.00	

Fecal incontinence in clothing usually after toilet training completed. Vast majority caused by chronic, functional constipation (retentive encopresis).

  I. Etiology

    A. Chronic, functional constipation. Stool accumulates in rectum, which subsequently leaks out through anus ("tip of iceberg"). Soiling is not volitional/intentional.

    B. Underlying pathology is rare: tethered spinal cord (secondary to occult spinal dysraphism), prior anal–rectal surgery, Hirschsprung's disease.

  II. Occurrence

    A. Stool incontinence, usually during day, of varying quantities.

    B. Soiling often has soft consistency and parents misinterpret this as diarrhea, child "can't make it to the bathroom in time."

    C. Parents commonly believe this is volitional or result of laziness.

    D. Important questions to ask:

      1. Age of toilet training, was process difficult?

      2. Frequency, consistency, size/amount of BM on toilet. Any blood? What time of day does it usually occur?

      3. Does child hide soiled clothing?

      4. How has family dealt with problem?

    E. Associated symptoms may include abdominal pain, abdominal distention, poor appetite, school avoidance.

    F. Ask about history of UTI and enuresis.

    G. Any possibility of sexual abuse?

  III. Clinical manifestations

    A. Common pediatric problem: boys affected more than girls.

  IV. Physical findings

    A. Abdomen may appear distended or full. Dull on percussion. Stool may be palpable in lower quadrants (smooth, movable mass).

    B. Anus may appear erythematous with stool around exterior. Observe for fissures. Digital exam may reveal decreased tone, copious stool in vault of varying consistency.

    C. Assess back for signs of occult spinal dysraphism: sacral dimple or hair tuft above gluteal crease, deviated gluteal crease.

    D. Assess muscle tone throughout.

V. Diagnostic tests

    A. Rarely necessary.

    B. Abdominal flat-plate x-ray can be useful to assess fecal load, tailor disimpaction.

    C. Plain x-ray of L/S spine if abnormal exam.

VI. Differential diagnosis

Constipation, 564.00	Tethered spinal cord, 724.9
Fecal incontinence, 787.6	Urinary incontinence, 788.30

    A. Majority of cases are from functional constipation.

    B. Tethered spinal cord: can result in fecal /urinary incontinence.

VII. Treatment

    A. All children with encopresis must first start with disimpaction ("cleanout"). Soiling will not resolve without this. Depending on amount of stool on x-ray exam, can give oral cathartics at bedtime for 1–3 nights in row and up to 1 Fleet enema bid for 1–3 days in row.

    B. After clean out, child immediately starts daily stool softening.

    C. Keep track of BMs, soiling episodes on calendar.

    D. High-fiber diet.

    E. Toilet retraining: child to sit on toilet after meals 2–3 times/day, work up to 5–10 minutes. Provide footstool. Ask child to "try" to have BM, to "practice," not expected to produce BM each time.

    F. Positive reinforcement only. No punishment for soiling. Soiling should be cleaned up swiftly with child's assistance and little attention paid to it.

VIII. Follow-up

    A. Encourage telephone contact. If continues to soil, may need further cleanout.

    B. Follow-up in clinic about 1 month after diagnosis.

    C. May need follow-up abdominal x-ray if results of cleanout are in doubt.

    D. Referral if patient not responding to treatment once compliance has been assured.

IX. Complications

Enuresis, 788.30
Urinary tract infection, 599.0

    A. Low self-esteem/shame.

    B. Child abuse.

    C. School avoidance.

    D. UTI (due to proximity of stool in clothing to urinary tract).

    E. Enuresis.

X. Education

   A. Stress to parents that child has not had control over soiling episodes.
   B. Relieve parental guilt over prior negative reinforcement.
   C. Explain to parent and child why soiling occurs, discuss normal defecation.
   D. Treatment will take at least 6 months. Parents are advised to be diligent about daily stool softening, toilet training during this time.
   E. Reassure about functional nature of chronic constipation.
   F. Advise parent to speak with school about problem so child will have better access to restroom at school, may need to provide written request.

GASTROESOPHAGEAL REFLUX DISEASE (GERD)

Gastroesophageal reflux, 530.81

Passage of stomach contents into esophagus. Gastroesophageal reflux (GER) is normal, physiologic process, can occur in healthy individuals. GERD refers to pathologic degree of GER, causing symptoms.

I. Etiology

   A. Infants (up to 18 months).
   1. Very common in infants, may be result of immaturity of lower esophageal sphincter (LES).
   2. Position of LES and feeding techniques may induce GER.
   3. GERD probably multifactorial.
   B. Children/adolescents.
   1. Probably multifactorial, exact cause not known.
   2. May be malfunctioning LES: inappropriate relaxation.
   3. Environmental/dietary influences may induce GER.

II. Occurrence

   A. About 50% of infants have recurrent vomiting in first 3 months, 67% of 4-month-olds, 5% of 10- to 12-month-olds.
   B. Increased incidence among premature babies, neurologically impaired children.

III. Clinical manifestations

   A. Infants: recurrent vomiting, regurgitation ("spit up"); usually effortless.
   B. Important questions to ask for affected infants:
   1. Type, quantity, frequency of feedings? How positioned during, after feeding?
   2. Quality, quantity, timing of emesis? Does baby cry/grimace with emesis?
   3. History of apnea?
   C. Children: regurgitation (reswallowed/spit up), possible vomiting, nausea, epigastric abdominal pain. Pain may be poorly localized. Can have any/all of these symptoms.
   D. Important questions to ask for affected children:
   1. Frequency, timing of symptoms including regurgitation with/without emesis.
   2. Abdominal pain: location, timing, frequency, quality.
   3. Any specific foods that provoke symptoms?
   4. Complete diet history including type and amount of beverages.
   5. Any dysphagia, food lodging, chronic throat clearing, dental decay?

E. For all age groups:
   1. History of hematemesis, melena, asthma, recurrent pneumonia, otitis media, sinusitis?
   2. Any decrease in appetite, poor weight gain, weight loss?

IV. Physical findings

A. Height, weight: plot on growth curve.
B. Full physical exam with attention to following:
   1. Abdomen: assess for tenderness, particularly over epigastrium.
   2. Rectal exam: obtain stool to test for occult blood.
   3. Mouth: assess for dental caries, enamel erosion.

V. Diagnostic tests

A. Upper GI series: only to rule out anatomic abnormalities. Not used to make diagnosis of GERD. Presence of GER on upper GI is common in all people. Must order in infants if forceful vomiting; in older children with frank vomiting, dysphagia.
B. Stool for occult blood: if positive, may indicate esophagitis.
C. Other tests by pediatric GI specialist if referral necessary (endoscopy, pH probe).

VI. Differential diagnosis

Gastritis, 535.5	Overfeeding, 783.6
Gastroesophageal reflux, 530.81	Pyloric stenosis, 537.0

A. GER: normal physiologic event. Infants with regurgitation who are otherwise well, growing normally, without pain.
B. GERD: infants who in addition to emesis have irritability during feeds, poor feeding/growth, recurrent lung problems. May be related to apnea. May have 1 or all of these symptoms. Recurrent GER symptoms in children >18 months is almost always considered pathologic (GERD).
C. Overfeeding.
D. Pyloric stenosis.
E. Gastritis.

VII. Treatment

A. Conservative management, infants: for GER, as adjunct to medical therapy in GERD:
   1. Smaller, more frequent feedings. Increase burping opportunities.
   2. Hold upright after feeds; do not place infant in car seat after feedings.
   3. Consider change to commercially available prethickened formula (Enfamil AR).
   4. Can add 1 teaspoon/ounce of cereal to bottle. Cross-cut nipple for easier flow.
   5. Elevate head of crib mattress. No extra bedding in crib. No prone positioning.
B. Conservative management, children: essential component along with medications.
   1. Smaller, more frequent meals. No skipping meals.

2. Avoid caffeine, carbonated drinks; fatty, fried foods; citrus; chocolate; peppermint.
3. Avoid, correct obesity.
4. Avoid tobacco and alcohol.
5. Elevate head of bed; no eating within 2 hours of bedtime.

C. Medical management.
1. Histamine-2 blockers (H_2 blockers): ranitidine (Zantac), famotidine (Pepcid).
2. Proton pump inhibitors (PPI): can try after 2-week trial of H_2 blockers if no response. Must give about 30 minutes before breakfast, do not skip meal.
   a. Lansoprazole (Prevacid): approved for use in children.
   b. Omeprazole (Prilosec).
   c. OTC antacids: not for long-term use. Only for temporary relief.

D. Surgery: fundoplication. Reserved for severe GERD that failed medical management.

VIII. Follow-up
A. Telephone contact after 2 weeks on H_2 blocker or proton pump inhibitor.
B. Return to clinic for increased symptoms, new symptoms.
C. Refer to pediatric GI specialist if symptoms severe/no response to initial treatments, lifestyle changes.

IX. Complications

Esophagitis, 530.10	Otitis media, 382.9
Failure to thrive, 783.41	Pneumonia, aspiration, 507.0
Nutritional deficits, 269.9	Sinusitis, 473.9

A. Esophagitis, stricture formation.
B. Failure to thrive, nutritional deficits.
C. Recurrent aspiration pneumonia.
D. May be related to recurrent otitis media, sinusitis.

X. Education
A. In otherwise healthy infant with normal growth, reassure parent: GER is common, most outgrow by first birthday.
B. Children: prognosis usually very good but unlikely to "outgrow."
C. Take medication exactly as prescribed. If helpful, medicate minimum of 2 months before discontinuing or stepping down therapy from PPI to H_2 blocker.
D. Nutritional guidance: avoid overfeeding, review all dietary restrictions/history at each visit.

HERNIA, INGUINAL

Abdominal distention, 787.3	Hernia, inguinal, 550.9
Abdominal masses, 789.3	Vomiting, 787.03
Abdominal tenderness, 789.6	

Protrusion of abdominal organ, usually bowel, into inguinal canal.

I. Etiology

A. Indirect: bowel protrudes through deep inguinal ring through inguinal canal lateral to inferior epigastric artery.

B. Direct: bowel protrudes between interior epigastric artery and edge of rectus muscle.

C. Incarcerated: hernia that cannot be returned or reduced by manipulation. Can become strangulated.

II. Occurrence

A. Most common surgical condition in children.

B. 60% are on right side.

C. Most common type is indirect (approximately 99%).

D. Approximately 50% present before 1 year of age, most seen in first 6 months.

E. Ratio of boys to girls, 4:1. Incidence approximate 10–20 in 1000 live births.

F. Higher incidence in premature babies, positive family history, cystic fibrosis, undescended testes, hypospadias, congenital dislocation of hip, and congenital abdominal wall defects.

III. Clinical manifestations

A. Bulge in inguinal region may extend to scrotum. Especially noticeable during crying/straining.

B. History of intermittent groin, labial/scrotal swelling.

C. Parents are usually first to notice.

D. Hernia reduces spontaneously when relaxed/sleeping.

E. Important questions to ask:

1. When was swelling/bulge first noticed? How often/when does it occur?

2. Does infant/child appear uncomfortable with it?

3. Any signs of intestinal obstruction such as vomiting, abdominal distention?

IV. Physical findings

A. Bulge at level of internal/external ring.

B. Scrotal/labial swelling.

C. Do not place finger in inguinal canal, done only for adult hernia exam.

D. In supine position, with legs and arms extended over head: wait for cry, which will increase intra-abdominal pressure. Should demonstrate bulge over external ring/scrotal swelling.

E. Have older children stand.

F. Palpate testes before palpation of inguinal bulge (retractile testes are common in infants and young children, can be mistaken for hernia).

G. Abdominal exam: assess for distention, masses, tenderness.

H. If swelling not apparent during exam, check for thickening of spermatic cord (silk sign) by palpating spermatic cord over pubic tubercle. Rubbing together area feels like silk.

V. Diagnostic tests

A. All girls with inguinal hernia should have rectal exam by experienced examiner; may need to order pelvic ultrasound.

B. Diagnosis otherwise made by history and physical exam.

VI. Differential diagnosis

Hernia, incarcerated inguinal, 550.1
Hydrocele, 603.9

  A. Inguinal hernia: scrotal swelling varies during day, increase in size with crying/straining.
  B. Incarcerated inguinal hernia: usually associated with discomfort, positive/negative abdominal distention. Bulge persists.
  C. Hydrocele: circumscribed fluid collection in scrotum; swelling does not change in size throughout day, gradually disappears over first year of life. Transillumination of scrotum cannot distinguish between hydrocele, inguinal hernia.

VII. Treatment
  A. Surgery: inguinal hernia does not resolve spontaneously, surgery usually elective shortly after diagnosis.
  B. Supports/trusses are not indicated, may be hazardous.

VIII. Follow-up
  A. Referral to pediatric surgeon when diagnosis of inguinal hernia made.

IX. Complications

Hernia, incarcerated inguinal, 550.1	Ischemia/infarction of testis, 608.83
Hernia, strangulated incarcerated, 552.9	Ovary/fallopian tube infarction, 620.8

  A. Incarcerated hernia: immediate referral for reduction under sedation.
  B. Strangulated incarcerated hernia: blood supply compromised: surgical emergency.
  C. Ischemia/infarction of testis: can occur in boys with undescended testicles, inguinal hernia.
  D. Ovary/fallopian tube infarction.

X. Education
  A. Uncomplicated indirect inguinal hernia: review signs, symptoms of incarcerated/strangulated hernia with family: abdominal distention, vomiting, pain, persistent bulge that does not reduce.
  B. Family understands importance of following through with surgical appointments.
  C. Operative repair necessary within first year of life due to increased incidence of incarceration after that time.

HERNIA, UMBILICAL

Abdominal distention, 787.3
Abdominal pain, 789.00
Hernia, umbilical, 553.1

Protrusion of part of intestine at umbilicus; defect is at abdominal wall, protruding bowel covered with skin, subcutaneous tissue.

I. Etiology
  A. Due to weakness/incomplete closure of umbilical ring.

II. Occurrence
A. Increased incidence among African American babies, low-birth-weight infants, females.

III. Clinical manifestations
A. Soft mass covered by skin that protrudes from umbilicus, usually with increased intra-abdominal pressure (crying/straining) or may be more persistent (ask parent about fluctuations in mass size/presence).
B. Size of defect varies from <1 cm in diameter to 5 cm.
C. Usually disappears spontaneously by 1 year of age. Larger hernias may resolve spontaneously by 5–6 years of age unless defect >2 cm.

IV. Physical findings
A. Examine infant in supine position.
B. Abdomen will reveal soft protrusion through umbilicus, usually easy to reduce through fibrous umbilical ring. Assess for abdominal distention.
C. Increase size may be visible with crying. Observe for signs of pain.

V. Diagnostic tests
A. None.

VI. Differential diagnosis

Hernia, strangulated umbilical, 552.1

A. Strangulated umbilical hernia (very rare): may show signs of intestinal obstruction such as pain, vomiting, persistent umbilical bulge that will not reduce.

VII. Treatment
A. Most resolve spontaneously.
B. Surgery reserved for hernias after 3–4 years of age, those causing symptoms (become strangulated), those becoming progressively larger after 1–2 years of age.

VIII. Follow-up
A. Assess hernia routinely at all visits. Immediate return if signs of incarceration.

IX. Complications

Incarceration umbilical hernia, 552.1

A. Incarceration: very rare.

X. Education
A. Instruct parent not to tape or bind umbilicus and on signs, symptoms of incarceration.
B. Reassure most resolve spontaneously.

INTUSSUSCEPTION

Abdominal pain, 789.0
Bilious vomiting, 787.1
Blood in stools, 578.1
Intussusception, 560.0
Lethargy, 780.79
Shock, 785.50
Vomiting, 787.03

Prolapse or "telescoping" of one part of intestine into lumen of adjoining intestine.

I. Etiology
  A. Can follow infections such as gastroenteritis, otitis media, URI, adenovirus.
  B. About 10% have "lead point" such as Meckel's diverticulum, polyp, duplication.
  C. May be alteration in intestinal peristalsis that provokes condition.

II. Occurrence
  A. Most common cause of intestinal obstruction 3 months to 6 years of age.
  B. 60% occur in children <1 year, 80% by 2 years. Rare in neonates.
  C. Incidence 1–4 in 1000 live births.
  D. Male-to-female ratio is 4:1.
  E. Peaks in spring and fall.

III. Clinical manifestations
  A. Sudden onset severe abdominal pain, usually periumbilical/lower abdomen, in previously well child.
  B. Pain colicky, paroxysmal occurring at frequent intervals.
  C. Child may appear well between episodes of pain at first.
  D. During pain, child flexes legs, pulls knees toward abdomen, cries.
  E. Vomiting common.
  F. Stools may appear normal in first few hours, after which little or no stool.
  G. Blood per rectum can occur within first 12 hours or up to 2 days after symptoms start. May be mixed with mucus described as "currant jelly stool."
  H. If symptoms unrecognized, may progress to lethargy, bilious vomiting, shock.

IV. Physical findings
  A. Weight, temperature, vital signs.
  B. Assess overall affect and activity level, observe during pain episode.
  C. Abdomen may be distended. Guarding during exam if having pain. About 70% may have palpable, ill-defined ("sausage-shaped") mass, may be mildly tender.
  D. Rectal exam may reveal bloody mucus.

V. Diagnostic tests
  A. Diagnosis usually made by history and physical exam.
  B. Barium enema: may show filling defect.
  C. Abdominal ultrasound can also detect intussusception.

VI. Differential diagnosis

Gastroenteritis, 558.9
Henoch-Schönlein purpura, 287.0
Meckel's diverticulum, 751.0

  A. Gastroenteritis.
  B. Meckel's diverticulum: painless, rectal bleeding from congenital appendage of ileum.
  C. Henoch-Schönlein purpura: associated with joint symptoms, purpura rash.

VII. Treatment
  A. Barium enema: hydrostatic/"air contrast" used to diagnose, treat intussusception.

    B. Untreated, condition almost always fatal.

    C. 10% recurrence rate after reduction by barium enema.

    D. Intussusception secondary to "lead point" from Meckel's diverticulum or polyp requires surgery.

VIII. Follow-up

    A. Immediate referral to tertiary care facility.

    B. Telephone or clinic follow-up after reduction.

IX. Complications

Dehydration, 276.5

    A. Dehydration, bowel necrosis, death.

X. Education

    A. Reassure parent that vast majority of cases have no specific lead point and are successfully treated with barium enema.

    B. Counsel family to call immediately if any signs of abdominal pain, rectal bleeding following reduction.

IRRITABLE BOWEL SYNDROME (IBS)

Abdominal distention, 787.3	Loose stools, 787.91
Abdominal pain, 789.00	Nausea, 787.02
Constipation, 564.00	Rectal fissures, 565.0
Hepatosplenomegaly, 571.8	Rectal fistula, 565.1
Irritable bowel syndrome (IBS), 564.1	Rectal skin tags, 455.9

Functional bowel disorder characterized by abdominal pain and changes in bowel function.

I. Etiology

    A. Thought to be combination of visceral hypersensitivity and possibly altered gut motility. May be due to alterations in enteric nervous system (ENS) and relationship to central nervous system (CNS).

    B. Stress/anxiety may induce/worsen symptoms but probably not root cause.

II. Occurrence

    A. Common cause of recurrent abdominal pain in older children and adolescents.

    B. About 6% of middle school students; 14% of high school students may fit criteria.

III. Clinical manifestations

    A. Abdominal pain/discomfort, usually lower abdomen or periumbilical; relieved by defecation/onset associated with change in frequency/appearance of stool.

    B. Otherwise well, without evidence of underlying structural/metabolic abnormalities.

    C. BMs may be predominantly loose, constipated, or fluctuate between the two.

    D. May pass mucus with stool.

E. Stool urgency, especially in morning; occasional feeling of incomplete defecation.
F. Abdominal bloating/distention, especially later in day.
G. Important questions to ask:
   1. Location, timing, frequency, duration, quality of pain.
   2. BM frequency, consistency, size. Straining? Mucus or blood? Stool urgency?
   3. Does BM relieve abdominal pain? Anything that helps or aggravates symptoms?
   4. Is patient on medications? Any OTC remedies?
   5. Sensation of abdominal bloating? What time of day?
H. Complete diet history including beverages. Any weight loss?
I. May have functional dyspepsia symptoms such as nausea. No vomiting.
J. Red flags in history indicating diagnosis other than IBS include growth failure, weight loss, joint symptoms, vomiting, blood in stool, fever, family history of inflammatory bowel disease (Crohn's or ulcerative colitis), dysphagia.

IV. Physical findings
A. Height, weight, temperature, vital signs.
B. Complete physical exam with attention to:
   1. Abdomen: assess for tenderness, masses, stool, hepatosplenomegaly.
   2. Rectal: assess for fissures, skin tags, fistula.

V. Diagnostic tests
A. No test to diagnose IBS.
B. Screening studies usually necessary to be sure no underlying pathology.
   1. Stool for occult blood, ova and parasite, giardia antigen.
   2. CBC, ESR.
   3. Consider lactose breath hydrogen test to rule out lactose intolerance.

VI. Differential diagnosis

Constipation, 564.	Inflammatory bowel disease, 558.9
Crohn's disease, 555.9	Recurrent abdominal pain syndrome, 789.
Gastroesophageal reflux, 530.81	Ulcerative colitis, 556.9

A. Constipation, GER.
B. Lactose intolerance: decreased lactase enzyme in small intestine causes malabsorption, subsequent diarrhea, abdominal pain, gas if excessive lactose ingested.
C. Recurrent abdominal pain syndrome.
D. Inflammatory bowel disease: Crohn's disease, ulcerative colitis: usually associated with growth delay/weight loss, anemia, diarrhea with/without blood, possibly joint pain, mouth ulcerations. Physical exam may reveal abnormal appearance to anus, abdominal tenderness.

VII. Treatment
A. High-fiber diet, consider starting fiber supplement (OTC). AAP recommends: child's age + 5 = grams of fiber/day.

B. Regular meals, avoid caffeine.

C. Ensure adequate rest and exercise.

D. Bloating/loose stools: reduce sorbitol and fructose in diet.

E. Predominantly constipation: add stool softener such as MiraLax, milk of magnesia.

F. Cognitive-behavioral therapy, such as relaxation and biofeedback.

G. Pharmacologic treatment reserved for continuing symptoms usually monitored by MD. Low-dose tricyclic antidepressants used with some success, probably due to effect on ENS. Antispasmodics used but little data at this time to support their use.

VIII. Follow-up

A. Return to clinic for any change/worsening of symptoms.

B. Refer to counselor as needed for relaxation therapy or biofeedback.

C. Refer to pediatric GI specialist if red flags or if treatment not successful.

IX. Complications

A. School absence/avoidance.

X. Education

A. Discuss IBS at first visit. Explain that although diagnosis of exclusion, real diagnosis.

B. Reassure if history consistent with IBS and physical exam and screening studies are negative further testing not necessary.

C. Discuss enteric nervous system and possible reasons for symptoms of IBS.

D. Explain importance of regular meals and exercise; both can help control symptoms.

E. Fiber supplementation may take 8 weeks to make difference.

F. Identify psychologic triggers such as family upset/school difficulties.

G. Insist on regular school attendance.

PYLORIC STENOSIS (PS)

Dehydration, 276.5	Pyloric stenosis, 537.0
Electrolyte imbalance, 276.9	Vomiting, 787.03
Peristalsis, 787.4	Weight loss, 783.21

Gastric obstruction at pylorus muscle.

I. Etiology

A. Unknown.

II. Occurrence

A. Most common form of nonbilious vomiting in infants.

B. Usually in infants after 2–3 weeks of age, up to 5 months of age.

C. About 3 per 1000 live births in US.

D. Male-to-female ratio = 4:1, especially firstborn males.

E. Caucasians > African Americans.

F. Increase incidence if mother had PS as infant (20% of her male offspring, 10% of female offspring will develop PS).

    G. Can be associated with other congenital defects (e.g., tracheoesophageal fistula).

III. Clinical manifestations

    A. Nonbilious vomiting. Vomiting progressively projectile, immediately after feeding.

    B. Can occur intermittently or with every feeding.

    C. Infant hungry after emesis.

    D. As condition worsens, increased fluid losses, electrolyte imbalance, weight loss.

IV. Physical findings

    A. Length, weight, temperature, vital signs.

    B. Assess overall hydration, activity level, signs of hunger.

    C. Abdomen: may palpate firm mass, approximately 2 cm in length, olive shaped. Usually to right of umbilicus in upper abdomen, toward midepigastrium. Easier to palpate after vomiting. Mass may not be palpable in early PS.

    D. Visible peristalsis may occur after feeding.

V. Diagnostic tests

    A. Abdominal ultrasound confirms majority of cases.

VI. Differential diagnosis

Gastroenteritis, 558.9	Inborn errors of metabolism, 277.9
Gastroesophageal reflux, 530.81	Overfeeding, 783.6

    A. GERD.

    B. Gastroenteritis.

    C. Inborn errors of metabolism.

    D. Overfeeding.

VII. Treatment

    A. Admit patient for rehydration/electrolyte management with referral to pediatric surgery (pyloromyotomy).

VIII. Follow-up

    A. Post-hospitalization office visit to ensure infant regaining weight, tolerating feeds.

    B. Follow-up with surgical team.

IX. Complications

Dehydration, 276.5
Failure to thrive, 783.41
Weight loss, 783.21

    A. Dehydration.

    B. Failure to thrive.

    C. Weight loss.

X. Education

    A. Reassure that infants do very well after surgical correction.

    B. Infant may resume normal feeding within 1–2 days postoperatively.

PEPTIC ULCER DISEASE (PUD)

Anemia, chronic iron-deficiency, 280.9	Irritability, 799.2
Family history of PUD, V12.71	Melena, 578.1
Gastrointestinal hemorrhage, 578.9	Peptic ulcer disease, 533.9
Hematemesis, 578.0	Periumbilical pain, 789.0
Hematochezia, 578.1	Vomiting, 787.03

Erosion or ulceration of gastroduodenal mucosa.

I. **Etiology**
   A. Imbalance between cytotoxic and cytoprotective factors.
      1. Cytotoxic: acid, pepsin, medications, infection.
      2. Cytoprotective: gastric mucous layer provides mechanical barrier.
   B. Primary PUD: mainly caused by *Helicobacter pylori* infection in adults.
      1. Route of transmission unknown, may be fecal–oral, acquired early in life.
      2. Can cause gastritis positive/negative peptic ulcer usually in >10 years of age.
   C. Secondary PUD: physiologic stress (burns, trauma), medications (NSAIDs, aspirin, corticosteroids), caustic ingestion (including alcohol), viral infections, Zollinger-Ellison syndrome, eosinophilic gastroenteritis (allergic inflammation), Crohn's disease.

II. **Occurrence**
   A. *H. pylori.*
      1. Increased risk for acquiring infection in developing countries, poor socioeconomic conditions, overcrowding.
      2. Possible ethnic/genetic predisposition: higher rate among Asian, African Americans, Hispanics.
      3. Less common in children, but may acquire infection in childhood that is asymptomatic until later.
      4. Among most common bacterial infections in humans.

III. **Clinical manifestations**
   A. Neonates (up to 1 month): usually presents with GI hemorrhage/perforation.
   B. Infants to 2 years: vomiting, irritability, poor growth, GI hemorrhage.
   C. Preschool: periumbilical pain, often postprandial, vomiting, GI hemorrhage.
   D. School age and older: epigastric abdominal pain that may awaken child from sleep. Acute/chronic GI blood loss (hematemesis, hematochezia, melena) may occur along with iron-deficiency anemia.
   E. Family history of PUD.
   F. Difficult to distinguish from other GI disorders such as GERD.
   G. Obtain full diet and medication history.
   H. Location, frequency, quality, duration, timing of pain. Does it wake child from sleep?
   I. Any regurgitation or vomiting? Hematemesis, coffee-grounds emesis?
   J. Frequency, consistency of stools. Any melena or hematochezia?

IV. Physical findings

A. Height, weight: plot on growth curve and compare with previous.

B. Temperature, vital signs.

C. Full physical exam with attention to following:

  1. HEENT: assess for dental caries, enamel erosion.

  2. Abdomen: assess for tenderness, masses, hepatosplenomegaly.

  3. Rectal: perform digital exam. Assess for fissures.

V. Diagnostic tests

A. Physical exam: CBC (anemia); comprehensive metabolic panel, amylase, lipase; urinalysis and urine culture.

B. Test stool for occult blood.

C. Upper GI series: to assess anatomy in child with vomiting. Little value in diagnosing ulcers or gastritis in children.

D. *H. pylori* serology: unreliable in children, not recommended.

E. Endoscopy with biopsies (test of choice) to diagnose *H. pylori* and PUD.

VI. Differential diagnosis

Crohn's disease, 555.9

Secondary peptic ulcer disease, 533.9

Helicobacter pylori infections, 041.86

A. *H. pylori* infections: reliable diagnosis in children by upper endoscopy.

B. Secondary PUD:

  1. Medication: history of NSAID, aspirin, corticosteroid use, and others.

  2. Trauma/stress PUD: history of burns, trauma, surgery.

  3. Caustic ingestion/ETOH.

  4. Crohn's disease: history may include growth problems, diarrhea, blood in stool.

VII. Treatment

A. *H. pylori:* 14 days of amoxicillin and Biaxin and at least 1 month of proton pump inhibitor (e.g., Prevacid).

B. Secondary PUD.

  1. Discontinue offending medication/caustic substance. If on corticosteroids to treat another disease, may wean or give acid-reducing medicine until therapy complete.

  2. Gastritis/PUD can be treated first with H_2 blocker (Zantac, Pepcid). If no response in 7–14 days, can increase therapy to PPI.

  3. History of upper GI bleed, melena, hematochezia requires referral to tertiary care facility/consultation of MD before therapy.

  4. Treat iron-deficiency anemia.

VIII. Follow-up

A. *H. pylori:* follow-up testing (repeat endoscopy) for patients symptomatic after treatment. Other methods can be unreliable or not approved for children.

B. Return to clinic 1 month after treatment started for nonspecific/suspected PUD.

C. Immediate return for any worsening symptoms.

IX. Complications

Anemia, chronic iron-deficiency, 280.9	Massive gastrointestinal bleed, 578.9
Gastric cancer, 151.9	Perforation, 531.6
Helicobacter pylori, 041.86	

   A. *H. pylori* (chronic colonization carries theoretical risk of developing gastric cancer).
   B. Massive GI bleed/perforation.
   C. Chronic iron-deficiency anemia.
X. Education
   A. *H. pylori* not common in children, communicability low. Increased risk among household contacts of others with this infection.
   B. Explain that because differentiating between GERD and PUD is difficult, if no response to treatment with acid-reducing medication, possible endoscopy may be necessary.
   C. Employ conservative management for symptoms, such as dietary restrictions.

PINWORMS (ENTEROBIASIS)

Perianal erythema, 695.9	Pinworms (enterobiasis), 127.4
Perianal irritation, 569.49	Sleeplessness, 780.52

I. Etiology
   A. Humans only known hosts for this obligate parasite; ingest embryonated eggs, which hatch in stomach. Larvae migrate to cecum area where mature into adult worms.
   B. Adult worms are about 1 cm in length. Females migrate by night to perianal region to deposit eggs.
   C. Ova mature after approximately 6 hours. Larvae viable for about 20 days.
   D. Eggs carried under fingernails, transmitted directly to another human or deposited in environment (dust, bed clothes) where others come in contact. Autoinfection/reinfection common; highly communicable.
II. Occurrence
   A. Highest prevalence in children 5–14 years of age.
   B. Increased incidence in crowded living conditions, among family members of infected patients, in institutions.
III. Clinical manifestations
   A. Anal pruritus, especially nocturnal (most likely from female pinworm depositing eggs).
   B. Sleeplessness.
   C. Perianal irritation/erythema may occur (most likely from scratching).
IV. Physical findings
   A. Child should appear well. Physical exam normal or nonspecific perianal irritation.

V. Diagnostic tests
   A. Cellophane tape test.
      1. Adult worms sometimes visualized in evening around anus using flashlight: white, thread-like moving worm.
      2. Essentially diagnostic, specimen rarely required.
VI. Differential diagnosis

Erythema, unspecified, **695.9**
Perianal streptococcal infection, **041.00**

   A. Perianal streptococcal infection: anal erythema, pain. No pruritus.
VII. Treatment
   A. Vermox: children >2 years, adults: 100 mg (chew, crush, swallow). Repeat in 2 weeks.
   B. Consider simultaneous treatment for household contacts (except pregnant women and children <2 years).
VIII. Follow-up
   A. As needed, not usually necessary.
   B. Consult with MD for patients <2 years.
IX. Complications

Perianal irritation, **569.49**

   A. Perianal irritation/discomfort; secondary bacterial infection from scratching.
   B. Rarely effects ectopic sites (i.e., female genital tract, appendix, peritoneal cavity, liver, spleen).
X. Education
   A. Teach parent proper technique for obtaining specimen if needed:
      1. Use only clear cellophane tape. Spread buttocks early in morning, before toileting, or at night and apply tape sticky side down to perianal area.
      2. Place tape sticky side down on clear glass slide.
      3. Teach proper precautions for handling communicable specimen.
   B. Infection highly contagious and reinfection is common.
   C. Discuss strategies to avoid reinfection.
      1. Keep fingernails very short. Frequent hand washing, especially with toileting.
      2. Wash bedclothes, underwear daily; handle with precaution. Bathe daily.
      3. Discourage child from scratching anus and from placing fingers in mouth.
   D. Infections are spread only human to human. Cannot be spread by pets.
   E. Eggs are viable in environment for several days or longer.
   F. Discuss importance of second dose of medication at 2 weeks.
   G. Reassure about benign nature of the infection.
   H. Treatment side effects include abdominal pain, diarrhea.

VIRAL GASTROENTERITIS

Abdominal cramps, 789.	Headache, 784.0
Dehydration, 276.5	Muscle aches, 729.1
Diarrhea, 787.9	Viral gastroenteritis, 008.8
Fever, 780.6	Vomiting, 787.03

Viral infection of GI tract.

I. Etiology

A. Caused by several viruses, mainly:
1. Rotavirus: highly contagious, incubation period 1–3 days. Spread by fecal–oral route. Most common viral cause.
2. Adenovirus: second most common cause, mainly children <2 years. Incubation period: 8–10 days.
3. Norwalk group: mainly older children, adults. Main cause of viral gastroenteritis epidemics. Highly contagious, fecal–oral route. From contaminated food, water, or person to person.

B. Osmotic diarrhea usually results from carbohydrate malabsorption, increased fluid/salts in intestines.

II. Occurrence

A. Rotavirus most common cause of severe, dehydrating diarrhea in infants/young children. Occurs mainly during winter months.

B. Adenovirus can occur year-round, slight increase in summer months.

C. Norwalk can occur year-round.

III. Clinical manifestations

A. Watery diarrhea most common symptom. Vomiting and fever common.

B. Rotavirus may cause severe, watery diarrhea for 5–7 days.

C. Adenovirus diarrhea may last for 1–2 weeks with/without vomiting at onset. May be associated with low-grade fever.

D. Norwalk may cause acute-onset vomiting, abdominal cramps, diarrhea for 1–2 days. Vomiting main symptom in children; can have fever, headache, muscle aches.

E. Pertinent history to obtain:
1. Onset of symptoms, sudden? Any sick contacts? Fever history?
2. Stools: consistency, frequency, quantity, history of melena/hematochezia.
3. Vomiting: frequency, quantity, quality. Contain bile or blood?
4. Abdominal pain, cramping: frequency, duration, relation to stools.
5. Complete diet and medication history.

IV. Physical findings

A. Weight, temperature, vital signs.

B. Assess hydration status and level of activity.

C. Complete physical exam with attention to abdomen (tenderness, guarding, masses) and rectal (perianal irritation, diaper rash from diarrhea).

V. Diagnostic tests

A. Not usually necessary.

B. Rotavirus/adenovirus diagnosed using commercially available kit.

C. If dehydrated: serum electrolytes.

VI. Differential diagnosis

Bacterial infection, 041.9

Giardia, 007.1

A. Parasite infection (giardia, campylobacter).

B. Bacterial infection.

VII. Treatment

A. Supportive care: prevent/correct dehydration.

VIII. Follow-up

A. Return to clinic if any increased symptoms or signs of dehydration.

IX. Complications

Dehydration, 276.5

Diaper rash, 691.0

A. Dehydration.

B. Diaper rash.

X. Education

A. Reassure family about self-limited nature of viral gastroenteritis.

B. Review signs/symptoms of dehydration with family.

C. Discuss communicability, precautions (hand washing, handling of soiled objects).

VOMITING, ACUTE

Abdominal pain, 789.00	Hematochezia, 578.1
Diarrhea, 787.91	Joint pain, 719.40
Dysuria, 788.1	Melena, 578.1
Headache, 784.0	Vomiting, acute, 787.03

Forceful expulsion of stomach contents through mouth. Highly coordinated reflex; can be symptom of disease within or outside GI tract.

I. Etiology

A. Common symptom of infection such as gastroenteritis. Can also be from infection outside GI tract such as UTI, otitis media, other systemic infections.

B. Different from regurgitation-type emesis (nonforceful), common sign of GERD.

C. Additional etiologies vary by age:

1. Infant: overfeeding, mechanical obstruction (pyloric stenosis, malrotation, volvulus), necrotizing enterocolitis, Hirschsprung's disease, intussusception, cow's milk protein allergy.

2. Child: appendicitis, sinusitis, toxic ingestions, gastritis, mechanical obstruction (foreign body, malrotation).

    3. Adolescent: appendicitis, sinusitis, toxic ingestion, inflammatory bowel disease (IBD), migraine, pregnancy, bulimia.

II. Occurrence
    A. Common pediatric symptom.
    B. Infection is one of most common medical causes of nonbilious vomiting in first year of life, usually acute gastroenteritis.

III. Clinical manifestations
    A. Usually forceful, may be preceded by nausea, increased salivation, retching.
        1. Describe vomiting and symptoms preceding it.
        2. How often is child vomiting? When did it first begin?
        3. Any bile staining or hematemesis?
        4. How soon after oral intake does vomiting occur?
    B. Ask about possible associated symptoms:
        1. Fever? How is it treated? Any headache, body aches, joint pain?
        2. Describe stools, any diarrhea? Any melena or hematochezia?
        3. Is child continuing to urinate? Any dysuria or frequency?
        4. Any URI symptoms, cough, ear, throat pain? Abdominal pain?
    C. Diet history:
        1. Type, quantity of fluids, foods.
        2. History of ingestion of contaminated food?
        3. Medications/drugs or toxic ingestion history?
        4. Exposure to others with similar symptoms?

IV. Physical findings
    A. Weight, compare with previous measurements.
    B. Temperature, vital signs.
    C. Assess level of activity, does child appear ill?
    D. Complete physical exam with attention to:
        1. Abdomen: assess for distention, guarding, tenderness, masses.
        2. Hydration status.
        3. Rectal exam: observe for any abnormalities, digital exam may be necessary to check for occult blood.
        4. CNS: assess fontanel. Assess for irritability, nuchal rigidity, Brudzinski and Kernig's signs, funduscopic exam.

V. Diagnostic tests
    A. If child appears ill, dehydrated: serum electrolytes, CBC.
    B. If bilious vomiting, consider upper GI series to rule out mechanical obstruction.
    C. Projectile vomiting in infant <5 months: abdominal ultrasound to rule out pyloric stenosis.
    D. Abdominal flat-plate x-ray: if ingested radiopaque foreign body/bezoar suspected.
    E. Urinalysis with specific gravity.
    F. Other tests to be determined by history, physical exam.

VI. Differential diagnosis

Bulimia, 783.6
Hirschsprung's disease, 751.3
Inflammatory bowel disease, 558.9
Medication overdose, 977.9
Metabolic, 277.9
Migraine, 346.9
Overfeeding, 783.6

Pneumonia, 486.
Pregnancy, 643.9
Pyloric stenosis, 537.0
Upper respiratory tract infection, 456,9
Urinary tract infection, 599.
Viral gastroenteritis, 008.8

   A. Infection: usually associated with fever/all ages: viral gastroenteritis, UTI, pneumonia, upper respiratory tract infections (otitis media, sinusitis, pharyngitis).
   B. Mechanical: pyloric stenosis, infants, malrotation/volvulus (infants, children: bilious vomiting, abdominal pain, anorexia), foreign body ingestion or bezoar (children), Hirschsprung's disease (infants: delayed passage of meconium, constipation).
   C. Metabolic: inborn errors of metabolism (infants, rare).
   D. CNS: migraine (children, adolescents: headache, photophobia, family history common), brain tumor (rare), labyrinthitis.
   E. Medication overdose, reaction, toxic ingestion (including lead).
   F. Overfeeding (infants): normal physical exam, review feeding techniques.
   G. Pregnancy: consider in postmenarchal girls.
   H. Bulimia.
   I. Inflammatory bowel disease (child, adolescent): Crohn's disease, ulcerative colitis. Hematochezia, melena, abdominal pain, diarrhea, weight loss, anemia.
VII. Treatment
   A. Treat, prevent dehydration.
      1. Mild-moderate dehydration: oral rehydrate solution 5 mL every 1–5 minutes plus replacement of estimated volume of emesis. Mild dehydration: goal 50 mL/kg + losses over 4 hours. Moderate: 100 mL/kg + losses over 4 hours, reassess hourly.
      2. Severe dehydration: ED or admission for IV fluids. Start with normal saline or lactated Ringer's solution at 10–20 mL/kg over 1 hour.
   B. As vomiting decreases, offer larger amounts of ORS at less frequent intervals.
   C. After rehydration, other fluids including milk, food may be reintroduced.
   D. Antiemetic medications are generally not warranted/recommended.
VIII. Follow-up
   A. No/mild dehydration: telephone next day.
   B. Moderate dehydration: see patient next day.
   C. Immediate return if increased symptoms, signs of dehydration.
   D. Severe dehydration requires visit following discharge from ED/hospital.
IX. Complications

Dehydration, 276.5
Mallory-Weiss tear, 530.7

A. Dehydration.

B. Mallory-Weiss tear (linear tear at gastroesophageal junction from repeated vomiting): fresh red blood in emesis after multiple episodes of vomiting.

C. Other complications depend on etiology.

X. Education

A. Most cases of acute vomiting are from viral gastroenteritis.

B. Can be successfully treated at home if no signs of or mild dehydration.

C. Review dehydration signs/symptoms with family, reassure most cases self-limited.

D. Repeated vomiting can induce reflux of bile into stomach resulting in bile staining.

BIBLIOGRAPHY

Aiken JJ: Inguinal hernias. In Behrman RE, Kleigman, RM, Jensen HB, editors: *Nelson textbook of pediatrics*, ed 17, Philadelphia, 2004, WB Saunders.

Baker SS, et al: Constipation in infants and children: Evaluation and treatment, *J Pediatr Gastroenterol Nutr* 29:612-626, November 1999.

Barr RG: Infant colic. In Hyman PE, editor: *Pediatric functional gastrointestinal disorders*, New York, 1999, Academy Professional Information Services, Inc.

Chelimsky G, Czinn S: Peptic ulcer disease in children, *Pediatr Rev* 22(10):349-355, October 2001.

Fleisher DR: Coping with colic, *Contemp Pediatr* 15(6):144-156 June 1998.

Gold BD, et al: *Helicobacter pylori* infection in children: Recommendations for diagnosis and treatment, *J Pediatr Gastroenterol Nutr* 31:490-497, November 2000.

Hyams J: Chronic and recurrent abdominal pain. In Hyman PE, editor: *Pediatric functional gastrointestinal disorders*, New York, 1999, Academy Professional Information Services, Inc.

Lake AM: Chronic abdominal pain in childhood: Diagnosis and management, *Am Fam Physic* 59(7):1823-1830, 1999.

Lasche J, Duggan C: Managing acute diarrhea: What every pediatrician needs to know, *Contemp Pediatr* 16(2):74-83, February 1999.

Leung AK, Sigalet DL: Acute abdominal pain in children, *Am Fam Physic* 67(11):2321-2326, June 2000.

Moyer MS: Gastritis and peptic ulcer disease in children, *Int Sem Pediatr Gastroenterol Nutr* 8(4):1-10, December 1999.

Murray KF, Christie DL: Vomiting in infancy: When should you worry, *Contemp Pediatr* 17(9):81-115, September 2000.

Pickering LK, Snyder JD: Gastroenteritis. In Behrman RE, Kliegman RM, Jensen HB, editors: *Nelson textbook of pediatrics*, ed 17, Philadelphia, 2004, WB Saunders.

Rudolph CD, et al: Pediatric GE reflux clinical practice guidelines, *J Pediatr Gastroenterol Nutr* 32, Suppl 2:S1-S31, 2001.

Sylvester F: Peptic ulcer disease. In Behrman RE, Kliegman RM, Jensen HD, editors: *Nelson textbook of pediatrics*, ed 17, Philadelphia, 2004, WB Saunders.

Wyllie R: Pyloric stenosis and congenital anomalies of the stomach. In Behrman RE, Kliegman RM, Jensen HB, editors: *Nelson textbook of pediatrics*, ed 17, Philadelphia, 2004, WB Saunders.

Wyllie R: Ileus, adhesions, intussusception, and closed-loop obstructions. In Behrman RE, Kliegman RM, Jensen HB, editors: *Nelson textbook of pediatrics*, ed 17, Philadelphia, 2004, WB Saunders.

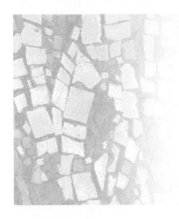

CHAPTER 27

Genitourinary Disorders

SHELLY J. KING

MALE GENITALIA DISORDERS

Absent testicle, 752.59	Hypospadias, 752.61
Congenital adrenal hyperplasia, 255.2	Intersexuality, 752.7
Cryptorchidism, 785.51	Retractile testicles, 752.52
Disorders of male genitalia, 608.9	

Cryptorchidism

I. Etiology/incidence
A. Cryptorchid testes can be absent, undescended, ectopic.
B. Can be result of chromosomal, hormonal, anatomic factors.
C. Majority (about 80%): palpable, are undescended or ectopic testes. Retractile testes: also palpable, sometimes misdiagnosed as undescended. Nonpalpable (20%) can be intra-abdominal, inguinal, absent testes.

II. Occurrence
A. Most common male congenital anomaly, affects nearly 1% of term infants.

III. Clinical manifestations
A. Risk of cryptorchidism increases in premature infant.
B. Bilateral nonpalpable testes or nonpalpable testes associated with hypospadias should be evaluated at birth for life-threatening intersex conditions such as congenital adrenal hyperplasia.
C. Parents may note retractile testicles in scrotum intermittently, especially after warm bath.
D. In case of absent testicle, contralateral testicle may be larger than expected.

IV. Physical findings
A. Often helpful to have child in cross-legged sitting position for exam.
B. Retractile testes can be placed into scrotum, remain there for short period.
C. Nonpalpable testes maybe ectopic, found in femoral or perineal regions.
D. Scrotum may be flat/underdeveloped on affected side.
E. Larger than expected testicle may represent absent or nonfunctioning testicle on contralateral side.

V. Diagnostic tests

A. Unilateral or bilateral palpable testes: no diagnostic testing indicated.

B. Bilateral nonpalpable testes or unilateral nonpalpable testes associated with phallic abnormality: evaluate with karyotype, endocrine testing, appropriate radiographic studies.

1. Human chorionic gonadotropin (hCG) stimulation test differentiates between anorchia and undescended testicles.

2. hCG can stimulate testosterone production in functioning testes and can also result in testicular descent.

VI. Differential diagnosis

Intersex conditions, 752.7

Retractile testes, 752.52

A. Retractile testes.

B. Intersex conditions.

VII. Treatment

A. If at 6 months of age testes remain undescended, intervention is necessary.

1. Type of treatment depends on testes' location, patient's age, association with other anomalies.

2. Reasons for treatment: reduced fertility, risk of tumor formation, trauma, torsion, repair of commonly associated defects such as inguinal hernia.

B. Placing testes into scrotum does not decrease risk of testicular cancer but does provide easy exam for early detection. Risk of testes cancer in cryptorchid male is 1 in 2000.

C. Orchiopexy or open surgery fixes testicle in scrotum and repairs hernia if needed. Laparoscopy can be used to locate nonpalpable testes or blind ending vessels. There is also laparoscopic approach to orchiopexy.

D. Hormone administration is not as successful as surgical approach but good option in high-risk patients and/or patients who have testes found in high scrotum or at external inguinal ring.

VIII. Follow-up

A. After surgery, examine incisions at 1 week, 1 month, 6 months postop.

B. Hormonal therapy: examine at 1 month, 6 months post-treatment (higher risk of reascension).

C. Yearly exam important; patient should be taught self-exam at puberty.

1. Asymmetry of testes needs further evaluation.

IX. Complications

Testicular atrophy, 608.3

A. Testicular atrophy is rated most serious complication of orchiopexy.

X. Education

A. All males need to be taught self-scrotal exam at puberty. Especially important with history of undescended testicle due to increased risk of cancer.

B. Prior to puberty, annual exam should be done. Scrotal pain needs to be evaluated immediately to rule out risk of testicular torsion, trauma, epididymitis, torsed testicular appendage.

Hydrocele

Hernia, 553.9
Hydrocele, 603.9
Intersexuality, 752.7

Scrotal swelling, 608.86
Vaginalis, 616.10

I. Etiology
A. Occurs when processus vaginalis (channel that allows testicle to move from abdomen to scrotum) remains patent.
B. Difference between hernia and hydrocele is size of patent processus vaginalis and its contents.
   1. Narrow channel only allows fluid from peritoneal cavity to pass, resulting in hydrocele.
   2. Inguinal hernia: much wider, can allow both fluid and intestinal contents to pass.

II. Occurrence
A. About 80% of infants are born with patent processus vaginalis; by end of first month of life, decreases to about 60%.
B. By 18–24 months of age, only 20–30% remain.
C. Rare in females: 6 males to 1 female.

III. Clinical manifestations
A. Females: rare, usually presents with soft bulge in labia or inguinal canal.
   1. Bulge can represent ovary or hernia.
   2. Intersex conditions (esp. testicular feminization): evaluate in female.
B. Males: parents complain of scrotal swelling in one or both sides. Can be continuous or intermittent, size can fluctuate.
   1. Parent may describe bluish hue to scrotum, often small in size in morning and growing larger during day as fluid accumulates.
   2. History is very important because may not be present at time of exam.

IV. Physical findings
A. Hydroceles typically transilluminate with penlight to scrotum.
B. Palpate testicle; if testicle cannot be palpated, can be seen by transillumination. If testes not seen or palpated, need scrotal U/S to differentiate.
C. Classified as communicating (patent processus vaginalis) or noncommunicating. Almost all congenital hydroceles are communicating. Noncommunicating hydroceles do not fluctuate in size.
D. Condition rarely painful unless associated with hernia that becomes incarcerated.

V. Diagnostic tests
A. If any concern regarding testes, ultrasound imaging is indicated.

VI. Differential diagnosis

Ectopic Testes, 752.51	Inguinal hernia, 550.9
Epididymitis, 604.90	Retractile testes, 752.52

    A. Inguinal hernia.
    B. Epididymitis.
    C. Retractile testes.
    D. Ectopic testes.
    E. Absent testes

VII. Treatment

    A. Generally safe to watch hydroceles until 18–24 months. After that age spontaneous resolution is uncommon.
    B. Earlier surgical intervention is indicated if hydrocele is large or associated with hernia. Increased risk of incarceration. Any abnormality of testes could lead to earlier surgical intervention.

VIII. Follow-up

    A. Child <18 months of age should be examined every 6 months. If no change, no intervention indicated until 18–24 months.
    B. If hydrocelectomy is performed, see patient 4 weeks postop to evaluate incision and scrotum. If exam is normal, can return to routine annual exam with health care provider.

IX. Complications

Hydrocele, 603.9	Testicular atrophy, 608.3
Incarcerated hernia, 552.9	Vaginalis, 616.10

    A. Complications from hydroceles are rare.
    B. Risk of incarcerated hernia in patients with wide patent processus vaginalis.
    C. Postoperative complications are rare; include recurrent hydrocele, testicular atrophy, lysis of vas deferens.

X. Education

    A. Although hydroceles and hernias are not really associated with increased risk of testicular cancer, discuss importance of self-scrotal exam.
    B. Teach parents importance of regular exam during observation period.
    C. If any scrotal pain, child needs to be seen immediately.

Epididymitis

Chlamydia, 079.98	Neisseria gonorrhea, 098.0
Disorders of male genitalia, 608.9	Neurogenic bladder, 596.54
Dysuria, 788.1	Orchitis, 604.90
Epididymitis, 604.90	Testicular torsion, 608.2
Exstrophy, 753.5	Urethral discharge, 788.7
Imperforate anus, 751.2	

I. Etiology

A. Epididymitis refers to edema, irritation of epididymis or lining of testicle.

B. Can occur from infectious/inflammatory cause.

C. Can be difficult to distinguish epididymitis from testicular torsion, because both can be quite painful.

D. Can be sexually acquired; *Neisseria gonorrhoeae* and *Chlamydia* are common pathogens.

E. Can be related to genitourinary abnormalities or urethra manipulation.

F. Rarely associated with heavy lifting or straining that result in efflux of urine into vas deferens. If urine is infectious, then bacterial epididymitis can occur; if not, chemical inflammation develops.

II. Occurrence

A. Rare in children before puberty unless child has genitourinary abnormality.

B. More commonly occurs in sexually active adolescents.

III. Clinical manifestations

A. Most likely to occur in postpubertal male and very young males.

B. Those with imperforate anus, exstrophy, neurogenic bladder, any conditions requiring intermittent catheterization are more prone to this type of infection.

IV. Physical findings

A. Include sexual history in postpubertal male.

B. Urethral discharge may be present.

C. Often slow onset of pain that continues to become more severe.

D. May have dysuria and see blood or discharge in urine.

E. Physical exam yields swollen and inflamed scrotum.

F. May complain of tenderness along epididymis.

G. If testicle is tender and swollen, may also have orchitis.

V. Diagnostic tests

A. Urine culture and urinalysis may be positive or negative for bacteria. If positive then x-ray evaluation by voiding cystourethrogram (VCUG) is indicated.

B. Scrotal ultrasound with Doppler flow is useful in differentiating epididymitis from testicular torsion. Ultrasound will show enlarged epididymis with increased blood flow unless edema is so severe it results in ischemia.

VI. Differential diagnosis

Bacterial epididymitis, **604.90**	Torsion of testicular appendage, **608.2**
Chemical epididymitis, **604.90**	Urinary tract infections, **599.0**
Testicular torsion, **608.2**	

A. Testicular torsion.

B. Chemical epididymitis.

C. Bacterial epididymitis.

D. Torsion of testicular appendage.

E. Urinary tract infection (UTI).

VII. Treatment

    A. Start 2 weeks of appropriate broad-spectrum antibiotic while cultures are pending. If necessary, change appropriately when cultures are final.

        1. Children not sexually active: cephalexin 40 mg/kg/24 hr in 3 divided doses. Can also use:

            a. Ampicillin 50 mg/kg/bid.

            b. Trimethoprim-sulfamethoxazole (TMP-SMX) (>2 months of age) 4 mg/kg and 20 mg/kg bid.

            c. Ciprofloxacin 15 mg/kg bid postpuberty.

    B. Ibuprofen for several days will help decrease inflammation, pain.

    C. Scrotal support and elevating scrotum will help resolve edema.

    D. If pain and edema are severe or not responding to treatment, consider IV antibiotics. Prolonged infection can result in damage to epididymis.

VIII. Follow-up

    A. If pain increases, see patient immediately.

    B. If condition is resolving, follow up in 2 weeks with repeat ultrasonography.

    C. If positive urine cultures, a voiding cystourethrogram (VCUG) should be done. Increased likelihood of genitourinary abnormalities in males with positive urine cultures.

IX. Complications

    A. Possible damage to vas deferens, epididymis with recurrent or untreated infection.

X. Education

    A. Preventive education especially when epididymitis is associated with sexually transmitted infections (STIs).

    B. Signs/symptoms of testicular torsion and acute scrotum indicate need for immediate attention by medical professional.

    C. Genitourinary abnormalities can be associated with urinary infections so patient will follow up with necessary testing.

Hypospadias/Chordee

Disorders of male genitalia, 608.9
Hypospadias, 752.61
Chordee, 607.89

I. Etiology/incidence

    A. Cause of hypospadias is unknown; genetic link is suspected (many families with multiple occurrences).

    B. Hypospadias is a congenital anomaly in which urethral meatus is not in its normal position at tip of penis.

    C. Spectrum defect ranging from mild to severe, depending on degree of chordee (bend of penis), location of urethral opening. Mild forms can be found during newborn circumcision; stop circumcision, foreskin used to repair defect.

II. Occurrence
    A. Occurs in 1/250 of males in US.
III. Clinical manifestations
    A. Difficult for older child to stand to urinate.
    B. If associated with chordee, future intercourse may be difficult.
    C. Parental anxiety/guilt common with genital malformation.
IV. Physical findings
    A. Urethral opening lies on undersurface of penis.
    B. Degrees of hypospadias: distal shaft refers to opening being closest to natural location.
        1. As opening gets closer to scrotum, condition becomes more severe.
        2. Referred to as midshaft, penoscrotal (located at penoscrotal junction), and perineal (located just beneath scrotum).
    C. Chordee or bend of penis is often present.
    D. Foreskin typically seen only on dorsal side of penis, gives "hooded" appearance.
    E. Penile glans has spade like appearance and cleft/blind ending pit may be seen at location where meatus would normally reside.
    F. Cryptorchidism may be associated.
V. Diagnostic tests
    A. Rarely necessary with hypospadias.
    B. Early referral to experienced pediatric urologist important: allay fears about child's masculinity, opportunity to assess for intersex disorders (uncommon but considered with severe hypospadias and hypospadias associated with cryptorchidism).
    C. In some of more extensive cases, urinary tract will need to be evaluated.
VI. Differential diagnosis

Intersexuality, 752.7

    A. Intersex disorders.
VII. Treatment
    A. Referral to pediatric urologist as soon after birth as possible (reassure parents after surgical intervention child's potency/fertility no longer affected; makes it easier to discuss problem with other family members).
    B. More than 200 surgical techniques described for hypospadias repair.
        1. Goals same in each repair; cosmetically normal-appearing penis, straight with urethral meatus at tip. Repairs are performed at 6 months of age.
        2. Patient should be able to stand to void.
        3. Selected cases may require preadministration of testosterone to enhance blood supply to genitalia.
        4. Most surgery is done on outpatient basis.
        5. Many approaches to postoperative dressing. Absorbable sutures are used in repairs, will not need to be removed.

      6. Stent may be left through urethra to drain bladder while urethra heals. Nonabsorbable suture may be used to hold stent in place, will need to be removed about 1 week postop.

VIII. Follow-up
    A. Seen in 1 week to inspect incision, remove any dressings, stent if necessary.
    B. Seen again 2–3 months later, after majority of edema is resolved, to ensure penis is straight, meatus is widely open.
    C. Some surgeons schedule visit after toilet training to visualize normal voiding stream; others see child after puberty to discuss surgery, alleviate fears.
    D. If ever difficulty voiding or UTI, patient should be seen immediately by pediatric urologist.

IX. Complications

GU hematoma, 863.80	Urethral stricture, 598.9
Meatal stenosis residual chordee, 607.89	Urethrocutaneous fistula, 599.1
Urethral diverticulum, 599.2	Wound infection, 958.3

    A. Experienced hypospadiac surgeon is important to minimize complications.
    B. Rate of complication varies according to severity of defect.
       1. Early postoperative complications: uncommon but include wound infection, urethrocutaneous fistula, hematoma.
       2. Late complications: urethral stricture, meatal stenosis residual chordee, urethral diverticulum.
       3. If secondary procedure necessary, not performed until tissues well healed—approximately 6 months after initial repair.

X. Education
    A. Important to educate newborn care providers not to circumcise if any penile defects: foreskin is used for repair.
    B. Understanding defect and its correction can alleviate parental fears. Reassure them child's masculinity not affected; structural problem that can be corrected surgically.
    C. Patient must understand potential for complications. Any difficulty voiding or urinary tract infection need follow-up with pediatric urologist.

FEMALE GENITALIA DISORDERS

Disorders of female genitalia, 629.9	Incontinence, 788.31
Dysuria, 788.1	Labial adhesions, 752.49

Labial Adhesions
  I. Etiology
    A. Labial adhesions are fusion of labia minora, occur as result of vulvar irritation, lack of estrogen.
    B. Possible causes: chronic inflammation, irritation secondary to infection, trauma, incontinence.

II. Occurrence

 A. Primarily in girls 3 months to 6 years of age.

III. Clinical manifestations

 A. Dysuria and incontinence are common complaints when efflux of urine is blocked and urine is trapped behind adhesions.

 B. Toilet-trained girls may complain of postvoid dribbling. Maternal estrogens seem to prevent this in newborns.

IV. Physical findings

 A. Labial adhesions appear as thin film that begins posteriorly and advance anteriorly.

 B. In more severe cases, cannot see vaginal introitus or urethral meatus.

 C. Presence of scarring that deviates from midline or more dense adhesions should raise question of repeat trauma/sexual abuse.

V. Diagnostic tests

 A. None.

VI. Differential diagnosis

Intersexuality, 752.7

Sexual abuse, 995.53

 A. Intersex conditions.

 B. Sexual abuse.

VII. Treatment

 A. Majority requires no treatment, resolve spontaneously.

 B. More significant adhesions that present with dysuria and postvoid dribbling can be treated with hormone cream or lysis of adhesions.

  1. Premarin cream: 0.625 mg applied with gentle pressure to midline twice a day for 10–14 days.

 C. Lysis of thinned adhesions can be done in office after EMLA cream application.

 D. More dense-appearing adhesions or those that have been broken down previously may be done more effectively and with less trauma in operating room. Critical to prevent readherence by applying barrier cream to raw surfaces twice a day for 6–8 weeks.

VIII. Follow-up

 A. No treatment: follow up with each well-child check, may become more severe with time (best obtained by urethral catheterization).

 B. If begins to complain of dysuria: careful collection of urine specimens because it is difficult to collect clean specimen by voiding when adhesions are present.

 C. After treatment: seen 4–6 weeks later to ensure no reoccurrence.

IX. Complications

Urinary tract infections (UTI), 599.0

 A. Biggest risk is reoccurrence due to poor parental compliance after adhesions have been taken down.

B. If painful voiding, child may delay voiding, empty more poorly resulting in true UTIs.

C. Prolonged use of estrogen can result in development of secondary sex characteristics.

X. Education

A. Importance of post-treatment management must be stressed to parents; most important in preventing further problems with adhesions. Sometimes difficult for parents, especially if child complains of discomfort when medication is applied.

B. Child should learn to void with legs widely separated to facilitate good bladder emptying and to keep labia separated during voiding.

C. If urine specimen necessary, take care to avoid contamination; done best by catheterization.

D. Parents understand length of Premarin treatment, possible side effects of prolonged or repeated use.

PEDIATRIC URINARY TRACT INFECTIONS

Constipation, 564.00	Nausea, 787.02
Diarrhea, 787.91	Poor feeding, 783.3
Dysuria 788.1	Suprapubic/urethral pain, 788.0
Fever, 780.6	Urinary frequency, 788.41
Flank pain, 789.0	Urinary tract infections, 599.0
Incontinence, 788.31	Vomiting, 787.03
Irritability, 799.2	

I. Etiology

A. Periurethral bacteria infect bladder, ureter, kidney. *Escherichia coli* most frequently identified pathogen.

II. Occurrence

A. Fairly common, majority are ascending.

B. Up to 6 months of age, more common in males than females, incidence of 2 cases per 100 live births.

C. After 1 year of age, much more common in females.

D. Approximately 3% of toilet-trained females will develop infection.

    1. Of children who develop infection, 17% will develop infection-related renal scarring

    2. Of those, 10–20% will have hypertension.

III. Clinical manifestations

A. Symptoms of UTI in infants often difficult to recognize.

B. Usually, generalized illness with fever, irritability, poor feeding, vomiting, diarrhea. Suspect when no other source for illness.

C. Older children complain of dysuria, suprapubic/urethral pain, urinary frequency, incontinence. Can also have fever, flank pain, nausea, vomiting if kidney is involved.

D. Foul-smelling urine, constipation (commonly associated, obtain stool history).

IV. Physical findings

A. Perform thorough exam.

B. May detect renal mass in infants with gross anatomic abnormalities such as obstruction or mass.

C. Costal-vertebral angle (CVA) tenderness seen while palpating flank of older children.

D. If dysuria is primary concern, perineal exam may show external irritation related to incontinence, vaginal voiding, labial adhesions.

E. Sometimes treated as UTIs: vaginitis and pinworms sometimes mistaken (because often present with dysuria).

F. Vaginal discharge: culture if present, may have suprapubic tenderness.

G. Males: scrotal exam to rule out epididymitis, especially in older males who may be sexually active.

   1. Look for urethral discharge, culture if present.

   2. UTIs <6 months of age are very uncommon, need evaluation.

   3. Abdominal exam may also yield large stool burden; constipation very common in children with UTIs.

V. Diagnostic tests

A. Collecting urine specimen is very important in documenting infection. Four techniques for obtaining a specimen are listed in Table 27-1.

TABLE 27-1 • Techniques for obtaining a specimen

Techniques	Use for specimen	Drawbacks
Bagged specimen (baggy attached to perineum)	Helpful in ruling out UTI	If positive, cath specimen needs to be obtained (false positives: 90%, especially if left on for >20 minutes)
Clean-catch midstream	Better collection Provides results of multiple organisms of small colony counts that are suggestive of contamination	Difficult for children (parents have a hard time cleaning, separating labia in girls); urine often hits perineum before reaching the cup.
Catheterized specimen	Most widely accepted technique for determining true UTIs	Some offices not set up to catheterize children
Urinalysis	Provides information on leukocytes and nitrates (positive nitrates is highly predictive of infection), urine culture should be sent to assess colony count, pathogens present, appropriate antibiotic treatment	
Suprapubic aspirate	Most reliable	Rarely utilized because of anxiety associated with placing needle through abdominal wall and into bladder; can be threatening to child, parent/care provider

B. X-ray evaluation: infants, febrile UTIs, males, recurrent UTIs, children who are not toilet trained (controversial, these children often hold urine for long periods and empty poorly; many providers will wait to see if there is reoccurrence before x-ray). Important that true infection is documented by catheterized culture when deciding what additional evaluation is necessary.

C. If criteria met, then VCUG and renal bladder ultrasound are ordered to evaluate urinary tract.

    1. Obstructions of urinary tract seen in 5–10%; 21–57% have vesicoureteral reflux.

       a. If tests are negative: no additional evaluation necessary unless further problems arise.

       b. If tests are positive: refer to pediatric urologist for evaluation, consultation, possibly treatment.

D. In case of febrile child, serum chemistries can identify elevation in creatinine or BUN, may implicate urinary tract. CBC with elevated WBC count can indicate bacterial infection.

VI. Differential diagnosis (see Table 27-2)

VII. Treatment

A. Goals: prevent renal damage, urosepsis, future infections.

    1. How goals are accomplished varies according to severity and age of patient.

B. Systemically ill infant is hospitalized

       a. Parenteral broad-spectrum antibiotics, usually aminoglycoside (i.e., gentamicin), ampicillin. Third-generation cephalosporins can also be used.

    2. Some situations can be managed with outpatient therapy:

       a. Parenteral ceftriaxone if child is taking fluids well, parents are reliable enough to contact provider if condition changes.

       b. Some older children can be managed as outpatients with cephalosporins, penicillins, sulfonamides. Antibiotic treatment is 7–10 days.

       c. Parent involvement is very important when managing patients outside hospital; provider must have confidence in family.

    3. Continue parenteral treatment until culture, sensitivity returns and clinical picture is improving. Then, place child on appropriate oral antimicrobial.

TABLE 27-2 • Urinary tract infections

Febrile UTIs	Afebrile UTIs
Obstruction of urinary tract, 599.6	Perineal irritation, 709.9/chemical irritation
Renal mass, 593.9	Labial adhesions, 752.49/vaginal voiding
Urosepsis, 599.	Pinworms, 127.4
Pelvic inflammatory disease, 614.9	Abuse (rare)
Sexually transmitted infections	Hematuria, 599.7/Hypercalciuria, 275.40

    4. Nitrofurantoin is not good antimicrobial in systemically ill patient, does not attain high serum concentrations.

C. Lower tract or bladder infections are referred to as uncomplicated UTI.

    1. Children: 3- to 5-day course of oral antimicrobials.

    2. Nitrofurantoin: good option provides high urinary concentration (other agents used: sulfonamides, cephalosporins, penicillins).

    3. Antibiotic prophylaxis: maintained after infection is treated to prevent infection from reoccurring before completion of x-ray evaluation.

        a. Nitrofurantoin: 1.2–2.4 mg/kg or TMP-SMX 2 mg/kg of trimethoprim 1 time a day are common choices.

        b. Cephalosporins (Keflex) or ampicillin: 1/4 treatment dose daily.

        c. Nitrofurantoin: do not use until >1 month of age.

        d. TMP-SMX: do not use until >2 months of age.

        e. Both Keflex and ampicillin can be used in newborn.

    4. Treatment must also include good oral intake of fluids, encouraging toilet-trained patient to void more frequently.

    5. If associated constipation, this must also be addressed.

        a. Prevents good urinary evacuation.

        b. Provides good medium for microbial growth.

        c. Dysfunctional elimination syndrome (poor emptying of bowel and bladder) is hallmark of UTIs in toilet-trained patients.

    6. Educate parent in treatment of problem.

        a. Urination on timed schedule usually every 2 hours with techniques for relaxation of external urinary sphincter.

        b. Voiding to completion with each attempt is vital to preventing further infections.

        c. Stool softeners are often necessary while working on dietary measures to prevent constipation.

    7. Perineal irritation.

        a. Scented soaps, bubble baths may irritate urethra, cause burning that results in disrupted urinary stream, poor emptying of bladder; discontinue in patients with recurrent UTIs.

        b. Covering perineum with barrier cream helps prevent burning caused from irritation especially with incontinence associated with infection.

VIII. Follow-up

A. Follow-up culture to prove infection has resolved.

B. If x-ray evaluation is positive or if infections are recurrent: urology consult preferably with pediatric urology group. Specialist can do postvoid ultrasound/other treatments to help patient learn to empty more effectively, correct any structural abnormalities if necessary.

C. More thorough education of problems associated with infection will help family and provider.

IX. Complications

Chronic cystitis, 595.2	Incontinence, 788.31
Hypertension, 401.9	Loss of renal function, 593.9

A. Serious risks, warrant effective management.
 1. Renal scarring, loss of renal function are most serious complications.
 2. Hypertension can result from renal scaring.
 3. Chronic cystitis can result in poor functional use of bladder, sometimes incontinence.

X. Education

A. Understand signs/symptoms of UTIs and need for treatment/evaluation.
B. Importance of daily antibiotic and/or stool softener (if prescribed); easy to forget to take medication.
C. Understand dysfunctional elimination and its treatment, primarily need to empty bladder frequently to completion, to avoid constipation.
D. Follow-up critical in management of UTIs due to risk of renal sequelae.

HEMATURIA

Alport syndrome, 759.89	Hemolytic uremic syndrome, 283.11
Anatomic abnormalities, 759.9	Hypercalciuria, 275.40
Benign familial hematuria, 599.7	Lupus erythematosus, 710.0
Calculi, 592.9	Purpura, 287.0
Disorders of renal parenchyma, 588.9	Sickle cell nephropathy, 583.81
Glomerulonephritis, 583.9	Urethralgia, 788.9
Hematuria, 599.7	Urinary tract infection, 599.0

I. Etiology/incidence

A. Gross hematuria (blood visible to naked eye) can originate from upper/lower urinary tract.
B. Causes: variable, include trauma, UTI, calculi, disorders of renal parenchyma, glomerulonephritis, Alport syndrome, hypercalciuria, benign exercise-induced hematuria, anatomic abnormalities, hemolytic uremic syndrome, sickle cell nephropathy, Henoch-Schönlein purpura, Goodpasture disease, lupus erythematosus, STIs (in postpubertal child).

II. Occurrence

A. Common in children (unlike adults): rarely associated with neoplasm (<1%).
B. Microscopic hematuria found on routine health exam by dipstick urinalysis in 0.5–2% of school-aged children.

III. Clinical manifestations

A. History important in determining diagnosis.
 1. Urinary frequency, fever, dysuria may indicate infection, most common cause of blood in school-aged child's urine.
 2. May describe recent trauma.
 3. Blood in other sites (i.e., sputum/stools) may indicate blood dyscrasia.

    B. Family history: familial diseases such as hypercalciuria, Alport syndrome, calculi, structural anomalies.

    C. Hemolytic uremic syndrome, one of most common causes of acute renal failure in children: preceded by gastroenteritis, bloody diarrhea.

        1. Question child regarding any joint pain, edema, tenderness.

        2. Any recent cold, upper respiratory symptoms? Sore throat/skin infection present?

    D. Acute nephritic syndrome: associated with gross hematuria, edema, hypertension, renal insufficiency.

        1. Post-streptococcal glomerulonephritis occurs 7–14 days after onset of strep infection.

        2. Winter months: commonly associated with strep pharyngitis.

        3. Summer months: more likely to be skin infections.

    E. When bleeding occurs, urine color is important.

        1. Brown/Coca-Cola-colored urine: more likely from kidney.

        2. Red/pink urine: more likely from bladder.

        3. Red blood spotting at end of urinary stream/in underwear: most likely from urethra.

IV. Physical findings

    A. A full body exam is done, looking for:

        1. Abdominal or renal mass.

        2. Presence of abdominal, CVA tenderness.

    B. Check child's underwear for blood, perineum for signs of trauma.

    C. Assess joints for edema, inflammation, tenderness.

    D. Edema of face, hands, or feet.

    E. Assess for signs of upper respiratory infection, pharyngitis, or other illness.

V. Diagnostic tests

    A. Urinalysis may reveal infection or proteinuria.

    B. Laboratory analysis: formal urinalysis, culture if thought to be infection; urine calcium/creatinine ratio; urine protein/creatinine ratio.

    C. Serum studies: CBC with differential and platelet count, complete metabolic panel, anti-streptolysin enzyme (ASO) or streptozyme, antinuclear antibody (ANA) and C3.

    D. Skin or throat cultures when appropriate.

    E. Sickle cell screen in all African American patients.

    F. Coagulation studies with history of bleeding from other sites.

VI. Differential diagnosis

> Hematuria (benign, essential, idiopathic), **599.7**
> Idiopathic hypercalcemia, **275.42**

    A. Pseudohematuria.

    B. Idiopathic hypercalcemia.

    C. Extrarenal hematuria.

    D. Exercise-induced hematuria.

VII. Treatment

    A. Systemically ill child with gross hematuria: admit while being evaluated.

B. If elevated ASO and low C3 (hypocomplementemia), refer to nephrologist to rule out/treat nephritis.

C. If abnormal ultrasound, referral to urologist to determine presence of structural anomalies.

D. With UTIs, refer to urologist and consider VCUG.

E. Abnormal ANA results, elevated ANA: consult rheumatology, nephrology; commonly associated positive crithidia may indicate lupus erythematosus.

F. Other blood dyscrasias: consult hematology.

G. Elevated serum creatinine, hypertension, peripheral edema, abnormal calcium/creatinine ratio, protein/creatinine ratio: refer to nephrologist. Renal biopsy/cystoscopy may be necessary to diagnose.

H. Urethralgia: hallmarked by blood at end of urinary stream or in underwear, can persist without negative consequence in child for years. Treatment is controversial: some use antibiotics, but not been proven effective.

I. If child develops hypertension or proteinuria, refer to nephrologist.

J. If chlamydia or gonorrhea is suspected:
  1. <9 Years of age: erythromycin 50 mg/kg/day qid (max 2 g/day)
  2. 9–15 Years of age: ceftriaxone 250 mg IM single dose followed by 7 days of doxycycline 200 mg/24 hr bid.
  3. >15 Years of age: azithromycin 1 gram in 1 dose.

VIII. Follow-up

A. Determined by disease, usually done by appropriate specialist.

B. Urethralgia without significant symptoms and benign familial hematuria without proteinuria and hypertension: monitor by checking urine and blood pressure every 6–12 months.

IX. Complications

Electrolyte imbalance, 276.9
Renal failure, 586.

A. Renal failure.

B. Significant electrolyte imbalance.

C. Follow-up with specialist very important for children with these complications.

X. Education

A. Parents must understand importance of having studies done and follow-up with specialists.

B. If medications prescribed, how and when to give and possible side effects.

C. Know signs/symptoms of progressive renal disease: edema, hypertension, increasing blood in urine, proteinuria, UTI, lethargy, pallor.

PROTEINURIA

Cold exposure, 991.9
Congestive heart disease, 428.0
Edema, 782.3

Hypertension, 401.9
Obstructive uropathy, 599.9
Polycystic kidney disease, 753.12

Febrile illness, 780.6   Proteinuria, 791.0
Glomerulonephritis, 583.9   Pyelonephritis, chronic, 590.80
Hematuria, 599.7   Tubular necrosis, acute, 584.5

I. Etiology

A. Renal insufficiency often associated with proteinuria.
B. Diagnosed by random urinalysis on well-child checkup or associated with serious illness.
C. Common causes of proteinuria include chronic pyelonephritis, febrile illness, glomerulonephritis, exercise induced, idiopathic, orthostatic, polycystic kidney disease, acute tubular necrosis, cold exposure, congestive heart disease, obstructive uropathy, pregnancy, drug induced, trauma.

II. Occurrence

A. Positive screening by dipstick: approximately 10% of 8- to 15-year-olds.
   1. Dipstick finding considered positive if it is = 1+ (30 mg/dL). False positives can occur with concentrated urine specimens; if specific gravity is >1.015, dipstick finding for protein needs to be higher than 2+.
B. If in doubt, look for other symptoms: hypertension, edema, hematuria.
C. Always best to confirm lower range and asymptomatic results by rechecking/confirming by protein-to-calcium ratio.

III. Clinical manifestations

A. Varies with diagnosis.
B. Glomerulonephritis presents with hematuria and proteinuria.
   1. Decreased glomerular filtration rate can result in sodium and water retention, oliguria, circulatory overload, edema, hypertension.
   2. Chronic glomerulonephritis results in failure to thrive, slow growth, fatigue.
C. Postural or orthostatic proteinuria: usually discovered on well-child check.
   1. Usually >8 years of age and totally asymptomatic.
   2. Exercise-induced proteinuria is seen after vigorous exercise, resolves with 48 hours rest.
   3. Febrile proteinuria resolves as temperature returns to normal.
D. Henoch-Schönlein purpura nephritis (a systemic vasculitis) presents with abdominal cramping, purpuric rash, joint pain.
   1. Bloody diarrhea occurs in 50% of patients.
   2. Hemolytic uremic syndrome, systemic lupus erythematosus can also present with purpura, inflammatory bowel.
   3. Known history of renal disease or strong family history of renal compromise.

IV. Physical findings

A. Urinalysis shows proteinuria ranging from trace to 4+, microscopic/gross hematuria.
B. May be associated infection indicated by elevated urine WBC, nitrites.
C. Blood pressure may be elevated.

    D. Edema (esp. periorbital) may be present.

    E. Patient complains of joint pain, stiffness. Joints swollen, inflamed on exam.

    F. Complaints of dysuria or frequency: signs of infection, CVA tenderness, flank pain may indicate obstruction or pyelonephritis.

V. Diagnostic tests

    A. In nonacute setting: obtain protein-to-creatinine ratio.

        1. If >0.2, repeat; if still elevated, obtain 12- or 24-hour urine.

        2. Supine and upright collection obtained to rule out orthostatic proteinuria. Nonpathologic proteinuria associated with posture, fever, or exercise usually yields results <1 g/24 hours.

        3. Renal ultrasound is normal.

    B. Pathologic proteinuria results from glomerular, tubular disorders of kidney.

        1. Protein-to-creatinine ratio is >0.2, 24-hour urine results are = 3 grams of protein in 24 hours.

        2. Renal ultrasound can show infectious or obstructive nephropathy.

        3. Complete metabolic panel, CBC with differential and platelets, ASO, C3, ANA help sort out the immunologic from the nephrologic causes.

        4. Throat and/or skin cultures can identify post-streptococcal glomerulonephritis.

VI. Differential diagnosis

    A. See Etiology.

VII. Treatment

    A. Treatment is dependent on type and severity of proteinuria, obstructive uropathy can be repaired surgically.

    B. Infectious uropathy: treat with antibiotics.

    C. Associated hypertension: may need short- or long-term treatment.

    D. Nephrology referral with edema and hypertension.

    E. If creatinine-to-protein ratio is >0.2, refer to nephrology for further evaluation.

    F. Systemically ill patients require hospitalization to determine cause.

VIII. Follow-up

    A. Follow-up may be lifelong depending on cause.

    B. Recheck asymptomatic proteinuria annually by dipstick analysis and blood pressure: if either is abnormal, referral or additional evaluation needed.

IX. Complications

Failure to thrive, 783.41
Hypertension, 401.9
Renal failure, 584.9

    A. Failure to thrive, renal failure, hypertension.

X. Education

    A. Know signs/symptoms of progressive disease process.

    B. Ensure routine urinalysis remains part of well-child check so early evaluation and treatment can be done.

    C. Follow nonpathologic proteinuria annually.

    D. Close observation for pathologic proteinuria.

BIBLIOGRAPHY

Behrman RE, et al: *Textbook of pediatrics*, ed 17, Philadelphia, 2004, WB Saunders.

Gearhart JP, Rink RC, Mouriquand PD: *Pediatric urology*, Philadelphia, 2001, WB Saunders.

Johnson KB, Oski FA: *Oski's essential pediatrics*, Philadelphia, 1997, Lippincott-Raven.

Oneil JA, Jr, et al: *Principles of pediatric surgery*, ed 2, St Louis, 2004, Mosby.

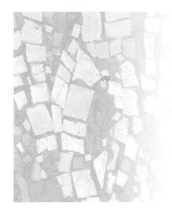

CHAPTER 28

Gynecologic Disorders

MARY LOU C. ROSENBLATT

AMENORRHEA

Primary: No episodes of spontaneous uterine bleeding by 16½ years. Evaluate for delayed puberty if no secondary sex characteristics by 14 years.

Secondary: After onset of menarche, absence of uterine bleeding for 6 months or time equal to 3 previous menstrual cycles. Regular monthly cycles not often seen until 1–2 years after menarche. Because evaluation of amenorrhea applies to all amenorrhea, not necessary to categorize workup as primary or secondary.

I. Etiology

A. External genital anomaly: androgen insensitivity (46,XY).

B. Internal genital anomaly:
  1. Vaginal agenesis.
  2. Imperforate hymen.
  3. Transverse vaginal septum.
  4. Agenesis of the cervix.
  5. Agenesis of the uterus.
  6. Gonadal dysgenesis.

C. Hypogonadotrophic hypogonadism:
  1. Stress.
  2. Weight loss or gain.
    a. Obesity.
    b. Eating disorders.

     c. Competitive athletics.

     d. Familial (ask ages of menarche for mother, sisters).

     e. Drugs (phenothiazines, oral contraceptives, Depo Provera, illicit drugs).

     f. Environmental changes (such as going away to college).

  D. Pregnancy.

  E. CNS tumor.

  F. Pituitary gland infarct, irradiation, surgery.

  G. Adrenal gland tumor, disease.

  H. Chronic diseases.

  I. Hypo- or hyperthyroidism.

  J. Autoimmune oophoritis.

  K. Ovarian failure, tumor, irradiation, or surgery.

  L. Polycystic ovary syndrome (PCOS).

  M. Asherman's syndrome (history of uterine surgery).

II. Occurrence

  A. Primary: 3/1000 girls have menarche after $15\frac{1}{2}$ years.

  B. Secondary: most common reason is pregnancy. Also consider stress, weight changes, eating disorders.

     1. 8–10% of 14–18 year olds report missing 3 consecutive menses in past year.

III. Clinical manifestations

  A. May have no signs or, depending on cause, may be specific signs, such as wide-spaced nipples, web neck, short stature of Turner's syndrome, obesity, acanthosis nigricans of PCOS, or wasting of anorexia.

  B. Evaluate galactorrhead/amenorrhea for prolactinoma and empty sella syndrome.

IV. Physical findings

  A. Physical exam to rule out nonreproductive system problems.

  B. Plot height and weight looking for Turner's syndrome, obesity, anorexia; explain need for genital exam.

  C. On external exam check for patent hymen.

  D. A cotton Q-tip can determine the length of the vagina.

  E. A one-finger vaginal-abdominal or rectal-abdominal exam may determine the presence of a cervix and uterus.

  F. Estrogenized vaginal mucosa is pink.

  G. A pelvic exam for sexually active teens to identify normal organ structure. Clitoromegaly is seen in the presence of excess androgens.

V. Diagnostic tests

  A. Testing indicated in stepwise progression based on history and physical exam.

  B. If any concern about sexual activity, obtain pregnancy test. Keep in mind admitting sexual activity may be difficult for some teens.

     1. Negative pregnancy test: follow stepwise progression again, starting with thyroid-stimulating hormone (TSH) and prolactin.

2. Pelvic ultrasound to look at pelvic structures may be needed.
3. Vaginal maturation index can be obtained to evaluate estrogenation of vagina.
4. Progestational challenge checks endogenous estrogen levels and competency of outflow tract.

VI. Differential diagnosis
A. See Etiology.

VII. Treatment
A. Cause of amenorrhea determines treatment.

VIII. Follow-up
A. Determined by the cause and treatment.
B. Referral may be needed in cases of anatomic or chromosomal abnormality, CNS tumor, eating disorder, or specialized management.

IX. Complications

Infertility, 628.9

A. Infertility may result from some causes of amenorrhea, making it important to listen to patient's questions, concerns and offer emotional support.

X. Education
A. Offer information relevant to the cause and treatment of the individual's diagnosis.

CHLAMYDIAL INFECTION

Abdominal tenderness, 789.6   Penile discharge, 788.7
Cervicitis, 616.0   Salpingitis, 614.2
Chlamydial infection, 079.98   Urethritis, 597.80
Epididymitis, 604.90   Vaginal discharge, 623.5
Hypertropic cervical ectopy, 622.6

I. Etiology
A. An obligate intracellular bacterial agent with at least 18 serologic variants.

II. Occurrence
A. Most common sexually transmitted infection (STI) in US with high rates among sexually active adolescents.

III. Clinical manifestations
A. Causes urethritis, cervicitis, epididymitis, salpingitis, perihepatitis, endometritis reactive arthritis.
B. Can lead to acute and chronic pelvic inflammatory disease (PID).
C. Incubation varies; about 1 week.

IV. Physical findings
A. May be no symptoms for males or females.
B. Females: mucopurulent vaginal discharge, hypertropic cervical ectopy, abdominal tenderness.
C. Males: penile discharge, abdominal tenderness, testicular tenderness.

V. Diagnostic tests
    A. Tissue culture.
    B. Nucleic acid amplification: highly sensitive from cervical, urethral, blind vaginal swabs, or urine.

VI. Differential diagnosis

Gonorrhea, **098.0**

    A. Other STIs, such as gonorrhea.

VII. Treatment
    A. Recommended regimens:
        1. Azithromycin 1 gram one dose PO *OR*
        2. Doxycycline 100 mg PO bid for 7 days.
        3. See CDC guidelines (see Bibliography) for alternative regimens or treatment guidelines for PID.

VIII. Follow-up
    A. Rescreen 3–4 months after treatment in high-risk population.

IX. Complications

Chronic pelvic pain, **625.9**	Infertility, **628.9**
Ectopic pregnancy, **633.90**	Pelvic inflammatory disease (PID), **614.9**

    A. PID.
    B. Ectopic pregnancy.
    C. Infertility.
    D. Chronic pelvic pain.

X. Education
    A. Abstain from sexual intercourse until 7 days after single-dose treatment or completion of 7-day regimen.
    B. Sex partner(s) need treatment.
    C. Risks associated with untreated infection to motivate completion of treatment.
    D. Avoid multiple partners.
    E. Educate about safer sex: use condoms every intercourse, limit number of sexual partners, carefully screen any potential partner.

DYSMENORRHEA

Abdominal pain, **789.00**	Headache, **784.0**
Diarrhea, **787.91**	Nausea, **787.02**
Dizziness, **780.4**	Nervousness, **799.2**
Dysmenorrhea, **625.3**	Pain with menses, **625.3**
Fatigue, **780.79**	Vomiting, **787.03**

Primary: pain associated with menstrual cycle without organic source.
Secondary: menstrual pain due to organic disease.

I. Etiology
    A. Primary: elevated prostaglandins, prostaglandin levels are higher in women with ovulatory cycles.

B. Secondary: due to pelvic pathology such as infection, structural abnormalities, endometriosis.

II. Occurrence

A. 60% of teens report pain with menses; 10–14% of those miss school days due to pain.

III. Clinical manifestations

A. Primary: may begin 6–36 months after menarche.

1. Lower abdominal pain; may radiate to thighs or back.
2. Nausea, vomiting, diarrhea, dizziness, nervousness, headache, fatigue may accompany.
3. Commonly pain starts within 1–4 hours of onset of menses, lasts 1–2 days. Pain may begin before menses and last from 2–4 days.

B. Secondary: pain with menses and associated symptoms. History should include sexual history, gastrointestinal and genitourinary systems history.

IV. Physical findings

A. Primary: normal physical exam.

B. Patients with STIs may have purulent cervical discharge, cervical motion tenderness, uterine tenderness, adnexal tenderness. Mass in adnexa could be cyst, ectopic pregnancy, tubo-ovarian abscess. Tender/nodular cul-de-sac may be found with endometriosis.

V. Diagnostic tests

A. For sexually active teens: pelvic exam to rule out STIs, gonorrhea and chlamydia tests, pregnancy test (if menses are irregular/missed).

B. Urinalysis if urinary symptoms.

VI. Differential diagnosis

Cervicitis inflammatory disease, 616.0	Inflammatory bowel disease, 558.9
Chlamydia, 079.98	Ovarian cysts, 620.2
Constipation, 564.00	Pelvic inflammatory disease (PID), 614.9
Cystitis, 595.9	Postsurgical adhesions, 614.0
Dyspareunia, 625.0	Pyelonephritis, 590.80
Endometriosis, 617.9	Uterine malformation, 752.3
Gonorrhea, 098.0	

A. Cervicitis or PID caused by agents such as gonorrhea, chlamydia.

B. Cystitis, pyelonephritis.

C. Inflammatory bowel disease.

D. Constipation.

E. Endometriosis: not common in adolescents but may be significant in adolescents with chronic pelvic pain. Pain may occur before and after menses, may include dyspareunia, pain on defecation, abnormal uterine bleeding.

F. Uterine malformation.

G. Ovarian cysts.

H. Postsurgical adhesions.

VII. Treatment

A. Primary: nonsteroidal antiinflammatory (NSAIDs), oral contraceptives.

B. Secondary: treat identified cause.

VIII. Follow-up
  A. If standard treatments such as NSAIDs or oral contraceptives do not relieve pain or if etiology is complex, refer to gynecologist.
  B. When infections are cause, treat and follow up per protocol.
    1. PID: inpatient or outpatient therapy, monitor for medication compliance.
    2. Gonorrhea or chlamydia: rescreen every 3–4 months.
IX. Complications

Dysmenorrhea, 625.3

  A. Primary dysmenorrhea should improve with either NSAID or oral contraceptive therapy. If not, consider other causes.
  B. Secondary dysmenorrhea: may have complications based on diagnosis (i.e., teens with PID may suffer from infertility, adhesions, or ectopic pregnancy).
  X. Education
  A. Take antiinflammatory agents with food; start as soon as symptoms occur.
  B. Hormonal contraception is useful when contraception is needed. Teach sexually active teens about safer sex.
  C. When infection is cause, partners need to be treated.

GENITAL HERPES

Genital herpes, 054.10
Genitalia lesion, 625.8

  I. Etiology
  A. Recurrent lifelong infection, 2 types: herpes simplex virus type 1 (HSV1) and herpes simplex virus type 2 (HSV2).
  B. HSV2 causes most genital HSV infection but increasing numbers of genital HSV are caused by HSV1.
  II. Occurrence
  A. 50 Million persons in US have genital HSV infection.
  III. Clinical manifestations
  A. Vesicular or ulcerative lesions of male or female genitalia.
  B. Infection can be more severe in immunocompromised individuals.
  C. Infections caused by direct contact.
  D. Incubation period: 2 days to 2 weeks. Virus persists for life in latent form.
  E. Recurrent infections shed virus for 3–4 days rather than 1–2 weeks in primary infection.
  IV. Physical findings
  A. Vesicular or ulcerative lesions of male or female genitalia.
  V. Diagnostic tests
  A. HSV culture provides best sensitivity when lesions are cultured before they begin to heal.

B. Type specific and nonspecific antibodies to HSV develop in weeks after infection and persist indefinitely, but do not differentiate between genital and orolabial infections.

VI. Differential diagnosis

Candidal inflammation, 112.9	Syphilis, 091.0
Excoriation, 919.8	Warts, 078.10
Folliculitis, 704.8	

A. Folliculitis.

B. Chancre of syphilis, warts, candidal inflammation, excoriation.

VII. Treatment

A. Primary infection: Oral acyclovir therapy begun within 6 days of onset of infection can decrease viral shedding by 3–5 days. Subsequent severity/ frequency of recurrences not affected by treatment. Topical antiviral drugs not recommended.

    1. Recommended regimens:

        a. Acyclovir 400 mg PO tid for 7–10 days *OR*

        b. Acyclovir 200 mg PO 5 times per day for 7–10 days *OR*

        c. Famciclovir 250 mg PO tid for 7–10 days *OR*

        d. Valacyclovir 1 g PO bid for 7–10 days.

B. Recurrent infections: acyclovir therapy started within 2 days of onset of recurrence may shorten clinical course by 1 day. Provide prescription so immediate therapy can begin in case of recurrence.

    1. Recommended regimens:

        a. Acyclovir 400 mg PO tid for 5 days *OR*

        b. Acyclovir 200 mg PO 5 times per day for 5 days *OR*

        c. Acyclovir 800 mg PO bid for 5 days *OR*

        d. Famciclovir 125 mg PO bid for 5 days *OR*

        e. Valacyclovir 500 mg PO bid for 3–5 days *OR*

        f. Valacyclovir 1 g PO qid for 5 days.

C. Suppressive therapy for recurrent infections (>6 episodes per year): can benefit from daily therapy. Acyclovir: safety and effectiveness for 6 years; valacyclovir or famciclovir for 1 year. Because outbreaks diminish in frequency over time, periodic discontinuation of therapy (i.e., yearly) may be helpful in reassessing need for therapy.

    1. Recommended regimens:

        a. Acyclovir 400 mg PO bid *OR*

        b. Famciclovir 250 mg PO bid *OR*

        c. Valacyclovir 500 mg PO daily *OR*

        d. Valacyclovir 1 g PO daily.

VIII. Follow-up

A. Follow patient's emotional adjustment to having HSV.

B. Test for other STIs.

IX. Complications

Genital HSV, 054.10
Skin-colored lesions, 709.8
Warts, 078.10

- **A.** Daily medication may not suppress recurrent outbreaks.
- **B.** Immune-suppressed patients may have prolonged/severe outbreaks requiring IV therapy.
- **C.** Transmission to neonate from infected mother is highest among women who acquire genital HSV near time of delivery.

X. Education

- **A.** Psychologic burden may be great. Counseling includes supportive groups, CDC website, written materials. If depression is identified, refer to mental health provider.
- **B.** Latex condoms may reduce transmission if used correctly.
- **C.** Patients should refrain from sexual contact if lesions are present.
- **D.** Sexual partners should be notified by patient.
- **E.** Sexual transmission may occur with asymptomatic viral shedding.
- **F.** Explain risk of neonatal infection to male and female patients; they should inform provider during pregnancy.

GENITAL WARTS

Genital warts, 078.19

I. Etiology

- **A.** Human papilloma viruses (HPVs) are DNA viruses and include >100 types: >30 types can infect genital tract.
- **B.** Types 16, 18, 45 associated with cervical cancer.

II. Occurrence

- **A.** Anogenital HPV occurs in >40% of sexually experienced adolescent females.
- **B.** HPV is etiology of 90% of cervical cancers.

III. Clinical manifestations

- **A.** May have no symptoms.
- **B.** When present, warts are epithelial tumors of skin/mucous membrane.
- **C.** Immunocompromised individuals may have larger quantity of warts.
- **D.** Incubation unknown; likely ranges from 3 months to several years.
- **E.** May regress spontaneously or may persist for years.

IV. Physical findings

- **A.** Skin-colored lesions with cauliflower-like surface may be several millimeters to several centimeters wide; may be painless or itch, burn, bleed; can be found on vagina, cervix, vulva, penis, anus, perianal area, scrotum.

V. Diagnostic tests

- **A.** May be seen with application of 3–5% acetic acid. Can be detected with viral nucleic acid (DNA, RNA) or capsid probes.

    B. A Papanicolaou (Pap) smear can detect abnormal cervical cells caused by virus, and viral probes can test cells for HPV.

VI. Differential diagnosis

Condyloma lata, 091.3
Molluscum contagiosum, 078.0

    A. Molluscum contagiosum.

    B. Condyloma lata (syphilis).

    C. Pink, pearly, penile papules.

VII. Treatment

    A. Recommended regimens:

        1. Patient applied:

            a. Podofilox 0.5% solution or gel.

            b. Imiquimod 5% cream.

        2. Provider administered:

            a. Cryotherapy with liquid nitrogen or cryoprobe.

            b. Podophyllin resin 10–25%.

            c. Trichloroacetic acid or bichloroacetic acid 80–90%.

            d. Surgery.

VIII. Follow-up

    A. Females: regular Pap smears to assess for cellular damage.

IX. Complications

    A. Recurrences common due to reactivation of virus. May persist for life. Duration of contagiousness unknown.

    B. Local treatment can damage normal surrounding skin.

X. Education

    A. Females: regular Pap smears to assess for cellular damage from HPV.

    B. Screen for other STIs.

    C. Partners should be informed.

    D. Teach safer sex.

GONORRHEA

Gonorrhea, 098.0

I. Etiology

    A. *Neisseria gonorrhoeae* is gram-negative, oxidase-positive diplococcus.

II. Occurrence

    A. 650,000 new cases of gonorrhea per year in US.

    B. 15- to 19-year-olds have highest incidence of infection.

    C. Co-infection with chlamydia is common.

III. Clinical manifestations

    A. Males tend to have symptomatic infections of urethra.

    B. Females may have cervicitis, PID, perihepatitis, bartholinitis.

    C. Rectal and pharyngeal infections may be asymptomatic.

    D. Disseminated infections occur in up to 3% of untreated persons.

      1. Bacteremia causes arthritis-dermatitis syndrome.

      2. More common in females infected within 1 week of menstrual period.

   E. Incubation is 2–7 days.

IV. Physical findings

   A. May be no symptoms.

   B. Males may experience penile discharge, dysuria.

   C. Females may have vaginal discharge, abdominal pain.

V. Diagnostic tests

   A. Culture is excellent but may require special handling.

   B. Nucleic acid amplification is highly sensitive; may be used with mucosal discharge/urine.

   C. Gram stain showing gram-negative intracellular diplococci are most useful in acutely ill patients.

VI. Differential diagnosis

Abdominal pain, **789.**	Penile discharge, **788.7**
Chlamydia, **079.98**	Vaginal discharge, **623.5**
Dysuria, **788.1**	

   A. Chlamydia may cause similar symptoms.

   B. Non-gonococcal urethritis (NGU): 40% of cases caused by chlamydia; 20–30% caused by *Ureaplasma urealyticum;* and 30–40% uncertain but may include HSV, *Trichomonas vaginalis, Escherichia coli,* and others.

VII. Treatment

   A. Dual treatment for chlamydia should be considered in populations where chlamydia is found with 10–30% of gonococcal infections.

   B. Recommended regimens for uncomplicated gonococcal infections of cervix, urethra, rectum:

      1. Cefixime 400 mg one dose PO, *OR*

      2. Ceftriaxone 125 mg one dose IM, *OR*

      3. Ciprofloxacin 500 mg one dose PO, *OR*

      4. Ofloxacin 400 mg one dose PO, *OR*

      5. Levofloxacin 250 mg one dose PO.

      6. PLUS, if chlamydial infection is not ruled out: azithromycin 1 g PO ×1 *OR* doxycycline 100 mg PO bid ×7 days.

VIII. Follow-up

   A. Test of cure for uncomplicated gonococcal infection not indicated.

   B. Persistent infection may be due to reinfected or untreated co-infection with chlamydia.

IX. Complications

Ectopic pregnancy, **633.90**	Pelvic inflammatory disease (PID), **614.9**
Infertility, **628.9**	Tubal scarring, **478.9**

   A. PID.

   B. Tubal scarring.

   C. Infertility.

   D. Ectopic pregnancy.

   E. Hematogenous spread causing skin and joint syndrome.

X. Education

   A. Partners need to be evaluated and treated.

   B. Encourage use of condom.

   C. Screen for other STIs (chlamydia, HIV, syphilis, hepatitis B).

SYPHILIS

Fever, **780.6**	Papular lesions, **709.9**
Headache, **784.0**	Rash, **781.2**
Lymphadenopathy, **785.6**	Syphilis, **097.9**
Malaise, **780.79**	Ulcers (chancres), **091.0**

I. Etiology

   A. Person-to-person transmission of spirochete, *Treponema pallidum*.

   B. Incubation is 10–90 days.

II. Occurrence

   A. Rare in much of industrialized world but problem in large urban areas and rural south of US.

III. Clinical manifestations

   A. Primary: painless, indurated ulcers (chancres) at site of inoculation, within 3 weeks of exposure.

   B. Secondary: 1–2 months later, generalized maculopapular rash (includes palms and soles), fever, malaise, headache, lymphadenopathy.

   C. Hypertropic, papular lesions (condyloma lata) in moist areas of vulva or anus.

   D. Latent: seroreactivity but no clinical manifestations of syphilis, may last years.

      1. Early latent: acquired in last year.

      2. Late latent: acquired >1 year or unknown duration.

   E. Tertiary: may be many years after acquiring infection; features major organ damage.

   F. Neurosyphilis: central nervous system (CNS) disease can occur during any stage of syphilis; examine cerebrospinal fluid in patients with neurologic involvement.

IV. Physical findings

   A. Primary: chancre at site of inoculation, painless ulcer.

   B. Secondary: maculopapular rash, generalized, including palms/soles, condyloma lata.

   C. Neurosyphilis: abnormal neurologic exam.

V. Diagnostic tests

   A. Positive darkfield exam is definitive for syphilis but may not be readily available.

   B. Nontreponemal tests (VDRL, RPR) are quantitative, testing activity, treatment response. Same lab should measure subsequent tests to ensure reliability. Tests may become negative 2 years after treatment.

   C. Treponemal tests (FTA-ABS, TP-PA) must confirm nontreponemal test.

   D. Tests usually positive for life. Other spirochetal disease causes positive tests (yaws, pinta, leptospirosis, rat-bite fever, Lyme disease).

VI. Differential diagnosis

Pityriasis rosea, **696.3**

    A. Rash of secondary syphilis can be confused with pityriasis rosea, making blood evaluation important for sexually active adolescents diagnosed with pityriasis.

VII. Treatment

    A. Recommended regimen for adults:

        1. Primary, secondary, and early latent:

            a. Penicillin G benzathine, 2.4 million units IM ×1 (preferred) *OR*

            b. If penicillin allergic, not pregnant: doxycycline 100 mg PO bid ×14 days *OR* tetracycline 500 mg PO qid ×14 days.

        2. Late latent, latent of unknown duration, tertiary or neurosyphilis, HIV positive and pregnant patients refer to CDC guidelines for treatment. Note: patients allergic to penicillin should be desensitized.

VIII. Follow-up

    A. Evaluate blood tests for early-acquired syphilis at 3, 6, and 12 months.

    B. Add 24-month test for persons with syphilis of >1 year duration.

IX. Complications

HIV, **V08.**	Stillbirth, **779.9**
Hydrops fetalis, **752.3**	Syphilis, **097.9**
Prematurity, **765.1**	

    A. Untreated syphilis causes damage to most body organs over time, infects partners.

    B. Co-infection with HIV, other STIs.

    C. Infected pregnant women pass along syphilis to fetus, resulting in stillbirth, hydrops fetalis, or prematurity. Infants may suffer numerous complications.

    D. Jarisch-Herxheimer reaction (acute, febrile reaction with headache myalgia) may occur in first 24 hours after treatment (occurs most with patients being treated for early syphilis). Antipyretics may be used but may not prevent this reaction.

X. Education

    A. Sexual partners must be treated. Public health department finds contacts anonymously.

    B. HIV status should be checked. If negative, rechecked in 3 months.

    C. Safer sex counseling.

TRICHOMONIASIS

Trichomoniasis, **131.01**
Vaginal discharge, **623.5**

I. Etiology

    A. *Trichomonas vaginalis* is a flagellated protozoan.

II. Occurrence

A. Primarily sexually transmitted, may coexist with other STIs.

III. Clinical manifestations

A. Most males have no symptoms.

B. Females may have profuse, pruritic, malodorous, yellow-green vaginal discharge or no symptoms at all.

C. Incubation period: 4–28 days.

IV. Physical findings

A. Females: frothy white, yellow-green vaginal discharge with erythematous vaginal mucosa and friable "strawberry cervix."

V. Diagnostic tests

A. On wet mount, trichomonad has jerky motion and lashing flagella.

VI. Differential diagnosis

Chlamydia, 079.98	Monilia, 112.9
Gonorrhea, 098.0	Pruritus, 698.9

A. Other STIs such as gonorrhea and chlamydia could be cause of discharge.

B. Monilia could be cause of pruritus.

VII. Treatment

A. Recommended regimen: metronidazole 2 g dose PO.

B. Alternative regimen: metronidazole 500 mg PO bid ×7 days.

VIII. Follow-up

A. None needed unless discharge persists.

IX. Complications

A. If no response to initial treatment, may repeat metronidazole 1 g bid ×7 days *OR* 2 g daily ×3–5 days.

B. In rare cases where infection persists despite treatment of patient and partner, CDC may be helpful in looking at resistance of organism.

X. Education

A. Treat partners even if no symptoms.

B. Patients should abstain from sex until he or she and partner are treated and asymptomatic.

C. Safer sex counseling.

D. Screen for other STIs.

E. No alcohol consumption for 48 hours due to disulfiram-like effects of metronidazole (flushing, pulsating headache, violent vomiting, restlessness).

VULVOVAGINITIS

Vaginal discharge, 623.5
Vulvovaginitis, 616.10

I. Etiology

A. Bacterial vaginosis is syndrome found in sexually active females caused by changes in vaginal flora. Normal vaginal ecosystem is disrupted by increases in *Gardnerella vaginosis, Mycoplasma hominis,* Ureaplasma species, anaerobic bacteria and marked decrease in lactobacillus species.

   B. Incubation is unknown.

II. Occurrence

   A. Common, may occur with other infections.

   B. Although not proven to be sexually transmitted, it is uncommon in sexually inexperienced females.

III. Clinical manifestations

   A. May have no symptoms.

   B. White, homogenous, adherent vaginal discharge with fishy odor.

IV. Physical findings

   A. White, malodorous vaginal discharge.

   B. Not associated with abdominal pain or pruritus.

V. Diagnostic tests

   A. 3 of following 4 criteria establish diagnosis:

   1. Homogenous, white, adherent vaginal discharge.

   2. Vaginal fluid pH >4.5.

   3. Fishy odor before or after adding 10% KOH (whiff test).

   4. Clue cells (squamous vaginal epithelial cells covered with bacteria, causing granular appearance) on microscopic exam.

VI. Differential diagnosis

Edema, 782.3
Erythema, 695.9
Vaginal discharge, 623.5

   A. Characterized by white, thick, pruritic discharge with pH < 4.5; pseudohyphae are seen under microscope when 10% KOH is added. Candida also causes erythema and edema of vulva-vagina.

   B. Rule out other STIs.

VII. Treatment

   A. Not necessary in asymptomatic women.

   B. Recommended regimens:

   1. Metronidazole 500 mg PO bid ×7 days *OR*

   2. Metronidazole 2.0 gm PO single dose.

   3. Metronidazole gel 0.75% one applicator intravaginally daily ×5 days *OR*

   4. Clindamycin cream 2%, one applicator intravaginally at bedtime ×7 days.

VIII. Follow-up

   A. Recurrence is common.

IX. Complications

HIV, V08.   Postpartum endometritis, 314.9
Pelvic inflammatory disease (PID), 614.9   Preterm labor, 644.2

   A. May be risk factor for PID, HIV, preterm labor, postpartum endometritis.

X. Education
   A. Not clearly sexually transmitted.
   B. Partner treatment does not affect recurrence.

BIBLIOGRAPHY

American Academy of Pediatrics: In Pickering LK, editor: *Red book: 2003 report of the Committee on Infectious Disease,* ed 26, Elk Grove Village, IL, 2003, American Academy of Pediatrics.

Centers for Disease Control and Prevention: Sexually transmitted diseases treatment guidelines 2002. *MMWR* 51(No. RR06):1-80, 2002.

Joffe A: Amenorrhea. In Hoekelman RA, editor: *Primary pediatric care,* ed 4, St Louis, 2001, Mosby, pp 975-977.

Neinstein SN: *Adolescent health care, a practical guide,* ed 4, Baltimore, 2002, Williams and Wilkins.

Peipert JF: Genital chlamydial infections, *N Engl J Med* 349:2424-2430, 2003.

Sanfillippo JS, et al: *Pediatric and adolescent gynecology.* Philadelphia, 2001, WB Saunders.

Speroff L, Glass RH, Kase NG: *Clinical gynecologic endocrinology and infertility,* ed 6, Philadelphia, 1999, Lippincott, Williams and Wilkins, pp 421-485.

CHAPTER 29

Endocrine Disorders

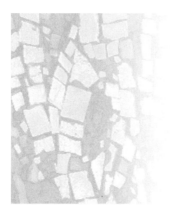

LINDA S. GILMAN

HYPERTHYROIDISM

Agranulocytosis, 288.0
Amenorrhea, 626.0
Blurred vision, 368.8
Breathlessness, 786.05
Cardiac enlargement, 429.3
Chills, 780.99
Cough, 786.2
Diaphoresing, 780.8
Diffuse enlarged goiter, 240.9
Emotional liability, 301.3
Enlarged thyroid, 240.9
Euthyroid, 244.9
Exophthalmia, 376.30
Fast heart rate, 785.0
Fatigue, 729.89
Fever, 780.6
Flushed moist skin, 782.62
Graves disease, 242.0
Heat intolerance, 992.6
Hyperthyroidism, 242.90
Insomnia, 780.52

Irritability, 799.2
Leukopenia, 288.0
Lid lag, 374.41
Lid retraction, 374.41
Loss of visual acuity, 369.9
Nervousness, 799.2
Palmer erythema, 695.0
Palpations, 785.1
Pedal edema, 782.3
Periorbital edema, 376.33
Proptosis, 242.0
Rash, 782.1
Skin reactions, 782.1
Sweating, 780.8
Tachycardia, 785.0
Thyroid bruits, 240.9
Thyroiditis, 245.2
Trembling hands, 780.1
Tremors, 781.0
Weight loss, 783.21
Widening pulse pressure, 785.9

Clinical syndrome resulting from excessive exposure on tissues of body to action of thyroid hormone.

I. Etiology

    A. Hyperthyroidism in childhood with few exceptions is due to autoimmune response to thyroid-stimulating hormone (TSH) receptors. This tissue response causes condition known as Hashimoto thyroiditis. Graves disease common cause of hyperthyroidism in children.

    B. Increases as adolescence approaches.

    C. No specific etiology known.

II. Occurrence

    A. About 5% of all patients are <15 years old.

        1. Peak incidence in adolescence at 12–14 years of age.

        2. 5 times higher in girls than boys.

        3. May be present at birth if mother thyrotoxic during pregnancy.

    B. Symptoms develop gradually, time between onset and diagnosis may be 6–12 months and longer in prepubertal children compared with adolescent.

III. Clinical manifestations

    A. Insomnia.

    B. Heat intolerance followed by diaphoresing.

    C. Weight loss, voracious appetite without weight gain.

    D. Increased sweating, palpations, tachycardia.

    E. Muscle weakness and fatigue.

    F. Light menses or amenorrhea.

    G. Hyperactive GI tract with vomiting or frequent stooling.

    H. Tremors, nervousness, irritability, hyperactivity, emotional liability.

    I. School work suffers.

    J. Breathlessness.

    K. Blurred vision.

IV. Physical findings

    A. Enlarged thyroid, thyroid bruits, thrills.

    B. Thinning of hair.

    C. Proptosis, exophthalmia, noticeable lid lag, lid retraction, periorbital edema.

    D. Diffuse enlarged goiter.

    E. Fast heart rate, cardiac enlargement, widening pulse pressure.

    F. Trembling hands, tremor of finger with extended arm.

    G. Staring gaze, loss of visual acuity.

    H. Flushed moist skin.

    I. Pedal edema.

    J. Palmer erythema.

    K. Increased deep tendon reflexes.

V. Diagnostic tests

    A. TSH produced by pituitary gland.

    B. Thyroid hormones (T_3, T_4).

    C. Iodine thyroid scan.

    D. Antithyroid antibodies test.

VI. Differential diagnosis

Pituitary tumor, 227.3

    A. Pituitary tumor.

VII. Treatment/management

    A. Refer to endocrinologist.

    B. Antithyroid agents:
      1. Methimazole (Tapazole): to induce remission.
      2. Propylthiouracil (PTU): to induce remission.
      3. Propranolol (Inderal): to decrease adrenergic hyperresponsiveness symptoms until gland-modifying agents take action.
    C. Subtotal thyroidectomy.
    D. Radioactive iodine (131-iodine).

VIII. Follow-up
    A. Monitor for adverse side effects of antithyroid drugs such as skin reactions, leukopenia, agranulocytosis.
    B. Most serious side effect: agranulocytosis, usually occurs in first 3 months of therapy.
    C. Report rash, fever, chills, cough that does not resolve in 1 week.
    D. When patient is euthyroid as determined by lab tests of TSH and T_4, a 6-month follow-up should be instituted to assess for risk of relapse.

IX. Complications

Agranulocytosis, 288.0	Hypersensitivity, 782.0
Glomerulonephritis, 583.9	Lupus-like syndrome, 710.0
Hepatic failure, 572.8	Thyrotoxicosis, 242.91
Hepatitis, 573.3	Vasculitis, 447.6

    A. Toxic reaction with drug therapy, most severe: hypersensitivity, agranulocytosis, hepatitis, hepatic failure, lupus-like syndrome, glomerulonephritis, vasculitis of skin, thyroid storm or thyrotoxicosis.

X. Education
    A. Initial adjustment to therapy: stress need to report side effects of therapy.
    B. Compliance to treatment: do not miss doses; if do, take missed dose as soon as possible.
    C. Side effects of medication.
    D. If after several weeks of therapy symptoms continue, may need increased dose of antithyroid medication.

HYPOTHYROIDISM

Abdominal distention, 787.3	Hypothyroidism, 244.9
Ankle swelling, 719.07	Hypothyroidism, congenital, 243.
Asymptomatic goiter, 240.9	Hypotonia, 781.3
Autoimmune destruction (Hashimoto thyroiditis), 245.2	Large for gestation infant, 766.1
	Lethargy, 780.79
Coarse sparse hair, 704.2	Mental retardation, 319.0
Cold intolerance, 780.99	Mild weight gain, 783.1
Constipation, 564.00	Noisy respirations, 784.49
Delayed dentition, 520.6	Poor feeding, 783.3
Delayed puberty, 259.0	Precocious puberty, 259.1
Depression, 311.	Prolonged jaundice, 782.4

Dry skin, 701.1	Sexual pseudoprecocity, 259.1
Dysphagia, 787.2	Short stature, 783.43
Feeding difficulties, 783.3	Sleep apnea, 780.57
Feet swelling, 729.81	Sleep disturbance, 780.50
Headaches, 784.0	Slow fetal growth, 764.9
Hoarseness, 784.49	Slowed pulse, 427.89
Hypoglycemia, 241.2	Visual problems, 368.8
Hypothermia, 991.6	

Condition resulting from deficient production of thyroid hormone or defect in hormonal receptor activity.

I. Etiology
A. Hypothyroidism may be congenital or acquired.
   1. Congenital hypothyroidism.
      a. Most commonly from inadequate production of thyroid hormone due to agenesis, dysplasia, ectopy of thyroid or autosomal recessive defects in thyroid hormone synthesis and defects in other enzymatic steps in T_4 synthesis and release.
      b. Most common preventable cause of mental retardation.
   2. Acquired hypothyroidism most commonly caused by autoimmune destruction (Hashimoto thyroiditis).

II. Occurrence
A. 1 case per 3500 population for congenital hypothyroidism.
B. Acquired hypothyroidism.
   1. Depending on diagnostic criteria, may be as high as 10% in young females. Higher incidence in females (2:1).
   2. Morbidity if congenital untreated results in profound growth failure, developmental cognitive delay (cretinism).
   3. When untreated in older children: growth failure, slow metabolism, impaired memory.

III. Clinical manifestations
A. Congenital.
   1. Constipation.
   2. Hypotonia.
   3. Hypoglycemia.
   4. Hypothermia.
   5. Poor feeding.
   6. Hoarse cry, noisy respirations.
   7. Large for gestation.
B. Acquired.
   1. Asymptomatic goiter.
   2. Hoarseness, dysphagia.
   3. Mild weight gain.
   4. Slow growth/delayed osseous maturation.
   5. Lethargy, sleep disturbance/sleep apnea.
   6. Cold intolerance.

7. Constipation.
8. Sexual pseudoprecocity.
9. Headaches.

IV. Physical findings
  A. Congenital.
  1. Large for gestation infant.
  2. Hypotonia, puffy face.
  3. Wide anterior, posterior fontanel.
  4. Prolonged jaundice.
  5. Abdominal distention.
  6. Feeding difficulties/slowed gastric motility.
  B. Acquired.
  1. Visual problems.
  2. Precocious puberty (young children).
  3. Dry skin.
  4. Slowed pulse.
  5. Delayed puberty.
  6. Coarse sparse hair.
  7. Delayed dentition.
  8. Ankle and feet swelling.
  9. Short stature.
  10. Depression.

V. Diagnostic tests
  A. Newborn screen for T_4: if low, then TSH drawn for definitive testing.
  B. Serum thyrotropin concentration/TSH.
  C. T_4 and T_3.
  D. Serum antithyroid globulin antibodies.
  E. Antithyroid peroxidase.
  F. Radionucleotide studies.
  G. Radioisotope-based thyroid scanning.

VI. Differential diagnosis

Bowel syndrome, chronic, 564.1	Iodine deficiency, 269.3
Cortisol excess, 255.8	Malnutrition, 263.9
Diabetes mellitus, 250.00	Precocious puberty, 259.1
Familial short stature, 783.43	Renal disease, 593.9
Growth hormone deficiency, 253.3	Turner's syndrome, 758.6

  A. Endemic goiter/nutritional iodine deficiency.
  B. Chromosomal abnormalities such as Turner's syndrome.
  C. Precocious puberty in young child.
  D. Familial short stature.
  E. Constitutional growth delay.
  F. Growth hormone deficiency.
  G. Chronic bowel syndrome.
  H. Renal disease.
  I. Malnutrition/gluten-induced enteropathy.

    J. Cortisol excess.

    K. Diabetes mellitus.

 VII. Treatment

    A. Levothyroxine (Levothroid, Levoxyl, Synthroid) synthetic drug identical to human T_4 is preferred thyroid hormone replacement.

    B. Neonates: initial doses 10–15 mcg/kg PO every am ac. Dosage titrated on basis of thyroid function tests q3 months until 2 years of age. Desired T_4 range: 10–15 mcg/dL.

    C. Children: 2–6 years of age: 5 mcg/kg PO every am ac; 6–12 years of age: 4–5 mcg/kg PO am ac.

    D. Adolescents: 100–150 mcg PO every am ac.

    E. With age, levothyroxine dose decreases on weight basis.

VIII. Follow-up

    A. Monitor for behavior change, school performance.

    B. Monitor serum TSH 2–3 months after change in dosage.

    C. Monitor for symptoms of hypothyroidism, hyperthyroidism.

 IX. Complications

    A. Noncompliance with treatment protocol.

  X. Education

    A. Educate parents on signs/symptoms of hypothyroidism and hyperthyroidism.

    B. Allow child to take responsibility for own care as soon as old enough (9–10 years of age).

SHORT STATURE

Constitutional growth delay, 253.3	Growth hormone deficiency, 253.3
Familial short stature, 783.43	Turner's syndrome, 758.6

Generally accepted definition is stature below 3rd percentile, or 2 standard deviations (SD) below mean, for age.

  I. Etiology

    A. Familial short stature.

    B. Constitutional growth delay.

    C. Growth hormone deficiency.

    D. Chromosomal disorder/Turner's syndrome.

 II. Occurrence

    A. Growth hormone deficiency estimated 10,000 to 15,000 children in US.

    B. Turner's syndrome 1 in 2500 female births.

    C. About 1 million children in US whose heights are >2 SD below mean for age.

III. Clinical manifestations

    A. Familial short stature.

      1. Growth pattern remains in its centile channel for height and weight.

      2. Family history of short stature, normal birth length/weight, normal growth rate with predicted adult height of 3rd percentile.

B. Constitutional growth delay.
   1. Bone age lower than chronological age.
   2. Family history reveals short stature in childhood, delayed puberty, eventual normal stature.
C. Growth hormone deficiency.
   1. Small child with immature face, chubby body build.
   2. Rate of growth of all body parts is slow.
D. Chromosomal disorder/Turner's syndrome:
   1. Short stature.
   2. Pubertal delay.

IV. Physical findings

A. Familial short stature.
   1. Clinical/laboratory evidence of systemic disease or endocrine insufficiency.
   2. Annual growth rate within normal limits, growth at or below but progressing parallel to 3rd percentile.
B. Constitutional growth delay.
   1. Child growing at normal or near normal rate, annual growth rate of 5 cm/year, small for age.
   2. Delayed skeletal maturity.
   3. Normal thyroid and growth hormone levels.
C. Growth hormone deficiency.
   1. Typical child with growth hormone deficiency is short, slightly overweight.
   2. When present at birth, infant may have hypoglycemia, prolonged unexplained jaundice.
D. Chromosomal disorder/Turner's syndrome.
   1. Short stature, short neck, webbing of neck, low posterior hairline, shield chest, wide carrying angle, short 4th and 5th metacarpals, narrow high arched palate, epicanthal folds, nail dysplasia, clinodactylism.

V. Diagnostic tests

A. Detailed history, physical, and depending on findings, the following tests:
   1. X-ray of left hand and wrist to assess skeletal maturity.
   2. Urinalysis to assess ability to acidify and concentrate urine.
   3. Blood tests to include:
      a. Urea nitrogen.
      b. Creatinine.
      c. CO_2.
      d. Electrolytes.
      e. Calcium.
      f. Phosphorus.
      g. Alkaline phosphatase.
      h. Thyroid hormone.
      i. TSH.
      j. Erythrocyte sedimentation rate (ESR).
      k. Somatomedin C.

    4. Female patients: karyotype for abnormalities of X chromosome.

    5. X-ray of skull: sella turcica size, abnormality of sella area.

VI. Differential diagnosis

Cardiac disease, 429.9	Nutritional deficiencies, 269.9
Celiac disease, 579.0	Pituitary dwarfism, 253.3
Cortisol excess, 255.8	Psychosocial dwarfism, 259.4
Diabetes mellitus, 250.00	Renal disease, 583.9
Endocrine short stature, 783.43	Second-generation anorexia, 783.0
Inflammatory bowel disease, 569.9	Skeletal dysplasia, 756.0
Intrauterine growth retardation, 764.90	

    A. Intrauterine growth retardation.

    B. Skeletal dysplasia.

    C. Nutritional deficiencies/second-generation anorexia.

    D. Intestinal/gluten-induced enteropathy(celiac disease).

    E. Chronic inflammatory bowel disease.

    F. Renal disease.

    G. Cardiac disease.

    H. Diabetes mellitus.

    I. Psychosocial dwarfism, endocrine short stature, pituitary dwarfism.

    J. Cortisol excess.

VII. Treatment

    A. Refer to pediatric endocrinologist for diagnosis and treatment.

    B. Growth hormone is continued as long as potential for growth exists and child responded to therapy, can expect to reach normal adult height.

VIII. Follow-up

    A. Monitor growth patterns in response to medications.

    B. Awareness of therapy including expected response and possible adverse reactions.

IX. Complications

Hyperglycemia, 790.6

Slipped capital femoral epiphysis, 732.9

    A. Growth hormone administration: hyperglycemia, increased incidence of slipped capital femoral epiphysis.

X. Education

    A. Provide guidance for physical, psychologic, social development.

    B. Assist short children, families to cope with living in bigger world.

DIABETES MELLITUS

Blurred vision, 368.8	Incontinence, 788.30
Cerebral edema, 348.5	Increasing blood pressure, 401.9
Decrease in activity, 780.99	Ketonuria, 791.6
Decreasing heart rate, 427.89	Lethargy, 780.79

Dehydration, 276.5	Mental confusion, 289.9
Diabetes mellitus, 250.00	Monilial vaginitis, 112.1
Diabetic ketoacidosis, 250.10	Nocturia, 788.43
Enuresis, 788.30	Polydipsia, 783.5
Fatigue, 780.79	Polyphagia, 783.6
Flushed face and cheeks, 782.62	Polyuria, 788.42
Fruity odor to breath, 784.9	Seizures, 780.39
Glucosuria, 791.5	Slow labored breathing, 786.09
Headache, 784.0	Vomiting 787.03
High blood glucose levels, 790.29	Weight loss, 783.21

Type 1 diabetes: metabolic syndrome (autoimmune disease) characterized by glucose intolerance causing hypoglycemia/lack of pancreatic hormone, insulin. Insulin is essential hormone, allows glucose to enter insulin-dependent tissue such as skeletal muscle, liver, fat cells. Lack of available insulin results in catabolism and development of diabetic ketoacidosis.

I. Etiology

A. Beta cell mass in islets of Langerhans of pancreas are gradually destroyed in genetically susceptible child.

B. Triggers such as environmental, dietary, viral, bacterial, or chemical that induce T-cell–mediated beta cell injury and production of humoral autoantibodies.

C. Pancreatic islet cell antibodies are found in 70–85% of newly diagnosed diabetes mellitus. Degree of beta cell destruction determined by first-phase insulin response during testing for glucose tolerance.

II. Occurrence

A. Annual incidence in US is about 12–15 new cases/100,000 of child population.

B. Continues to be peak ages for presentation of diabetes mellitus: 5–7 years of age, at time of puberty; however, growing number of children present between 1 and 2 years of age.

III. Clinical manifestations

A. Polydipsia, polyphagia, enuresis in toilet-trained child.

B. Polyuria, nocturia.

C. Blurred vision.

D. Weight loss, vomiting.

E. Fatigue, decrease in activity.

F. Cerebral edema in diabetic ketoacidosis warning signs:
   1. Headache.
   2. Lethargy.
   3. Incontinence.
   4. Seizures.
   5. Pupillary changes.
   6. Decreasing heart rate.
   7. Increasing blood pressure.

G. Cerebral edema occurs in 1–5% of those with diabetic ketoacidosis.

IV. Physical findings
   A. Ketonuria, ketonemia, glucosuria.
   B. Vomiting.
   C. Dehydration.
   D. Slow labored breathing, flushed face and cheeks.
   E. Mental confusion, lethargy.
   F. Fruity odor to breath.
   G. High blood glucose levels.
   H. Monilial vaginitis in adolescent females.

V. Diagnostic tests
   A. Fasting plasma glucose, casual plasma glucose.
   B. Urine for ketones and glucose.
   C. Electrolytes and pH.
   D. Blood urea nitrogen.
   E. CBC.

VI. Differential diagnosis

Hypoglycemia, 251.2	Salicylate intoxication, 535.40
Intracranial lesions, 784.2	Sepsis, 038.9

   A. Hypoglycemia.
   B. Salicylate intoxication.
   C. Sepsis.
   D. Intracranial lesions.

VII. Treatment
   A. Multidisciplinary approach involving family with pediatric endocrinologist, PNP, diabetic nurse educator, social worker, nutritionist.
   B. Educate child, family in stabilizing blood sugars, diabetes management. Due to complexity of illness, management requires incorporation into daily life (Box 29-1).
   C. Treatment replaces insulin child is unable to produce, is corner stone of management.
   D. Insulin dosage is tailored to child's blood glucose and HbA1c levels (Table 29-1). Diabetic control: based on HbA1c levels, clinical symptoms. HbA1c levels provide information on glycemic control during past 60 days.
   E. Insulin is categorized by peak of onset.
   F. Various insulin injection devices available (Box 29-2).

VIII. Follow-up
   A. Review medical, nutritional, insulin therapy, daily blood glucose monitoring (Table 29-2).
   B. Follow up every 3 months to review management plans, physical/psychosocial needs (Table 29-3).

BOX 29-1 • Blood Glucose and Ketone Monitoring

- *Before breakfast*
- *Before lunch*
- *Before Dinner*
- *Bedtime*
- Nighttime: midnight, 0300
- Postprandial: 2 hours
- Pre-snack
- After school
- Intermittent: midmorning, during illness, pre- or postexercise, during travel or changes in routine
- Ketone: blood or urine. Sustained hyperglycemia, during illness, with CSI

Times in italics are routine and minimal time for blood glucose monitoring.
From Kaufman F: Type 1 diabetes mellitus, *Pediatr Rev* 24:9, 2003.

IX. Complications

Eating disorders, 307.50	Neuropathy, 357.2
Ketoacidosis, 250.10	Retinopathy, 362.10
Nephropathy, 583.9	Vaginal yeasts infections, 112.9

   A. Ketoacidosis.
   B. Vaginal yeast infections.
   C. Retinopathy.
   D. Nephropathy.
   E. Neuropathy.
   F. Lipid profile.
   G. Eating disorders.

X. Education

   A. Prevention of diabetic ketoacidosis.
   B. Knowledge of onsets of action, peak action, duration of action of 5 types of insulin (Table 29-4).
   C. Recognition of hypoglycemia and hyperglycemia.
   D. Management of hypoglycemia/evening protein or fat snack to prevent hypoglycemia.
   E. Prevention of long-term complications.
   F. Role of exercise in management/exercise improves glucose utilization.
   G. Insulin therapy and monitoring of glucose levels (Boxes 29-3 and 29-4).
   H. Meal planning, nutrition/eating meals and snacks within 1 hour of usual time.
   I. School issues and coping skills.
   J. Monitoring weight/maintain ideal body weight.

TABLE 29-1 • HbA1c and glycemic targets

	HbA1c	Premeal (mg/dL [mmol/L])	Postmeal (mg/dL [mmol/L])
Infants, toddlers	<7.5 to 8.5	100 to 180 (5.6 to 10)	<200 (11.1)
School-aged children	<8.0	70 or 80 to 150 (3.9 or 4.4 to 8.3)	<200 (11.1)
Teens	<7.5	70 to 140 or 150 (3.9 to 7.7 or 8.3)	<180 (10)

From Kaufman F: Type 1 diabetes mellitus, *Pediatr Rev* 24:9, 2003.

BOX 29-2 • Insulin Injection Devices

Insulin syringes
- Regular or short needles
- 0.3, 0.5, 1.0 mL

Indwelling catheters

Pen devices
- Disposable
- 0.5-unit increments
- Combined with glucose meter

Automatic injection devices

Jet injectors

Insulin pumps

From Kaufman F: Type 1 diabetes mellitus, *Pediatr Rev* 24:9, 2003.

TABLE 29-2 • Principal adjustments in basic or set insulin dose

Rapid-, short-, intermediate-, or long-acting insulin is adjusted after a pattern has been identified over 3–7 days.
  Increase or decrease by 0.5, 1.0, 1.5, or 2.0 units (10% of dose).

Time of test	Change this insulin
2 or 3 Insulin Injections	
Before breakfast	Evening intermediate- or long-acting
Before lunch	Morning rapid- or short-acting
Before dinner	Morning intermediate- or long-acting
Before bedtime	Evening rapid- or short-acting
In the night	Evening intermediate- or long-acting
Multiple Insulin Injections	
Same as above except:	
Before dinner	Lunch rapid- or short-acting
Insulin Pump	
Change bolus dose if blood glucose abnormal	<2–3 hours after the meal
Change basal dose if blood glucose abnormal	>3 hours after the meal
Recheck to be sure the changes made return blood glucose levels to the target range.	

From Kaufman F: Type 1 diabetes mellitus, *Pediatr Rev* 24:9, 2003.

TABLE 29-3 • The outpatient visit for patients with diabetes

Physical examination	Frequency recommendations
Weight, height, body mass index (BMI)	Every 3 months/assess changes in percentile
Sexual maturity rating stage	Every 3 months/note pubertal progression
Blood pressure	Every 3 months/target <90th percentile for age
Eye	Dilated funduscopic examination every 12 months after 5 years of diabetes
Thyroid	Every 3 months/presence of goiter, signs of thyroid dysfunction
Abdomen	Every 3 months/presence of hepatomegaly, fullness, signs of malabsorption, inflammation
Foot, peripheral pulses	Every 3 months inspection/after 12 years of age, thorough
Skin, joints, injection sites	Every 3 months/injection sites, joint mobility, lesions associated with diabetes
Neurologic	Every 12 months/signs of autonomic changes, pain, neuropathy

Laboratory test	Frequency
HbA1c	Every 3 months
Microalbuminuria	Every 12 months after puberty or after 5 years of diabetes
Urinalysis, creatinine	At presentation and with signs of renal problems
Fasting lipid profile	After stabilization at diagnosis and every few years
Thyroid function tests, including antithyroid antibodies	Every 12 months
Celiac screen	At time of diagnosis, if symptoms, at puberty
Islet antibodies	At diagnosis

From Kaufman F: Type 1 diabetes mellitus, *Pediatr Rev* 24:9, 2003.

TYPE 2 DIABETES

Acanthosis nigricans, 701.2	Polydipsia, 783.5
Dyslipidemia, 272.5	Polyuria, 788.42
Dysuria, 788.1	Sleep apnea, 780.57
Family history of type 2 diabetes, V18.0	Type 2 diabetes, 250.00
Hypertension, 401.9	Vaginal infection, 616.10
Obesity, 278.00	Weight loss, 783.2

Chronic metabolic disorder characterized by insulin resistance.
  I. Etiology
    A. Most common clinical factor for type 2 diabetes is obesity/body mass index (BMI) > 85% for age and sex.
  II. Occurrence
    A. Female-to-male ratio is 1.7:1 regardless of race. Youth between 8–19 years of age.

TABLE 29-4 • Onset of action, peak action, and duration of action in five types of insulin

Insulin preparation	Onset of action (hours)	Peak action (hours)	Duration of action (hours)	Maximal duration (hours)
Rapid-acting				
Lispro	¼–½	1–2	3–5	4–6
Aspart	¼–½	1–2	3–6	5–8
Short-acting				
Regular	½–1	2–4	3–6	6–8
Intermediate-acting				
NPH (isophane)	2–4	8–10	10–18	14–20
Lente (zinc suspension)	2–4	8–12	12–20	14–22
Long-acting				
Ultralente (extended zinc suspension)	6–10	10–16	18–20	20–24
Basal				
Glargine	1–2	None	19–24	24

From Kaufman F: Type 1 diabetes mellitus, *Pediatr Rev* 24:9, 2003.

III. Clinical findings
    A. Obesity.
    B. Polyuria.
    C. Polydipsia and weight loss.
    D. Vaginal infection as chief complaint.
    E. Dysuria.
    F. Family history.
    G. Sedentary lifestyle, sleep apnea.

IV. Physical findings
    A. Obesity.
    B. Acanthosis nigricans: darkened thick velvety pigmentation in skin folds.
    C. Hypertension.
    D. Dyslipidemia.
    E. Vaginal infection.

V. Diagnostic tests
    A. Clinical impression with urinalysis.
    B. Plasma insulin.
    C. C-peptide concentrations.

BOX 29-3 • Insulin Dosage Adjustment Algorithms

Insulin doses need to be adjusted for the following:
1. Correct for abnormal blood glucose level (correction algorithm)
    - Amount of insulin given per correction algorithm can be determined by taking into account age or insulin dose

Insulin Dosage	Age (2.8 mmol/L) that Blood Glucose Is Elevated	Amount/50 mg/dL
<5 units	<5 years old	0.25 units
5–10 units	6–9 years old	0.50 units
10–20 units	10–12 years old	1 unit
>20 units	Teens	1.5–2 units

    - Insulin dosage can also be determined by insulin sensitivity by using the 1800 or 1500 Rule. The 1800 Rule is used for rapid-acting insulin and the 1500 Rule for short-acting insulin. Insulin sensitivity is determined by dividing 1800 or 1500 by the total daily dose of insulin to determine how many mg/dL (mmol/L) that 1 unit of insulin decreases the glucose level.
2. Account for exercise and activity
    - Decrease insulin dose, add carbohydrate, or both.
    - For activity lasting $\frac{1}{2}$ to 2 hours, child probably will need to take 10 to 15 g of carbohydrate for every $\frac{1}{2}$ to 1 hour.
    - Occasionally, activity can elevate blood glucose levels. Usually occurs in afternoon for children taking 2 or 3 insulin injections per day or if CSII is disconnected for >1.5 to 2 hours.
    - With repeated strenuous physical activity, total daily insulin dose may need to be decreased by 10% to 20%.
3. Match carbohydrate intake (insulin : carbohydrate ratio or carbohydrate supplement)
    - Divide 450 by total units of insulin used per day to determine number of grams of carbohydrate that requires 1 unit of insulin.
4. Anticipate a change in the usual regime (anticipatory supplement)

From Kaufman F: Type 1 diabetes mellitus, *Pediatr Rev* 24:9, 2003.

  D. Autoantibodies to islet cell.
  E. Glutamic acid decarboxylase and tyrosine phosphatase helpful in distinguishing between type 1 and type 2 diabetes.

VI. Differential diagnosis

Type 1 diabetes, 250.01

  A. Type 1 diabetes.

VII. Treatment

  A. Whenever possible, manage child with multidisciplinary team.
  B. Treat underlying cause of disorder: obesity.
  C. Increase physical activity/moderate exercise is primary importance.
  D. Diet should aim for gradual, sustained weight loss (eat smaller portions, lower caloric foods).

BOX 29-4 • Advances in Glucose Monitoring

Very small blood samples required.
Forearms can be used for preprandial samples.
Results available in 5–45 seconds.
Glucose meters can fit in a pocket.
Glucose meters can store glucose values.
Glucose values can be displayed in a variety of forms and graphs.
Continuous or near-continuous glucose monitoring.

The Medtronic MiniMed system:
- Uses a glucose oxidase system.
- Measures subcutaneous glucose levels every 5 minutes.
- Is worn for up to 3 days.
- Glucose results analyzed retrospectively.

The GlucoWatch system:
- Uses iontophoresis.
- Measures glucose content of interstitial fluid every 20 minutes.
- Is worn for up to 12 hours.
- Contains alarms to detect hyper- and hypoglycemia.
- Gives real-time value.
- Is associated with minor skin irritation in some individuals.

From Kaufman F: Type 1 diabetes mellitus, *Pediatr Rev* 24:9, 2003.

    E. Treat hypertension if it exists.
VIII. Follow-up
    A. Routine health visits including dilated eye exam, foot exams, blood pressure, lipids, albuminuria.
    B. Assistance with lifestyle changes.
IX. Complications

Type 1 diabetes, ketoacidosis, 250.11

    A. Type 1 diabetes, ketoacidosis.
X. Education
    A. Lifestyle changes: most important, challenging issues.
    B. Near normalization of blood glucose and glycohemoglobin.
    C. Control lipids.
    D. Set outcome goals of mutual agreement.
    E. Review medication usage and insulin or oral medication if prescribed.

STEROID USE WITH ATHLETES

Acne, **706.1**	Mood swings, **296.99**
Aggressiveness, **301.3**	Ovulation, inhibition of, **628.0**
Alopecia, **704.00**	Prostate hypertrophy, **600.90**
Breast atrophy in females, **611.4**	Seborrhea, **706.3**

Depressed libido, **799.81**	Skin sensation, disturbance of, **782.0**
Depression, **311.**	Sustained penile erection/priapism, **607.3**
Early male baldness, **704.00**	Testicular atrophy, **608.3**
Headaches, **784.0**	Torn or ruptured tendons, **845.09**
Hirsutism, **704.1**	Voice change, **784.49**
Hypercholesterolemia, **272.0**	Weight gain, **783.1**
Hypertension, **401.9**	Weight loss, **783.21**
Jaundice, **782.4**	Water retention, **782.3**
Menses abnormalities, **626.4**	

Anabolic, androgenic steroids: synthetic hormones used to develop bulk, muscle strength.

I. Etiology
A. Administration of or use by competing athlete for sole intention of increasing performance in artificial, unfair manner.
B. Anabolic and androgenic steroids mimic action of hormones normally present.
C. Anabolic compounds stimulate building of muscle.
D. Androgenic compounds stimulate development of masculine characteristics.
E. Steroids refer to class of drugs, known as performance-enhancing drugs.
F. In males, testosterone is produced by testes and adrenal gland.
G. In females, testosterone is produced only by adrenal gland; much less testosterone than males.

II. Occurrence
A. The prevalence of self-reported use of anabolic steroids in adolescence has a range from 5% to 11% of males and up to 2.5% in females.
B. Athletes in nonschool sports as well as nonathletes have been shown to represent a significant portion of the user population.

III. Clinical manifestations
A. Improbable gains in lean body mass, muscle bulk, definition.
B. Behavioral changes/mood swings.
C. Advanced stages of acne on chest and back.
D. Headaches.
E. Depressed libido.
F. Early male baldness.
G. Sustained penile erection/priapism.
H. Deepening voice with laryngeal changes.
I. Menses abnormalities.
J. Inhibition of ovulation.
K. Depression, aggressiveness combativeness.

IV. Physical findings
A. Yellowing of eyes/jaundice.
B. Oily skin.
C. Water retention in tissue.
D. Unexplained weight gain or loss.

E. Breast development in males.

F. Testicular atrophy.

G. Seborrhea.

H. Hypertension.

I. Increased total cholesterol.

J. Prostate hypertrophy.

K. Weakened tendons resulting in tearing or rupture.

L. Damage to growth plate at end of bones, permanently stunting growth.

M. Baldness/alopecia.

N. Clitoral enlargement.

O. Hirsutism.

P. Breast atrophy in females.

Q. Acne.

V. Diagnostic tests

A. Urine for steroids.

B. Electrolytes.

C. Alkaline phosphatase.

D. Serum glutamic-oxaloacetic transaminase (SGOT), serum glutamic-pyruvic transaminase (SGPT).

E. Liver enzymes.

F. Cholesterol profile.

G. CBC.

VI. Differential diagnosis

Bipolar disease, 297.7

Brain tumor, 784.2

Pituitary gland dysfunction, 253.9

A. Bipolar disease.

B. Brain tumor.

C. Pituitary gland dysfunction.

VII. Treatment

A. Discontinuance of steroids, psychologic counseling.

VIII. Follow-up

A. Emphasize benefits of proper training and nutrition.

B. Provide effective role models for athlete.

C. Evaluate hypertension, lipids.

IX. Complications

Coronary heart disease, 414.00

Liver tumors, 573.8

A. Anabolic steroid psychologic addiction (addiction syndrome).

B. Epiphyseal plate closure if adolescent continuing to grow while taking steroids.

C. Liver tumors.

D. Risk of coronary heart disease directly related to low-density lipoprotein.

BOX 29-5 • Resources on the Internet

American Academy of Pediatrics, Committee on Sports Medicine and Fitness: Adolescents and Anabolic Steroids: A Subject Review (RE9720): http://aapolicy.aapublications.org/cgi/reprint/pediatrics; 99/6/904.pdf
Steroid Use in Adolescents: http://darkwing.uoregon.edu/~iishp/Nelson3.html
Type 2 Diabetes in Youth: www.diabetesinmichigan.org/Type2youthHC.htm

---

X. Education
A. Risks of steroid use; long-term health effects of continued use.

BIBLIOGRAPHY

Binns H, Ariza J: Guidelines help clinicians identify risk factors for overweight in children, *Pediatr Ann* 33:1, 2004.

Kaufman F: Type 1 diabetes mellitus, *Pediatr Rev* 24:9, 2003.

LaFrancchi S: Disorders of thyroid gland. In Behrman R, editor: *Nelson textbook of pediatrics,* Philadelphia, 2000, WB Saunders.

Pinhas-Hamiel O: Type 2 diabetes: Not just for grownups anymore, *Contemp Pediatr* 18:1, 2001.

Samuels C, Cohen L: Understanding growth patterns in short stature, *Contemp Pediatr* 18:6, 2001.

Sperling A: Diabetes mellitus in children. In Behrman R, editor: *Nelson textbook of pediatrics,* Philadelphia, 2000, WB Saunders.

Witchel S, Finegold D: Endocrinology. In Zitelli B, Davis H, editors: *Atlas of pediatric physical diagnosis,* St Louis, 2002, Mosby.

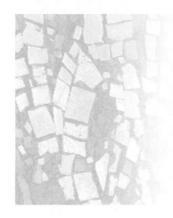

CHAPTER 30

Musculoskeletal Disorders

MIKI M. PATTERSON

INJURIES: SPRAIN, STRAIN, OVERUSE

Ankle sprain, **845.00**	Ligament tear, **848.9**
Dislocation, **839.8**	Sprain, **848.9**
Finger sprain, **842.10**	Wrist sprain, **842.00**
Fracture, **829.0**	

I. Etiology
   A. Damage or disruption to tendon (attaches muscle to bone), ligament (attaches bone to bone), from overstretching, exertion, repetitive application of excessive forces.

II. Occurrence
   A. Wrist, finger, ankle sprains are common among children.

III. Clinical manifestations
   A. Limp or pain with extremity or joint use.
   B. Feel tearing or heard a "pop" during activity or with trauma.

IV. Physical findings
   A. Pain, tenderness to palpation, swelling, discoloration (ecchymosis or erythema).

V. Diagnostic tests
   A. Radiograph in 2 planes to ensure no fracture and to assess bony relationships. May need views of unaffected side to compare ossification centers and normal alignment.
   B. Physical exam: stress joints to varus, valgus, anterior, posterior. If a "give" is felt (i.e., at a knee or ankle joint "opening up"), refer patient to orthopedist. Palpation over physis should be pain free.

VI. Differential diagnosis

Dislocation, **839.8**	Ligament tear, **848.9**
Fracture, **829.0**	Neurologic deficit, **781.99**

   A. Fracture, dislocation, ligament tears, neurologic deficit, vascular condition.

VII. Treatment

A. P.R.I.C.E. and medication for pain as needed: **P**rotect, **R**est, **I**ce, **C**ompression, **E**levation:

1. *Protect:* with splint/brace or relief of weight bearing with crutches.
2. *Rest:* do not use extremity.
3. *Ice:* apply ice immediately for 10–20 minutes then every 3–4 hours for the first 24–48 hours.
4. *Compression:* with ace wrap; do not pull tightly when wrapping; compression will decrease amount of blood allowed to seep from injured tissues and decrease range of motion at joint.
5. *Elevation:* above level of heart will decrease swelling accumulating from gravity.
6. Identify and alter factors that contributed to overuse.
7. May continue to do activities that do not cause pain.
8. Pain relievers such as ibuprofen or narcotic, if needed.

VIII. Follow-up

A. Return in 1 week to ensure resolution of majority of pain, swelling and return of function.
B. Pain and swelling after 2 weeks requires further workup.

IX. Complications

Compartment syndrome, 958.8
Skin abrasion, 919.

A. Missed fracture.
B. **Caution:** Salter fractures (through the growth plate) may not be visible on x-ray; if physis is tender, treat as fracture (Figure 30-1).

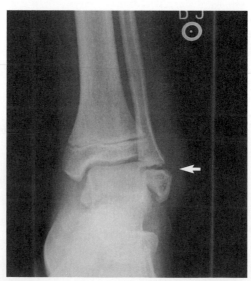

FIGURE 30-1 • Salter I fracture. Note the increased width compared with the distal tibial physis.

   C. Compartment syndrome.

   D. Skin breakdown (presents as burning sensation under brace or splint; results from ischemia of tissue; pressure should be relieved immediately).

X. Education

   A. Teach family to call immediately for any burning or worsening of **pain,** neurovascular changes such as **paresthesias** (numbness or tingling), **pallor, paralysis, pulselessness,** cyanosis. These 5 P's are signs of compartment syndrome.

     1. Considered a surgical *Emergency.*

     2. Most important: worsening pain and tightness.

     3. Compartment syndrome is accumulation of pressure in tissues, not relieved with elevation.

     4. Most common areas: calves, forearms, hands, feet.

   B. Range of motion, stretching should be pain free before beginning strengthening rehabilitation exercises then gradual return to regular activity.

INJURIES: FRACTURE, DISLOCATION

Dislocation, 839.8	Fracture, 829.0
Ecchymosis, 459.89	Point skin tenderness, 782.0
Erythema, 695.9	

I. Etiology

   A. Damage/disruption to bone or joint, respectively, from trauma, exertion, overuse.

   B. Most common causes: child abuse and neglect, sports, falls, motor vehicle, pedestrian/bicycle events.

II. Occurrence

   A. All age groups can be affected.

   B. Fractures are most common presentation of child abuse; 70% fractures in children <6 months are inflicted.

   C. Fractures suggestive of nonaccidental trauma in children: metaphyseal, rib (seen in 5–20% of abused), scapular/distal clavicle/night stick (midshaft ulna), vertebral fracture or subluxation, fingers in nonambulating child, humerus (except supracondylar) in those <3 years of age, bilateral/multiple fractures in different stages of healing as well as complex skull.

III. Clinical manifestations

   A. Feel tearing or heard "pop" or "crack."

   B. Most affect function.

   C. Findings suspect for abuse:

     1. Fracture in child <1 year of age.

     2. Unknown or unwitnessed injury.

     3. Delay in seeking medical attention.

     4. Changing story of how injury occurred.

     5. Fracture does not fit mechanism described (i.e., twisting an extremity will result in spiral fracture, whereas direct blow produces transverse fracture).

IV. Physical findings

A. Pain, point tenderness, swelling, ecchymosis or erythema, loss of function, obvious deformity.

V. Diagnostic tests

A. Radiographs in 2 planes: AP and lateral or both obliques.

B. May require CT scan or MRI for complex injuries (i.e., pelvis or spine).

VI. Differential diagnosis

Sprain, 848.9

A. Sprain.

VII. Treatment

A. Protect with immobilization/splinting, compression, ice, elevation.

B. Do not use extremity.

C. Pain medication (typically narcotic) such as acetaminophen (Tylenol) with codeine at 1 mg per kg of body weight every 4–6 hours for small children or hydrocodone (Vicodin), oxycodone (Percocet), or morphine by weight for those >100 lbs.

D. Dislocation and displaced fractures refer stat to orthopedist. Should be NPO if surgical intervention is imminent possibility.

VIII. Follow-up

A. Should be per orthopedist.

B. Many will not allow use of extremity for period of time while healing.

C. Muscles will spasm around fracture to try to pull bone ends together for healing.

D. Fractures without fixation move for 10–14 days after injury while granulation occurs (even in casts).

E. Frequent x-rays may be needed to ensure alignment of fractures.

F. In 2–6 weeks: callus develops, bone ends become "sticky," pain is reduced.

G. Consolidation begins at 3 weeks in infants, may take 3–6 months in older children, adults.

H. Weight bearing, casting, splinting, bracing, or full use are all related to fracture configuration, healing, patient specifics.

I. Remodeling of bone that occurs in children <8 years of age allows acceptance of angulated fractures.

J. Increased circulation to fractured bone causes some overgrowth (basis for 1-cm overlap of fractured femurs in young children).

IX. Complications

Compartment syndrome, 958.8
Loss of alignment, 781.2
Skin abrasion, 919.

A. Compartment syndrome.

B. Loss of alignment.

C. Shortening, angulation, delayed or nonunion of fracture.

D. Skin breakdown.

E. Neurovascular problems.

F. Infection.

G. Missed abuse.

X. Education.

A. Same as for sprains.

B. Family should seek medical attention for neurovascular changes or pain inside cast/splint/brace.

BACK PAIN

Back pain, 724.5

I. Etiology

A. See Differential diagnosis (next section).

II. Occurrence

A. Most common in preadolescent and adolescent.

III. Clinical manifestations

A. Complaint of back pain, sometimes night pain (red flag), with/without numbness or tingling.

IV. Physical findings

A. May or may not have:

1. Deformity of spine.

2. Pain with motion.

3. Positive straight leg raise sign.

4. Tight hamstrings (unable to sit upright with legs extended straight out in front).

5. Neurologic changes or skin lesions.

V. Diagnostic tests

A. Radiographs: AP and lateral thoracolumbar and/or lumbosacral spine.

B. Other testing as exam or history indicates (i.e., bone scan, MRI, labs: CBC w/diff, erythrocyte sedimentation rate [ESR], antinuclear antibodies [ANA], rheumatoid factor, or HLA-B27).

VI. Differential diagnosis

Ankylosis spondylitis, 720.0	Reiter syndrome, 099.3
Degenerative disk disease, 722.6	Scheurmann kyphosis, 737.10
Discitis, 722.90	Scoliosis, 737.30
Inflammatory bowel disease, 569.9	Sickle cell crisis, 282.60
Osteoma, 213.9	Spondylolisthesis, 756.12
Psoriatic arthritis, 696.0	Spondylolysis, 756.11

A. Overuse (heavy backpacks).

B. Fracture, spondylolysis (defect or separation of pars interarticularis), and spondylolisthesis (anterior slippage of vertebral body) typically occur at L-5 (Figure 30-2).

C. Scheurmann kyphosis (anterior wedging >5 degrees of 3 or more adjacent vertebrae).

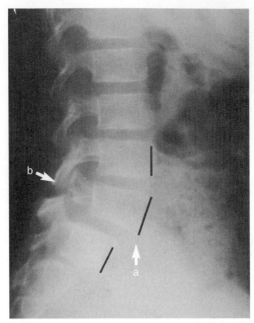

FIGURE 30-2 ● *(a)* Spondylolisthesis (slipped forward) L-5 on S-1 with *(b)* spondylolysis (fractured).

    D. Scoliosis (see later discussion).
    E. Degenerative disk disease, infection, diskitis.
    F. Inflammatory conditions, such as ankylosis spondylitis, psoriatic arthritis, inflammatory bowel disease, Reiter's syndrome (morning stiffness is hallmark sign).
    G. Neoplastic such as osteoid osteoma (hallmark sign: night pain or constant pain independent of motion).
    H. Other: sickle cell crisis, functional illness, referred pain such as kidney infection or menstrual cramping.
  VII. Treatment
    A. Depends on diagnosis: rest, nonsteroidal anti-inflammatory drugs (NSAIDs), stretching, abdominal strengthening, proper posture and backpack use, or referral to orthopedist.
  VIII. Follow-up
    A. Symptoms should improve in 2 weeks for overuse or strains.
  IX. Complications
    A. Missed diagnosis (see Differential diagnosis).
  X. Education
    A. Demonstrate exercises to help ensure done correctly.
    B. Work with family on medication schedule.
    C. If symptoms persist or new symptoms occur, call health care provider.

SCOLIOSIS

Scoliosis, 737.30

Abnormal lateral curvature of spine, typically with vertebral rotation.

I. **Etiology**
   A. Idiopathic 90% (most common) unknown etiology, familiar pattern has been noted.

II. **Occurrence**
   A. Idiopathic: 3–5% in adolescents screened; males = female.
   B. 0.6% Require treatment; however, females are treated more often (1%) than males (0.1%).

III. **Clinical manifestations**
   A. Does not typically cause back pain (<14%).

IV. **Physical findings**
   A. Difficult fitting clothes.
   B. S- or C-shape curve of spine.
   C. Prominent: scapular, ribcage, paraspinal musculature (especially on forward bend test) or breast.
   D. Asymmetric waistline or shoulder level.
   E. Plumb line dropped from C-7 does not correlate with gluteal crease.

V. **Diagnostic tests**
   A. Inspection with minimal clothing.
   B. Radiographs: scoliosis series, which is standing PA and lateral views of entire spine on 1 cassette (Figure 30-3).

VI. **Differential diagnosis**

Cerebral palsy, 343.9	Neurofibromatosis, 237.70
Emotional disturbance, 313.9	Polio, 045.1
Muscular dystrophy, 359.1	Spina bifida, 741.9
Myopathies, 359.9	Vertebra fracture, 805.8

   A. Congenital: embryonic malformation.
   B. Paralytic: polio, muscular dystrophy, cerebral palsy, spina bifida, myopathies, neurofibromatosis.
   C. Traumatic: fracture of vertebrae.
   D. Hysterical: rare, nonstructural, result of emotional disturbance.

VII. **Treatment**
   A. Orthopedic referral all curves >10°.
   B. Orthopedic treatment for curves 10–20° observation.
   C. Curves 20–40°: bracing (controversial) to prevent further curvature.
   D. Curves >40°: surgical intervention, posterior spinal fusion with segmental instrumentation occasionally requires anterior release.

VIII. **Follow-up**
   A. Per orthopedics: until skeletal maturity (about 1 year after menstruation for girls).

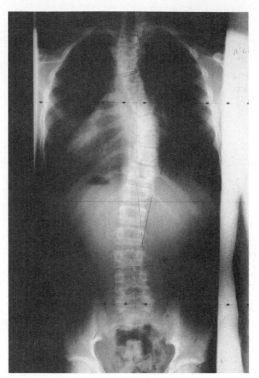

FIGURE 30-3 • Scoliosis radiograph.

IX. Complications

Lumbar back pain, 724.2

A. Progressive untreated scoliosis may result in significant deformity, cardiopulmonary compromise, debilitating lumbar back pain.

X. Education

A. If braces and/or exercises ordered, ensure compliance.
B. Bracing helps delay progression of curve.
C. Frequent skin inspection necessary with brace use.
D. Continue usual activities if pain free in brace.

HIP PAIN

Hip pain, 719.45

I. Differential diagnosis

A. Infection: septic arthritis, osteomyelitis, Lyme disease, psoas abscess, appendicitis.
B. Inflammatory: transient synovitis, systemic arthritis, juvenile rheumatoid arthritis (JRA), Kawasaki disease, idiopathic chondrolysis.

C. Orthopedic conditions: Legg-Calvé-Perthes disease, avascular necrosis (AVN), slipped capital femoral epiphysis (SCFE), stress fracture, apophyseal injuries, trochanteric bursitis, muscular strain.
D. Neoplastic: osteoid osteoma, leukemia, solid tumor, primary pigmented villonodular synovitis (PVNS), or sickle cell crisis pain.

SEPTIC HIP/SEPTIC ARTHRITIS

Appendicitis, 541.0	Osteomyelitis, 730.20
Avascular necrosis, 733.40	Pigmented villonodular synovitis
Chondrolysis, 733.99	(PVNS), 719.20
Juvenile rheumatoid arthritis, 714.30	Psoas abscess, 015.0
Kawasaki disease, 446.1	Septic arthritis, 711.0
Legg-Calvé-Perthes disease, 732.1	Sickle cell crisis, 282.60
Leukemia, 208.9	Slipped capitol femoral epiphysis, 732.2
Lyme disease, 088.81	Systemic arthritis, 716.9
Muscular strain, 848.9	Transient synovitis, 727.00
Osteoma, 213.9	Trochanteric bursitis, 726.5

Infection in joint; hip joint is infected second only to knee in children.
I. **Etiology**
   A. Bacterial infection spread hematogenously or from osteomyelitis of the femoral head.
   B. Most common organisms are *Staphylococcus* and *Streptococcus.*
II. **Occurrence**
   A. Males = females; infancy to 6 years.
III. **Clinical manifestations**
   A. Hip pain.
   B. Refusal to bear weight.
   C. Fever.
   D. Ill-appearing child with extreme pain and resistance to hip motion. Infection builds up pressure in hip capsule and can impede blood flow.
IV. **Physical findings**
   A. Fever >98.6°F (37°C), typically lie with hip flexed and externally rotated.
   B. Infants may be irritable with pseudoparalysis of lower extremity.
V. **Diagnostic tests**
   A. Elevate WBC and ESR.
   B. Ultrasound or radiographs demonstrate widening of joint space.
   C. Diagnosis confirmed with CT or ultrasound-guided aspiration.
VI. **Differential diagnosis**

Septic sacroiliac joint, 711.08

   A. Septic sacroiliac joint.

VII. Treatment
  A. Emergent referral to hospital for surgical drainage of hip joint.
  B. Intravenous antibiotics tailored to culture results.
  C. Keep child NPO.
VIII. Follow-up
  A. Per orthopedics, usually 1–2 weeks postop and 3–6 months to follow hip maturity.
IX. Complications

Joint destruction, 718.9
Osteomyelitis, 730.20
Septicemia, 038.9

  A. Septicemia, osteomyelitis, joint destruction.
X. Education
  A. Prepare family for child's hospitalization and treatment with IV antibiotics.

DEVELOPMENTALLY DISLOCATED HIP

Breech birth, 763.0
Dislocated hip, 835.00
Hip dysplasia, 755.63

Broad spectrum of hip dysplasia regarding dislocated or dislocatable or subluxing femoral head in relation to acetabulum at birth or early development.
  I. Etiology
    A. Genetic, intrauterine position, postnatal positioning.
  II. Occurrence
    A. Most common hip disorder in children.
    B. 1 in 100 infants have hip instability at birth and true dislocation is seen in 1 of 1000 births.
    C. Ratio: 6 female to 1 male.
    D. Left hip > right.
    E. Higher frequency in firstborn children.
  III. Clinical manifestations
    A. Breech birth commonly associated with this condition.
    B. Difficulty diapering (abducting leg).
    C. Older children may have awkward Trendelenburg gait, leg length discrepancy, pain with ambulation.
  IV. Physical findings
    A. Difficult in infants due to variety of levels of hip dysplasia.
    B. Unequal thigh skin creases/gluteal folds.
    C. Limited abduction.
    D. Positive Barlow's maneuver (to see if dislocatable with femur flexed and midline: adduct 10° gentle pressure posterior feel click with telescoping) (Figure 30-4).
    E. Positive Ortolani's maneuver (abducting hip, feel it clunk back into place) (Figure 30-5).

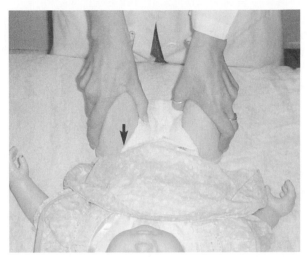

FIGURE 30-4 • Barlow's maneuver: knees flexed and brought to midline with gentle downward pressure to see if hip "clunks" out posteriorly.

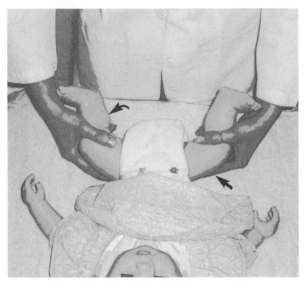

FIGURE 30-5 • Ortolani's maneuver: abduct hip while pushing up posteriorly with fingers trying to pop hip into the socket. A click is a positive finding.

    F. Galeazzi's test (prone with knees flexed and heels at buttock): positive when knee heights are different (Figure 30-6).

V. Diagnostic tests

Arthrogryposis, 728.3	Leg length discrepancy, 736.81
Congenital anomalies, 759.9	Septic hip, 711.08

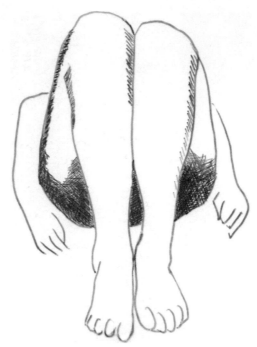

FIGURE 30-6 • Positive Galeazzi test. Note knee height difference.

    A. Ultrasound of hips. Radiographs less helpful because femoral heads have not ossified.

  VI. Differential diagnosis

    A. Congenital anomalies, arthrogryposis, septic hip, leg length discrepancy.

  VII. Treatment

    A. Refer to orthopedist.

    B. Treatment goal: reduce femoral head to anatomic position.

    C. May need Pavlik harness, hip spica cast, or surgical intervention.

VIII. Follow-up

    A. Reexamine hips each visit.

  IX. Complications

Degenerated changes, 721.90	Scoliosis, 737.30
Dysplasia, 755.63	Unstable gait, 781.2
Low back pain, 724.2	

    A. Delayed treatment affects normal growth of hip joint.

    B. If untreated: residual dysplasia, limited range of motion, unstable gait, pain, functional scoliosis, low back pain, early degenerated changes.

  X. Education

    A. Report any range-of-motion or neurovascular changes.

    B. Important to hold and cuddle baby even in braces and casts.

TRANSIENT SYNOVITIS

Fever, low-grade, 780.6
Transient synovitis, 727.00
Urinary tract infection, 599.0

I. Etiology
A. Unknown theory of post-traumatic or allergic cause.
B. Infection frequently assumed because 32–50% follow upper respiratory tract infection.

II. Occurrence
A. 0.2–3% Children 3–8 years of age; 6:1 male-to-female ratio.

III. Clinical manifestations
A. Pain and limp.

IV. Physical findings
A. Symptoms present <1 week to 1 month.
B. Fever absent or low grade. Do not appear severely ill.

V. Diagnostic tests
A. Negative CBC and ESR.
B. Ultrasound positive: effusion.

VI. Differential diagnosis

Legg-Calvé-Perthes disease, 732.1
Osteomyelitis, 730.20
Septic arthritis, 711.0

A. Septic arthritis MUST be ruled out. Osteomyelitis, Legg-Calvé-Perthes disease.

VII. Treatment
A. Conservative.
B. NSAIDs, rest, return to activity as tolerated.

VIII. Follow-up
A. If concerned, follow up in 1–2 days to be sure symptoms are resolving.

IX. Complications

Legg-Calvé-Perthes disease, 732.1
Septic arthritis, 711.0

A. Missed septic arthritis (rare).
B. 1–2% May develop Legg-Calvé-Perthes disease.

X. Education
A. Any fever >101.1°F (38.4°C) or ill appearance of child should prompt reexamination.

HIP PAIN: LEGG-CALVÉ-PERTHES DISEASE

Hip pain, 719.45
Legg-Calvé-Perthes disease, 732.1
Transient synovitis, 727.00

Idiopathic AVN of femoral head in children.

I. Etiology

A. Unknown cause of avascularity; however, multiple theories include trauma, transient synovitis, systemic abnormalities, vascular disturbances from intraosseous venous hypertension and venous obstruction.

II. Occurrence

A. 1 in 1200 general population.

B. 4:1 male- to-female ratio.

C. Typically 4–8 years of age.

D. Bilateral in only 15%, report of being associated with attention deficit hyperactivity disorder (ADHD).

III. Clinical manifestations

A. Pain of groin, medial thigh, or knee.

IV. Physical findings

A. Pain with weight bearing.

B. Limited internal rotation or abduction of hip.

C. Muscle spasm may have atrophy of thigh, calf, or buttock from disuse.

D. Leg length inequality.

V. Diagnostic tests

A. Radiographs: AP pelvis and frog lateral hips.

B. Initial x-rays may be normal; may need CT to see early changes.

C. Four stages:

1. Initial: interruption of blood supply, "crescent sign" areas of hyper- and hypodense appearance of femoral head.
2. Fragmentation: epiphysis appears fragmented.
3. Reossification: normal bone density returns, deformity becomes apparent.
4. Healed: healing complete, residual deformity common.

VI. Differential diagnosis

Knee fracture, 822.0	Slipped capital femoral epiphysis (SCFE), **732.2**
Septic hip, 711.08	Transient synovitis, **727.00**

A. Knee problem, fracture.

B. Transient synovitis.

C. Septic hip, SCFE.

D. Neuromuscular condition.

VII. Treatment

A. Refer to orthopedist.

B. Goal: prevent femoral head deformity, alter growth disturbances.

C. Generally try to unload femoral head while allowing motion.

D. Abduction brace and bed rest, home traction with legs progressive abduction.

E. Surgical adductor release or derotational femoral or pelvic osteotomies and spica body cast occasionally needed.

VIII. Follow-up

A. Per orthopedics.

B. Patients will be followed long term, bed rest with traction, bracing and surgery performed as indicated.

IX. Complications

Degenerated changes, 721.90
Unstable gait, 781.2

    A. May not show on initial films.
    B. Delayed treatment affects normal growth of hip joint.
    C. Residual deformities (coax magna), limited range of motion, unstable gait, pain, early degenerated changes seen with treated and untreated.

X. Education

    A. Progressive until body replaces "dead" femoral head with new bone; younger it occurs, longer body has to replace collapsing bone and remodel femoral head.
    B. No pressure should be put on rebuilding bone, but should be able to move in joint for shaping.

HIP PAIN: SLIPPED CAPITAL FEMORAL EPIPHYSIS

Slipped capital femoral epiphysis, 732.2

Femoral neck "slips" (displaces anteriorly) at physis (growth plate), leaving femoral head behind in acetabulum (Figure 30-7).

I. Etiology

    A. Unknown; however, suspect multifactorial cause, biomechanical, obesity, endocrine, metabolic, trauma, genetics, and other causes (i.e., kidney disorders or radiation).

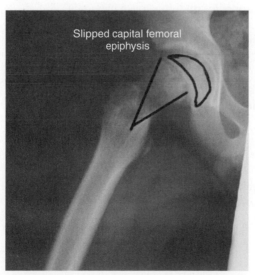

FIGURE 30-7 • Slipped capital femoral epiphysis. Note the appearance of ice cream falling off the cone.

II. Occurrence:
  A. Most common hip disorder of adolescents, 3 of 100,000 are 8–17 years of age.
  B. Males (10–17 years of age) affected 2–3 times more than females (8–15 years of age).
  C. Left hip most often affected; bilateral 25–70%.

III. Clinical manifestations
  A. Hip, groin, medial thigh, knee pain sometimes for months.
  B. May be brought on by very minor trauma (chronic/acute/or acute on chronic).
  C. Antalgic gait (limp to keep weight off painful extremity) or inability to bear weight.

IV. Physical findings
  A. Range of motion may be limited depending on severity of slip, may have limited internal rotation and abduction of the hip.

V. Diagnostic tests
  A. Radiographs: AP pelvis and true lateral (not frog lateral because may cause more femoral head displacement).

VI. Differential diagnosis

Appendicitis, 541.
Hip pain, 719.45
Testicular torsion, 608.2

  A. Knee problem.
  B. Infection.
  C. Inflammation.
  D. Referred pain such as appendicitis, testicular torsion.
  E. Other orthopedic conditions or malignancy.

VII. Treatment
  A. Immediate referral to orthopedist.
  B. DO NOT allow further weight bearing because femoral head can "slip" further.
  C. Surgical intervention with "pinning" by screw(s) to fuse physis between femoral head and neck.

VIII. Follow-up
  A. Orthopedics typically allow partial weight bearing with crutches for 6–8 weeks.
  B. Return in 2 weeks for wound check, staple removal.
  C. Follow healing clinically and radiographically for several months/year.

IX. Complications

Avascular necrosis, 733.40	Degenerative changes, 721.90
Chondrolysis, 733.99	Malunion, 733.81

  A. Missed on x-ray 25%.
  B. Avascular necrosis.

C. Chondrolysis (acute hylan cartilage necrosis).

D. Loss of range of motion.

E. Limb shortening.

F. Early degenerative changes.

G. Malunion.

X. Education.

A. High incidence of recurrence of other hip.

B. Parents or child should report any similar findings and be seen immediately.

KNEE PAIN: OSGOOD-SCHLATTER DISEASE

Knee pain, 719.46
Osgood Schlatter disease, 732.4

Painful swelling of tibial tubercle, caused by traction and resulting in apophysitis.

I. Etiology

A. Overuse by chronic repetitive knee flexion.

II. Occurrence

A. 11–14 years of age during rapid growth.

B. Males > females, but ratio changing with increased female participation in sports.

C. Frequently bilateral.

III. Clinical manifestations

A. Pain with running, jumping, kneeling. Resolves/fades with rest.

IV. Physical findings

A. Pain anterior knee, warmth, swelling and tenderness over tibial tubercle, especially with resistive knee extension (kicking motion) or squatting.

V. Diagnostic tests

A. Radiographs of knee: AP and lateral and 10-degree obliques to rule out tumor or fracture.

B. Classic prominent tibial tubercle above physis (Figure 30-8).

VI. Differential diagnosis

Knee fracture, 822.0
Sinding-Larsen-Johansson disease, 732.4

A. Tumor.

B. Fracture.

C. Sinding-Larsen Johansson disease (apophysitis of distal pole of patella).

VII. Treatment

A. Limit activities, especially sports, ice at end.

B. Hamstring and quadriceps stretching and strengthening.

C. Knee immobilizer or cylinder casting for severe pain for brief periods.

D. Ibuprofen.

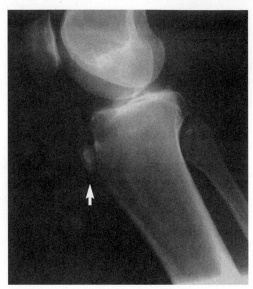

FIGURE 30-8 • Osgood-Schlatter disease: apophysitis of the tibial tubercle.

VIII. Follow-up

A. Teach patients, families to decrease activity, wear knee immobilizer when painful.

B. Follow up until skeletal maturity seen in closure of physis or growth plate.

IX. Complications

Apophysis deformity, 738.9
Enlargement of tibial tubercle, 718.86
Tibia fracture, 823.80

A. Enlargement of tibial tubercle (bony prominence).

B. Pain may continue into adulthood.

C. Fracture of tibial tubercle.

D. Premature closure of apophysis causing recurvatum deformity.

X. Education

A. "Bump" made because body thinks there is injury to bone which is being pulled apart at growth plate by patella; tendon bump will NOT go away.

B. Continued use while painful, typically increases size of "bump"; this is cosmetically unappealing for most and may interfere with kneeling. Condition ceases to exacerbate on skeletal maturity.

PHYSIOLOGIC GENU VARUM (BOW LEGS)

Genu varum, 736.42

I. Etiology

A. Physiologic genu varum or bowing is part of normal development.

II. Occurrence

A. Most common cause of bowlegs in toddlers.

B. Varum is greatest at 6 months of age, may progress to neutral by 18–24 months of age.

C. Adult physiologic valgus (knock knee): about 8°, typically reached by 5–6 years of age.

III. Clinical manifestations

A. Pain-free bowing appearance to legs of toddler.

IV. Physical findings

A. Gentle curve to entire leg.

B. Normal knee flexion, extension without pain.

C. Normal progression: 15° genu varum at birth (Figure 30-9); 0° (straight) 18–24 months; 10–12° genu valgum (knock knees) at 30 months to 4 years; 0° (straight) to 4–6° genu valgum normal at 4–6 years.

V. Diagnostic tests

A. Radiographic bowing of entire limb, no acute angulation seen (Figure 30-9).

B. Medial proximal tibial physeal changes suggestive of pathology (Blount's disease), refer to orthopedist.

VI. Differential diagnosis

Achondroplasia, 756.4	Osteogenesis imperfecta, 756.51
Blount's disease, 732.4	Osteomyelitis, 730.20
Chondrodysplasia, 756.4	Renal failure, 593.9
Leg fracture, 827.0	Rickets, 268.0

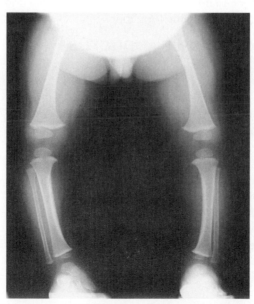

FIGURE 30-9 • Physiologic genu varum. Normal "beaking" of distal femur and proximal tibial metaphysis.

    A. Blount's disease, vitamin D-resistant rickets, renal failure, chondrodysplasia, achondroplasia, osteogenesis imperfecta, osteomyelitis, neoplasm, fracture.

VII. Treatment

    A. Generally resolve spontaneously.

    B. Refer to orthopedics for obvious asymmetry, clear progressive deformity or if associated with pain.

    C. Osteotomy and correction of angulation may be performed using internal or external fixation devices.

VIII. Follow-up

    A. Return visits every 3–6 months.

IX. Complications

Blount's disease, 732.4
Tibia vara, 732.4

    A. Tibial vara or Blount's disease (abrupt deformity medial proximal tibia).

    B. May be seen <5 years of age but more common in adolescents.

    C. Female > male.

    D. Bilateral 80%.

    E. Higher incidence in obese and African American children.

    F. Will not correct with age.

X. Education

    A. Reassurance of normal finding.

    B. Encourage child not to sleep or sit with legs tucked underneath; position might delay spontaneous correction.

IN-TOEING: METATARSUS ADDUCTUS

Metatarsus abductus varus, 754.53

I. Etiology

    A. Unknown, theory of intrauterine position.

II. Occurrence

    A. Most common childhood foot problem.

    B. 1 in 5000 births.

    C. 1:20 in sibling.

    D. Males, twins, preterm infants have higher incidence.

    E. Seen 1st year of life; left > right often bilateral.

III. Clinical manifestations

    A. Medial deviation of forefoot on hindfoot, in-toeing gait.

IV. Physical findings

    A. C-shaped foot.

V. Diagnostic tests

    A. No radiographs needed for infants.

    B. Children >4 years of age should have standing foot films, 3 views.

VI. Differential diagnosis

Spastic anterior tibialis, 781.0
Talipes equinovarus, 754.51

   A. Spastic anterior tibialis.
   B. Talipes equinovarus (clubbed foot).

VII. Treatment

   A. Most will correct with normal use.
   B. Severe deformity: refer to orthopedist for stretching, serial casting of flexible conditions, surgical intervention is rare.

VIII. Follow-up

   A. Per orthopedics until deformity is corrected.
   B. Serial casting may be done weekly. Have parents remove semirigid cast night before appointment. Teach to stretch then apply new cast with orthopedist holding position.

IX. Complications

   A. Cast/skin complications.
   B. Neurovascular problems.
   C. Incorrect position, especially if cast slips and toes are no longer visible (common with infants).

X. Education

   A. Most resolve spontaneously.
   B. Return to orthopedist if circulation problems, irritability (i.e., suspect cast is bothering child), or if child kicks cast off.

IN-TOEING: TIBIAL TORSION

Tibial torsion, 736.89

I. Etiology

   A. Normal development in utero, genetic influence.

II. Occurrence

   A. Birth 0–20° internal tibial rotation normal: 90% correct with growth, adults achieve 0–20° of external rotation.

III. Clinical manifestations

   A. Curved appearance to tibia or in-toeing or out-toeing gait.
   B. If knees are pointing forward, feet may either point in (internal tibial torsion) or out (external tibial torsion); becomes less noticeable with running.

IV. Physical findings

   A. Thigh-foot angle (Figure 30-10). Child prone with knee bent at 90° angle of imaginary line drawn down thigh and middle of foot. Normal 0–30° external.
   B. Foot progression angle is angle of foot compared to line extended in front of ambulating child. Best observed from directly behind patient (Figure 30-11).

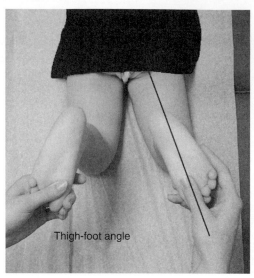

FIGURE 30-10 • Thigh-foot angle. A line drawn along the axis of the femur bisects the foot.

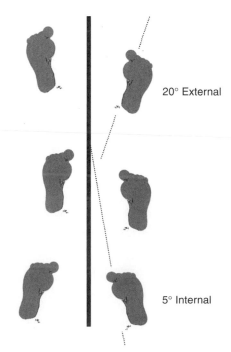

FIGURE 30-11 • Foot progression angle: normal variations.

V. Diagnostic tests
A. None if <8 years of age and symmetrical pain-free appearance.
B. If needed, standing leg length x-ray (scanogram) done on long cassette.
VI. Differential diagnosis

Hip dysplasia, 755.3

A. Developmental dysplasia of hip, neuromuscular conditions.
VII. Treatment
A. Observation.
B. None unless unilateral or severe or remains after age 8.
C. Tibial osteotomy rare but may be performed for severe cases.
VIII. Follow-up
A. If persists at 8 years of age, refer to orthopedist.
IX. Complications
A. Rare and related to surgical intervention.
X. Education
A. Reassurance and handouts.
B. Despite grandparents' insistence, braces are not effective. Studies show same improvement or correction through normal growth without braces.
C. Many athletic children, adults have tibial torsion; does not result in any increased incidence of arthritis or interfere with activity.

IN-TOEING: FEMORAL ANTEVERSION

Femoral anteversion, 755.63

I. Etiology
A. Normal and appears when child begins walking, causing ligaments to get looser; thus hips are allowed more internal rotation esp. in children 2–6 years of age.
II. Occurrence
A. Normal in 2- to 4-year-olds, usually corrects spontaneously by age 8.
III. Clinical manifestations
A. In-toeing gait.
B. Children tend to "W" sit pain free.
IV. Physical findings
A. Knees and toes point inward when standing.
B. Able to internally rotate hips up to 90 degrees.
V. Diagnostic tests
A. None.
VI. Differential diagnosis

Hip dysplasia, 755.63
Tibial torsion, 736.89

A. Tibial torsion, hip dysplasia.

VII. Treatment
   A. Discourage "W" sitting.
   B. Observation unless functional deformity after 8 years old.
   C. Refer to orthopedist for unilateral, severe, or painful deformity.
   D. Surgical intervention with femoral derotational osteotomy.

VIII. Follow-up
   A. Yearly if not progressive.

IX. Complications
   A. None unless surgical intervention.

X. Education
   A. Normal, child will grow out of it. Braces or shoe modification are ineffective.

FOOT PROBLEMS: TALIPES EQUINOVARUS (CLUBBED FOOT)

Clubbed foot, 754.51

Talipes equinovarus, 754.51

Rigid fixed foot deformity with inverted heel, forefoot adduction, and down-facing toes.

I. Etiology
   A. Unknown; possibly genetic, mechanical, chemical embryologic insults.

II. Occurrence
   A. Age: newborn.
   B. 2:1 males to females.
   C. 1.24 in 1000 live births.
   D. Increased incidence in families where parents/siblings have same disorder.

III. Clinical manifestations
   A. Tight Achilles tendon, joint capsule, medial ligaments.
   B. Short angulated talus, thin atrophic muscles.

IV. Physical findings
   A. Small foot and calf, with rigid equinus deformed foot with heel in varus.
   B. Prominent crease in arch of foot.
   C. Adducted forefoot.

V. Diagnostic tests
   A. Clinical exam of newborn, radiographs are of little use.

VI. Differential diagnosis

Arthrogryposis, 728.3

Calcaneovalgus, 755.67

Spastic hemiplegia, 342.1

   A. "Positional clubbed foot," arthrogryposis, spastic hemiplegia, calcaneovalgus.

VII. Treatment
   A. Refer to orthopedist. Serial casting and surgical intervention may be necessary.

VIII. Follow-up
   A. Per orthopedist.

B. Treatment soon after birth: weekly visits for manipulation and casting by orthopedist experienced in this form of treatment.

C. If rigid deformity, surgical intervention may be necessary; may entail heel cord and joint capsule releases and casting typically at 6 months of age.

D. Casting or braces may be used for a period of time; follow-up is ongoing because deformity may recur until about age 7.

IX. Complications

Leg length discrepancy, 736.81

A. Progressive deformity, leg length discrepancy, surgical complications.

X. Education

A. Affected foot will always be smaller but may function near normal after correction.

PES PLANUS: FLATFOOT

Pes planus: flatfoot, 734.

I. Etiology

A. Flexible normal (asymptomatic) genetic etiology or rigid (symptomatic) tarsal coalition (fusion of calcaneus with talus or navicular) common cause.

II. Occurrence

A. Normal occurrence <2 years of age due to medial fat pad. Rigid is rare.

III. Clinical manifestations

A. Flat foot while standing; normal arch that returns while sitting and hanging over exam table is flexible pes planus.

B. Bilateral.

C. Hereditary expression.

D. May cause some discomfort for older children.

IV. Physical findings

A. Loss of normal plantar arch while standing.

B. Limited subtalar joint motion for rigid pes planus.

C. Look at parents' feet!

V. Diagnostic tests

A. If rigid: radiographs, standing 3 views of both feet, CT or MRI looking for coalition.

VI. Differential diagnosis

Arthritis, 716.97
Arthrogryposis, 728.3
Foot fracture, 825.20

A. Overuse.

B. Arthrogryposis.

C. Neuromuscular condition.

D. Arthritis.

     E. Infection.

     F. Trauma/fracture.

VII. Treatment

     A. Refer rigid to orthopedist, orthotics may decrease symptoms of older child with flexible pes planus.

     B. Apply before sling.

VIII. Follow-up

     A. May require further workup or referral if not pain free after 1 month.

IX. Complications

     A. None known.

X. Education

     A. Proper shoe wear. Sneakers with built in arch preferred.

NURSEMAID'S ELBOW: RADIAL HEAD SUBLUXATION

Nursemaid's elbow, 832.0

I. Etiology

     A. Traction along axis of extended pronated arm resulting in radial head subluxation with annular ligament displacement.

     B. Typically "pulling" child's hand/arm to prevent from falling or pulling away or swinging child by arms.

II. Occurrence

     A. Most common elbow injury of children age 1–4 years.

     B. Female > males.

     C. Left > right.

III. Clinical manifestations

     A. Will not use arm.

     B. Holds arm close to body with elbow slightly flexed and pronated (palm down).

IV. Physical findings

     A. Restricted supination of elbow.

     B. Typically nontender or swollen; however, exhibits distress if tries moving elbow.

V. Diagnostic tests

     A. Radiographs AP and lateral of elbow if questionable success of reduction (Note: many times these are reduced when arm is rotated to get lateral x-ray.)

VI. Differential diagnosis

Elbow fracture, 813.01

     A. Fracture.

VII. Treatment

     A. Reduction maneuver.

        1. Child in parent's lap.

   2. Flex child's elbow to 90° with gentle pressure of thumb over radial head.
   3. Fully or "hyper" pronate wrist then fully supinate wrist and typically click will be felt and child will stop resisting (Figure 30-12).
   B. Sling and refer to orthopedists if child fails to use arm.
VIII. Follow-up
   A. Call or visit to ensure child is using arm normally within 1 week.
 IX. Complications
   A. Unreduced radius.
  X. Education
   A. Teach parents mechanism of injury to prevent reoccurrence (30–40%).

GROWING PAINS

Growing pains, 781.99

   I. Etiology
   A. Unknown theory of periosteal irritation.
  II. Occurrence
   A. Peak in 3–5 and 8–12-year-olds.
 III. Clinical manifestations
   A. Muscular pain (not joint): thighs, calves, behind knee.
   B. Typically late afternoon, early evening after physically active day.
   C. Can wake child from sleep.

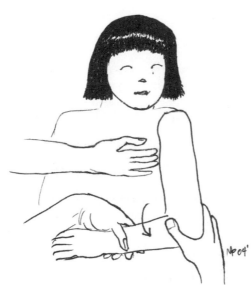

FIGURE 30-12 • Reduction maneuver for "nursemaid's elbow." Flex elbow to 90 degrees, fully pronate wrist (palm down) then with gentle pressure over radial head supinate the wrist (palm up).

IV. Physical findings

A. None.

V. Diagnostic tests

A. Only if suspicious, x-ray to exclude fracture/lesion.

VI. Differential diagnosis

A. Diagnosis of exclusion:

1. No fever.
2. Not in joint.
3. No swelling, erythema, warmth.
4. No trauma.
5. No weight loss, rashes, unusual fatigue or behavior.

VII. Treatment

A. Massage, heat, acetaminophen/ibuprofen.

VIII. Follow-up

A. Follow up if lasts >24 hours at time.

B. Follow up if child does not respond to medications and massage.

IX. Complications

A. None.

X. Education

A. Normal, may come and go, child is not "faking."

COSTROCONDRITIS

Costochondritis, 733.6

I. Etiology

A. Diagnosis of exclusion.

II. Occurrence

A. Unknown.

III. Clinical manifestations

A. Insidious and persistent lasting hours to days.

B. Worse with position change and deep breathing. May be diffuse or localized. Common after repetitive new activity of upper trunk and arms.

IV. Physical findings

A. Skin lesions, chest wall syndrome tests, "crowing rooster," "horizontal arm flexion," "hooking maneuver" diagnostic: if pain is reproduced, test is positive (Figure 30-13).

B. Chest expansion test (tape measure around chest at 4th intercostal level max) exhale then inhale = 5-cm excursion; <2.5 cm abnormal.

V. Treatment

A. NSAIDs, rest.

VI. Diagnostic tests

A. Radiographs of chest to rule out fracture or tumor.

B. CT, bone scan (most sensitive to rule out arthropathies, tumors, infection).

C. ESR, ANA, rheumatoid factor purpose to rule out: cardiopulmonary, abdominal sources associated with rheumatologic condition or assess structure of chest wall.

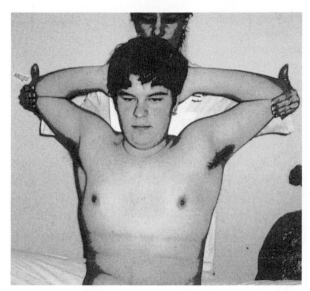

FIGURE 30-13 • "Crowing rooster" elbows are pulled back and up to expand chest. A positive test is when pain is reproduced with this maneuver.

VII. Differential diagnosis

Ankylosing spondylitis, 720.0
Fibromyalgia, 729.1
Sternoclavicular hyperostosis, 733.3

    A. Cardiopulmonary.
    B. Esophagus, head, neck, and interior chest wall.
    C. Ankylosing spondylitis.
    D. Sternoclavicular hyperostosis.
    E. Infection.
    F. Fibromyalgia.

VIII. Follow-up

    A. Within 2 weeks to document resolution of symptoms.

IX. Complications

    A. Missed diagnosis.

X. Education

    A. Call for changes in symptoms.

OSTEOPOROSIS

Osteoporosis, 733.00

I. Etiology

    A. Bony calcium deficit from various causes including lack of intake while prepubertal, absorption or metabolic origin.

II. Occurrence
A. Disease of childhood with severe adulthood complications.

III. Clinical manifestations
A. Majority (50–66%) of total body calcium is deposited to bone by end of puberty.

B. Earlier in females than males.

C. Highest velocity of increased bone mineral content within 9–12 months of menarche.

IV. Physical findings
A. Stress fractures, fractures with minimal trauma or no findings in childhood.

V. Diagnostic tests
A. Lack of calcium in past 3-day diet history.

B. Poor dietary habits.

C. High suspicion in lactose-intolerant or anorectic children.

VI. Differential diagnosis
A. None.

VII. Treatment
A. Increase dietary calcium intake or supplementation.

VIII. Follow-up
A. Continue to assess calcium intake, stress importance to prepubertal/pubescent children.

IX. Complications

Degenerative joint changes, 721.90
Dowager's hump (kyphosis), 737.10
Fractures, 829.0

A. Fractures.

B. Dowager's hump (kyphosis).

C. Early adulthood degenerative joint changes.

X. Education
A. 3 Servings of milk, cheese, yogurt daily: 1200 mg of calcium.

BIBLIOGRAPHY

American Academy of Pediatrics: Clinical practice guideline: Early detection of developmental dysplasia of the hip, *Pediatrics* 105(4):896-905, 2000.

Brooks WC, Gross RH: Genu varum in children: Diagnosis and treatment, *J Am Acad Orthopaedic Surgeons* 3(6):326-335, 1995.

Clark MC: Approaches to child with a limp, 2003; retrieved February 24, 2004, from *www.uptodate.com/appliction/topic/print.asp?file=ped_em/15821.*

Gregory PL., Biswas AC, Batt ME: Musculoskeletal problems of the chest wall in athletes, *Sports Med* 32(4):235-250, 2002.

Lincoln TL, Suen PW: Common rotational variations in children, *J Am Acad Orthopaedic Surgeons* 11(5):312-320, 2003.

Mason KJ: Pediatric/congenital disorders. In Schoen DC, editor: *Core curriculum for orthopaedic nursing,* Pitman, NJ, 2001, Anthony J Janetti, pp 238-300.

Moore BR, Bothner J: Radial head subluxation (nursemaid's elbow), 2003; retrieved February 24, 2004, from *www.uptodate.com/appliction/topic/print.asp?file=gen_pedi_em/22673.*

Nigrovic PA, Wilking AP: Overview of hip pain in childhood, 2002; retrieved February 23, 2004, from *www.uptodate.com/appliction/topic/print.asp?file=gen_pedi/21233&type= P&selected.*

Schoen DC, editor: *Core curriculum for orthopaedic nursing,* ed 4, Pitman, NJ, 2001, Anthony J Janetti.

Shelton YA, Mortimer E: Orthopaedic problems in the pediatric patient. In Steinberg G, Akins C, Baran D, editors: *Orthopaedics in primary care,* ed 3, Philadelphia, 1999, Lippincott Williams & Wilkins.

Wise CM: Clinical evaluation of musculoskeletal chest pain, 2001; retrieved February 24, 2004, from *www.uptodate.com/appliction/topic/print.asp?file=muscle/7511.*

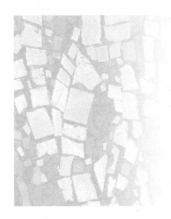

CHAPTER 31

Neurologic Disorders

SUSAN M. ROWLEY

ENCEPHALITIS

Altered consciousness, 780.09	Lethargy, 780.79
Confusion, 298.9	Seizure, 780.39
Encephalitis, 323.9	Stiff neck, 723.5
Headache, 784.0	Vomiting, 787.03
Irritability, 799.2	

I. Etiology

A. Inflammation of brain generally manifesting as brain dysfunction as a result of invasion or infection of brain tissue.

B. Type or source of infection.

C. Presenting symptoms will vary depending on cause and extent of involvement.

  1. Type: viral, aseptic, postinfectious, or autoimmune.

  2. Specific agent:

    a. Arboviruses (mosquito- and tick-borne).

    b. Herpes viruses (herpes, varicella, Epstein-Barr, cytomegalovirus [CMV]).

    c. Aseptic (unknown cause or presumptive unknown viral).

  3. Mode of invasion by agent with predilection to cause brain inflammation and dysfunction; direct inoculation (rabies, arboviruses, herpes simplex virus [HSV], enteroviruses) versus entities with predilection to secondary invasion of brain tissue; postinfectious (measles, varicella, influenza).

  4. Mode and site of inoculation: mouth/nose/lungs (varicella zoster virus [VZV], measles, mumps); genitalia (HSV); bowel (enteroviruses, echoviruses, cysticercosis) or via bite of an insect or animal (arthropod diseases, rabies).

  5. Immune response problems (immunocompromised, e.g., CMV encephalitis in HIV) or overreactive immune response (autoimmune: postinfectious encephalomyelitis).

6. Encephalitis secondary to underlying primary illness (e.g., Lyme or Lyme encephalitis).

II. Occurrence

A. Sporadic, such as opportunistic illness in immunocompromised hosts such as those with AIDS or cancer (e.g., CMV, chickenpox).

B. Seasonal: related to warm weather, outdoor activities.

C. Regional: sector prevalence.

D. Environmental: occupation, recreation, habits.

E. Age related: increased susceptibility in young, infirm, or elderly.

III. Clinical manifestations

A. Symptoms of specific brain involvement may include:

    1. Altered consciousness, irritability, sleepiness, lethargy, confusion, altered cry, stiff neck, seizure activity, headache, or cranial nerve dysfunction.

    2. Vomiting.

IV. Physical findings

A. Altered vital signs.

B. Rash.

C. Fever.

D. Meningeal irritation signs. Check specifically for:

    1. Brudzinski's sign (flexion of neck to chest causes flexion of both legs and thighs).

    2. Kernig's sign (recumbent leg cannot be extended with hip joint flexed at right angle).

E. Abnormal RTRs or emergence of primitive reflexes.

F. Abnormal sensory muscle strength, tone exam.

G. Abnormal cerebellar exam.

V. Diagnostic tests

A. If suspicious of encephalitis, may refer for spinal tap and/or admission depending on practice setting and ability to perform thorough workup.

B. Cerebrospinal fluid (CSF) analysis if intracranial pressure (ICP) not present.

C. CBC, erythrocyte sedimentation rate (ESR), urine, electrolytes, toxic screen.

D. Blood for antibodies.

E. Culture of blood, feces, nasopharyngeal swab.

F. EEG.

G. Head imaging study such as CT (quicker to rule out bleed or mass) or MRI to look for more subtle changes.

VI. Differential diagnosis

Autoimmune disorder, 279.4	Metabolic disorder, 277.9
Demyelinization, 341.9	Seizure disorder, 790.39
Intracranial hemorrhage, 432.9	

A. Infections/febrile illness of original or superimposed source.

B. Toxins, ingested or inhaled.

C. Seizure disorders with postictal state.

D. Masses or lesions.

E. Autoimmune disorder.

F. Demyelinization.

G. Metabolic disorders, especially inherited disorders now manifested by stress of acute illness.

H. Intracranial hemorrhage.

VII. Treatment

A. Hospitalization for initial effective treatment, which includes symptomatic and supportive care.

1. Antiemetics, antipyretics.
2. Fluids, electrolytes, IV therapy.
3. Increased ICP monitoring and management if needed.
4. Management to specific antivirals or antibiotics.
5. Specific medications for identified/suspected pathogens, therapies for underlying derangements caused by brain dysfunction over specific organ systems.

B. Antiviral therapy initiated promptly if treatable viral agent (e.g., herpes) is suspected, because may decrease morbidity and mortality and not be especially harmful.

VIII. Follow-up

A. Continued evaluation for sequelae; with regard to mental function and ability imperative.

B. Long-term follow-up may necessitate social, psychologic, school, vocational assistance, and family assessment and support.

IX. Complications

Herpes encephalitis, 054.3	Rabies, 071.
Immunodeficiency, 279.3	Rocky Mountain spotted fever, 082.0

A. Complications vary from mild to severe; can include coma to death.

B. Some entities are known for relatively high rate of complete recovery (Rocky Mountain spotted fever) to high rate of morbidity (herpes encephalitis) to definite mortality if untreated (rabies).

C. Immunocompromised state or immunodeficiency, whether innate, drug induced, or other disease related, alter these factors within given individual.

X. Education

A. For insect-borne sources.

1. Tick transmission.
    a. Clear brush, trim trees, and keep lawns mowed.
    b. Avoid or when in wooded areas, wear clothing with cuffs, long pants tucked in, apply DEET preparations sparingly, but not to face and hands.
    c. Inspect body after return inside.
    d. Remove tick immediately by using tweezer/fingers covered and remove as close as possible to tick's mouth.
2. Mosquito transmission.
    a. Clear standing water sources.
    b. Use insecticides when outdoors.

3. Body fluid transmission.
   a. Avoid shared vessels or utensils and crowded conditions.
   b. Use sexual, genital, and oral barrier methods.
   c. Use good hand washing and surface cleansing.
   d. Avoid contaminated needles and blood products.
   e. Use air filtration systems.
4. Environmental transmission.
   a. Wash hands.
   b. Boil water. Treat water or use only bottled water in endemic countries.
   c. Thoroughly cook contaminated meats.
   d. Thoroughly wash fruits and vegetables or avoid foods from endemic areas.
   e. Avoid contact with vector/host animals.
   f. Seek prompt care/evaluation for symptoms if living in or recently traveled to endemic areas.

HEADACHE

Benign paroxysmal vertigo, 386.11	Migraine, 346.9
Blurred vision, 368.8	Motion sickness, 994.6
Cyclic vomiting, 536.2	Nausea with vomiting, 787.01
Dizziness, 780.4	Photophobia, 368.13
Fatigue, 780.79	Presence of aura, 346.0
Headache, 784.0	Torticollis, 723.5
Irritability, 799.2	Vertigo, 780.4
Mental confusion, 298.9	

I. Etiology
   A. Complex series of events and processes involving several mechanisms of chemical or excitation response in brain related structures.
   B. Process of vasodilatation/vasoconstriction, trigeminal nerve irritation, thalamic threshold alterations, and alterations in specific brain chemicals have been implicated.
   C. May be idiopathic, genetically linked, or arise from structural sources.
   D. Intimately intertwined with variety of correlates such as concomitant illness, hormonal changes, sociodemographic factors, lifestyle factors, medications, substances, and environmental influences.

II. Incidence
   A. One of the most common presenting complaints to emergency departments.
   B. Varies with increasing incidence with age.
      1. By 15 years of age, 3 times as many have frequent nonmigranous headaches as migraine.
      2. By 3 years of age, 3–8% report headaches.
      3. By 5 years of age, 19.5% report headaches.
      4. Age 7, 37–57% report headaches; <15 years of age, 25% have significant headaches. Accounts for 10% of school absences.

C. More than half of persons suffering from migraine who meet International Headache Society criteria never received medical diagnosis of migraine.
D. As presenting complaint, headaches often are mixed in type and often represent mixture of underlying headache entities such as:
1. Tension.
2. Various migraine types: common (without aura) or complex (with aura), though complex are rare in children.
3. Chronic daily headaches (CDHs): may be medication overuse headaches (MOHs).
4. Other substance overuse (e.g., caffeine, marijuana): rebound headaches.
5. Increasing evidence that depression and increased rates of addictive personality characteristics surface in those with chronic headache into adulthood.

III. Clinical manifestations

A. Known correlates of diagnoses with migraine, particularly torticollis, cyclic vomiting, benign paroxysmal vertigo, and motion sickness.
B. Most evaluation is history to ascertain: if probable benign condition or a concerning condition representing serious pathology if exam is abnormal, especially neuro exam, then is concern for pathologic conditions leading to headache.
C. Assess for:
1. Level of head pain. Use pain scale.
2. Irritability, mental confusion, fatigue.
3. Blurry/altered vision.
4. Presence of aura, vertigo, dizziness, photophobia, phonophobia.
5. Nausea/vomiting.

IV. Physical findings

A. May have none if not having cephalgia at time of exam.
B. Demeanor of pain (prefer quiet, dark, not moving or is lively, functional).
C. Altered vital signs indicative of pain (e.g., increased HR, B/P, RR).
D. Abnormal neuro exam: heightens probability that pathology may be present.

V. Diagnostic tests

Controversial, but may consider:
A. CBC, ESR.
B. Electrolytes, thyroid function, toxin screen.
C. EEG not generally recommended. May not help unless child has altered consciousness.
D. If increased ICP is suspected or there are neuro exam abnormalities, an urgent CT imaging with/without contrast is indicated to outline a particular pathology. Perform CT before LP to R/O mass lesion and herniation.
E. Absence of increased ICP and normal urgent CT: lumbar puncture is warranted if there is papilledema to rule out or to aid diagnosis and treat pseudotumor cerebri or if meningitis or encephalitis is concern.
F. MRI is the preferred study for non-urgent cases to delineate structure and formation.

VI. Differential diagnosis

Anemia, 285.9	Hypothyroidism, 244.9
Brain tumor, 239.6	Intracranial bleed, 432.9
Glaucoma, 365.9	Intracranial pressure, 781.99
Head trauma, 959.01	Metabolic disorder, 277.9
Hypertension, 401.9	Stroke, 436.
Hyperthyroidism, 242.90	

- **A.** Hypertension.
- **B.** Anemia.
- **C.** Thyroid problems particularly hypothyroidism/hyperthyroidism.
- **D.** Toxins, infections.
- **E.** Metabolic inborn or acquired errors.
- **F.** Increased ICP may include shunt malfunction if shunt is present.
- **G.** Stroke, tumor/masses, intracranial bleed.
- **H.** Trauma.
- **I.** Glaucoma.

VII. Treatment

- **A.** If there is underlying pathology, treat the pathology.
- **B.** Adequate on-going treatment, whether pathologic or ideopathic, consists of prevention (prophylaxis) and acute management.
  1. Prevention recommendations for most common headache types in children:
     a. Nonpharmacologic.
        - Adequate rest/sleep.
        - Adequate, balanced nutrition.
        - Avoidance and discontinuation of caffeine, marijuana, other ingested/inhaled substances with withdrawal symptom potential.
        - Avoidance and discontinuation of overusage of pain relievers.
        - Adequate hydration.
        - Stress management/relaxation techniques used on a regular basis.
        - Support groups or counseling.
     b. Pharmacologic medications: antihistamines, antihypertensives, calcium channel blockers, antidepressants, antiseizure medications (Table 31-1).
  2. Acute management.
     a. Nonpharmacologic.
        - Rest, quiet, darkness.
        - Cool or warm cloths on forehead; warm baths/showers.
        - Stress management/relaxation techniques.
        - Biofeedback.
        - Massage, acupressure, aromatherapy.
     b. Pharmacologic: nonsteroidal antiinflammatory drugs (NSAIDS), Triptans, OTC analgesic combination medications, prescription combination medications, prescription ergotamines.

TABLE 31-1 • Prevention medications for headaches

Remember that dosages needed for headache and migraine prophylaxis are generally lower than that needed for its primary use category, so start with lowest dose and gradually increase to efficacy without side effects. Make adjustments after 2–4 weeks and use trials of 4–6 months if efficacy is evident.

Medication	Dosage ranges/ recommendations	Indications and advantages of use	Precautions and disadvantages of use
Beta blockers: Inderal (propanolol)	■ 1–2 mg/kg/d up to 4 mg/kg/d ■ Begin at 10 mg at bedtime, may work up to 40 mg at bedtime, rarely is 60 mg/d needed for adult size patients (divide the higher doses bid) ● 2 mg/kg; or <35 kg, 10–20 mg up to tid; >35 kg, 20–40 mg up to tid ■ Wean when discontinuing	■ Long-term experience ■ Efficacy documented at low doses: ● relatively few side effects (advantage to keep doses low and give only at bedtime) ● safe for younger children if BP and HR not already low for age	■ Avoid use with: Depression, may aggravate symptoms RAD/asthma Vagal tendencies Very athletic with low HR ■ May cause sexual dysfunction, especially in males ■ Pregnancy Category C ■ Discontinue if not effective after 4–6 weeks
Calcium channel blockers: Calan (verapamil)	■ Begin at 40 mg/d; may work up to 80–120 mg tid ■ General dose 4 mg/kg/d divided tid ■ Wean when discontinuing	■ Works best with migraines with aura, which are rare in children ■ Little toxicity if used in children without cardiac abnormalities	■ Avoid with those with hypotension ■ Caution with CYP 3A4 medications ■ Pregnancy Category C
Tricyclic antidepressants: Elavil (amitriptyline) Pamelor (nortriptyline)	■ Amitriptyline: start with smallest dose size of ½ of 10 mg or 10 mg or 1 mg/kg/d at bedtime. Increase gradually by 10 mg after 1–2 weeks on each dose. Teens may need 25 mg to start if adult size. ■ Nortriptyline: begin with 10 mg/d, may increase to 30 mg/d if tolerated ■ Wean when discontinuing	■ Both helpful in depression or sleep disturbances as aid in sleep initiation, quality ■ Amitriptyline works well to help with initial coverage of daily acute medication overuse (rebound)	■ Caution with underlying cardiac abnormalities; consider ECG first and episodically while used ■ As with all tricyclics, caution with possible suicide from overdose; limit the supply and caution re: access to med ■ Can lead to daytime drowsiness, interference with ADLs

Continued

TABLE 31-1 • Prevention medications for headaches—cont'd

Medication	Dosage ranges/ recommendations	Indications and advantages of use	Precautions and disadvantages of use

Antiseizure medications: Depakene/ Depakote (valproates) Topamax (topiramate) Neurontin (gabapentin)	■ Valproates: begin with 10–15 mg/kg/d, may give at bedtime only or bid to tid. Rarely >30 mg/kg/d is needed. >16 years: usual initial dose is 250 mg bid.
	 ■ Topiramate generally begun at 15 mg (sprinkle) for school-age child or 25 mg (sprinkle or tablet) for older youth/teens; or 1 mg/kg/d and no greater than 25 mg/d for at least the first week. May gradually increase by 1–3 mg/kg/d at 1–2 week intervals. Max 5–9 mg/kg/d bid (antiseizure doses), which are rarely needed.
	 ■ Gabapentin initial dose is 10 mg/kg/d or one 100-mg capsule at bedtime. Comes in solution also of 250 mg/5 mL. May gradually increase to 25–35 mg/kg/d (antiseizure doses) if necessary.
		■ Valproates can have level measured (therapeutic level for seizures 40–100)
		 ■ Depakote: FDA-approved for migraines in those ≥16
		 ■ Topiramate has potential for decreasing appetite.
		 ■ Gabapentin: few side effects or interactions
			■ "Toxicity" of anticonvulsants: "drunklike" behavior, warrants a decrease/discontinuation of medication
			 ■ Valproates: liver function and platelet monitoring initially and episodically (q3–6mo)
			   • Pregnancy Category D
			   • May have more GI symptoms (e.g., upset stomach, diarrhea, weight gain)
			   • May have hair loss
			 ■ Topiramate: acute myopia and angle-closure glaucoma reported, so ensure routine vision care
			   • Kidney stones also reported so ensure adequate fluids
			   • Pregnancy Category C
			 ■ Gabapentin is pregnancy Category C

Antihistamine: Periactin (cyproheptadine)	■ 0.25–0.4 mg/kg or 2–4 mg at bedtime and may work up to bid or tid	■ Works best for toddler and early school-age child ■ May be useful for those with allergies	■ Can have antihistamine side effects of dry mouth and drowsiness ■ Less effective for older children and teen

C. Remember: to break cycle of chronic daily headaches, offending overused acute agent must be stopped and future acute medications not used > twice per week.
- PO steroids may be tried or ergots via IV in overuse scenario.
- Prevention medications may be needed as well.
- Hospitalization may be required initially if the IV route of medication is needed.
- Amitriptyline PO is one agent recommended for prophylaxis in medication/substance overuse circumstance, may be started OP (Table 31-2).

VIII. Follow-up
A. For continuing symptomatology and medication adjustment: once per month or every several months for visits (initiation, treatment takes months to assess).
B. If cause is acute, symptomatic and therapeutic care of etiology is needed.
C. Reevaluation is warranted any time initial premise and diagnosis do not fit or symptoms persist or worsen with time or new symptoms emerge.

IX. Complications

Activity disruption, 780.99
Drug addiction, 304.9

A. Long-term tendency toward addictive substances.
B. Side effects of medications.
C. Disruption of daily living activities(e.g., school, extracurricular activities, work).

X. Education
A. Stress management, coping methods tailored to age of child and concern.
B. Importance of adherence to nonpharmacologic and pharmacologic regimes.
C. Measure change over weeks generally rather than days.
D. Excellent websites: www.headachecare.com and www.achenet.org.

HEAD TRAUMA

Alterations of level consciousness, 780.09   Nausea, 787.02
Confusion, 298.9   Skull fracture, 803.0
Head trauma, 959.01   Vomiting, 787.03
Intracranial pressure, 781.99

I. Etiology
A. Any alteration in integrity of cerebral structure or surrounding/supportive head structures.
B. Process can be short term or permanent.
C. Level of recovery determined by degree of insult.
D. Children have unique ability to "reassign" functions from one location in brain to others; therefore, sometimes able to perform old functions via new pathways (plasticity) (Figures 31-1, 31-2, and 31-3).

TABLE 31-2 • Acute headache and migraine medications for youth

Remember use > twice per week (per 1 or 2 doses up to max per 24 hours regime) for extended periods of time for headache often leads to rebound. Effect of medications not already containing caffeine may be boosted by taking in non-cola caffeine with medication, if nausea and vomiting do not feature predominantly.

NSAIDS:

Tylenol (acetaminophen) (can be combined with codeine)	Acetaminophen: 10–15 mg/kg/dose q4–6h prn	■ OTC ■ Tylenol available in suppository for those with nausea/vomiting; has less GI upset potential ■ Acetaminophen may be allowed during pregnancy	■ Acetaminophen does not have antiinflammatory effect, often less effective
Motrin, Advil (ibuprofen) Aleve (naproxen sodium)	Ibuprofen: 5–10 mg/kg/d q6–8h prn with greater efficacy seen in 10 mg/kg/d range with max of 800 mg dose up to tid Naproxen sodium: 220 mg 1–2 tabs at onset, may repeat once more in 24 hours. Generally reserved for those 75–100 lbs		■ Ibuprofen and naproxen sodium not recommended in pregnancy ■ Best taken with food ■ Discourage narcotic use because of later dependency potential
Combination Medications: "Migraine" OTC: Motrin and Advil with "migraine" label is still ibuprofen 200 mg	Excedrin migraine is combination of 250 mg acetaminophen, 250 mg aspirin, with 65 mg caffeine. Reserve for those ≥25 kg or using 10 mg/kg/d guideline. Max 8 tablets/d over 2 days if adult size	■ Works very well for some because it offers combination relief	■ Do not use when otherwise ill because of Reye's syndrome's association with aspirin ■ Can cause gastric upset ■ Not recommended during pregnancy
Midrin (prescription and controlled substance) combination of isometheptene mucate 65 mg, dichloralphenazone	Reserve for those >35 kg to follow 10 mg/kg acetaminophen guideline, then only 1 at onset with only 1 repeat in 12 hrs. If adult size, may use 2 initially	■ Aids the initiation of therapeutic sleep ■ Useful in breaking prolonged headache	■ Often disrupts ADLs ■ Gastritis may accompany ■ Not contraindicated with pregnancy, but is with nursing mothers

100 mg, acetaminophen 325mg (sympathomimetic + sedative + analgesic)	with 1 q1h up to 5 in 12 hours (rare; more than 3 tolerated before falling into deep sleep)		
Triptans Imitrex, Maxalt, Amerge, Axert, Zomig, Relpax, Frova	■ Most child studies with imitrex, but can follow lowest dose guidelines for others. Imitrex: 5–10 mg nasal spray (1 or 2 sprays) or initial 25-mg dose tablet for school age. Adult-size: Repeat once after 2 hours, but no more than 40 mg/d. Other preparations ok for adult size patients. Do not use >4 times in 30 days	■ Multiple types of preparations including nasal spray, disintegrating tablets, injections and tablets ■ Only acute medication that specifically targets migraine chemistry	■ Contraindicated in those with underlying cardiac abnormalities or hypertension, so consider witnessed first dose and/or ECG first and repeat episodically if still using ■ Do not use with basilar or hemiplegic migraine ■ Do not use within 24 hours of ergots ■ Vascular changes may be perceived as uncomfortable, some do not tolerate them ■ Pregnancy Category C
Ergot alkaloids Migranal, Cafergot, DHE or DHEA	■ Migranal: nasal spray contains caffeine 4 mg/mL or 0.5 mg/spray of dihydroergotamine mesylate; currently for adult size patients 1 spray each nostril; may repeat 15 minutes later; but max of 6 sprays per 24 hours or 8 sprays per week ■ Cafergot: tablet or suppository. Due to high nausea and vomiting complaints, no longer recommended ■ DHE: used IV inpatient to break chronic headache or rebound headache cycles	■ Nasal spray availability or suppository can be advantageous ■ Ergots have historically been very effective medications for pain relief	■ Caution with cardiac disease: consider ECG or observation with first dose ■ Do not use within 24 hours of triptans ■ Pregnancy Category X ■ Interacts with propranolol, nicotine ■ Can cause cardiac valve fibrosis with chronic use

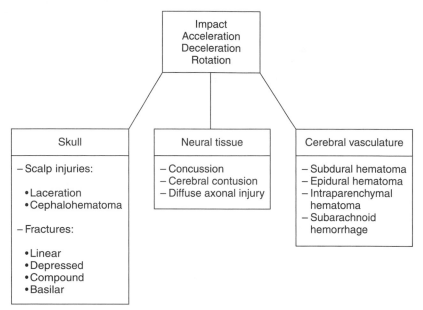

FIGURE 31-1 • Head trauma injury forces. (From Woestman R, et al: Mild head injury in children, identification, clinical evaluation, neuroimaging, and disposition. *J Pediatr Health Care* 12(6): 290, 1998.)

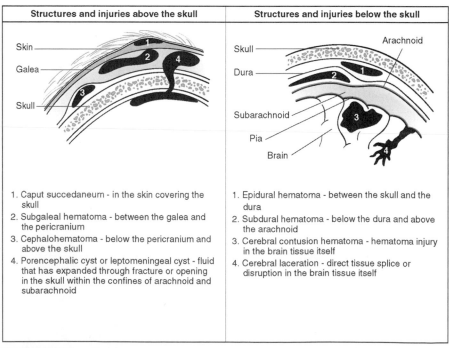

FIGURE 31-2 • Head injury by type and location.

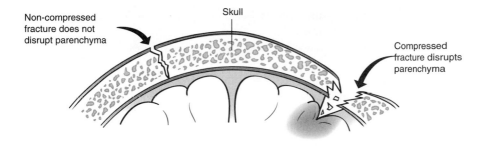

FIGURE 31-3 • Fracture types.

E. Generally, injuries to external soft tissue structures above scalp resolve over time.
F. Exception is leptomeningeal cyst, which needs surgical intervention.
G. 75% of skull fractures in children are simple linear fractures and do not need intervention.

II. Occurrence

A. Concussion is most common mild head injury type.
B. Age related. For example: cephalohematoma related to birth mechanics; subdural hematoma related to shaken baby syndrome; skull fracture related to fall from bike without helmet in school-age child; concussion related to motor vehicle accident in teen.
C. Sports-related head trauma estimated to cause 300,000 mild to moderate concussions.
D. Motor vehicle accidents (MVAs) cause 1 of 3 injury-related deaths among those >12 years, and among those 0–19 years motor vehicle injuries are highest cause of traumatic brain injury .
E. Gender variation: males 2–3 times more frequent compared to females, likely related to more risk-taking behaviors found in males.

III. Clinical manifestations

A. Gradation of effects from mild to severe.
B. No obvious findings reported other than history of trauma (Figure 31-2).
C. Subtle (closed head trauma): may have mild, transient confusion, nausea.
D. Minor (no alteration of consciousness, no vomiting or symptoms of dysfunction of bodily systems) to major with alterations of level of consciousness, vomiting, increased ICP, major derangements in bodily functions.
E. Obvious skull fracture, extrusion/alterations of brain contents.

IV. Physical findings

A. Assess for:
   1. Altered state of consciousness/sensory function, disordered thinking or abilities.
   2. Alteration in cranial nerve function, especially pupil response, tracking, doll's eyes, papilledema, abnormal cerebellar findings.

3. Abnormal posture or tone, weakness, abnormal reflexes or appearance of primitive reflexes.
4. Head circumference or palpation for abnormalities.
5. Nausea, vomiting.
6. Skin condition such as cool, clammy, mottled.
7. Increased or decreased ICP signs.
8. Abnormal loss of fluids either clear or bloody from nose or ears, ecchymosis behind ears (Battle sign), periorbital ecchymosis (raccoon sign).
9. Ask how injury was sustained: was consciousness lost? If so, how long? Did child vomit after event (more common in children than adults)? Headache and its quality, any seizures/abnormal movements?
10. Utilize Glasgow Coma Scale or Modified Glasgow Coma Scale (Table 31-3).

V. Diagnostic tests
   A. Skull films, CT scan, MRI.
   1. Skull films may be used if fracture seems more likely.
   2. CT for ease of obtainment, speed, ability to assess for blood and soft tissue damage as well as CSF shifts, but sometimes reserved for

TABLE 31-3 • Glasgow Coma Scale and modified Glasgow Coma Scale

Glasgow Coma Scale		Modified Glasgow Coma Scale for children <2 years of age	
Sign	Score	Sign	Score
Eye opening		Eye opening	
Spontaneous	4	Spontaneous	4
To verbal command	3	To speech	3
To pain	2	To pain	2
No response	1	No response	1
Best motor response		Best motor response	
Obeys verbal commands	6	Normal spontaneous movements	6
Localizes pain	5	Withdraws to touch	5
Withdraws to pain	4	Withdraws to pain	4
Flexion response to pain	3	Flexion response to pain	3
Extension response to pain	2	Extension response to pain	2
No response	1	No response	1
Best verbal response		Best verbal response	
Oriented	5	Smiles, listens, follow objects	5
Confused	4	Irritable cry, consolable	4
Inappropriate words	3	Inappropriate persistent cry	3
Nonspecific sounds	2	Agitated, restless	2
No response	1	No response	1

From Woestman R, et al: Mild head injury in children, identification, clinical evaluation, neuroimaging, and disposition, *J Pediatr Health Care* 12(6):290, 1998.
Data for Glasgow Coma scale from Teasdale G, Jennett B: Assessment of coma and impaired consciousness: a practical scale, *Lancet* 2:81-84, 1974.
Modified Glasgow Coma Scale for children <2 years of age adapted from Wong DL: The child with cerebral dysfunction. In Wong DL, editor: *Whaley & Wong's essentials of pediatric nursing,* St Louis, 1993, Mosby, pp 932-983.

Glasgow Coma Scales of 14–15 or <16 for cost effectiveness and morbidity probability.

3. MRI generally reserved for long-term assessment due to time, cost, potential need for sedation.

B. EEG may be warranted if seizures or depressed consciousness.

C. Laboratory tests: hematocrit (to assess blood loss urgently).

VI. Differential diagnosis

Loss of consciousness, **780.09**

Seizure, **780.39**

Syncope, **780.2**

A. History of head trauma antecedent to findings and how many times.

B. Infection.

C. Inherited disorders.

D. Syncope or seizures, which may have led to loss of consciousness and head trauma secondary to primary cause rather than other way around.

VII. Treatment

A. Assessment of ABCs needed urgently, otherwise outpatient instruction for guardian/parent or admission for Glasgow Coma Scales of 9–13, suspected child abuse etiology or CT positive for pathology.

B. Urgent treatment or hospital treatment and management may consist of:

1. Management of increased ICP.

2. Parenchymal and/or bony damage repair or blood evacuation.

3. Chemical derangement correction.

4. Nutritional support.

5. Anticonvulsants.

VIII. Follow-up

A. For minor trauma, child may go home, if supervision by parents is reliable. Give home instruction sheets, follow-up next day at least via phone call.

B. For more severe head trauma: admission, consult, refer to specialists as needed.

IX. Complications

Altering pulse, **427.89**   Edema, **782.3**

Dilated pupil, **379.43**   Yawning, **786.09**

A. Immediate concerns can include rapid decline of function to death. Warning signs of impending herniation can be:

1. Unequal pupils, fixed/unresponsive pupils, absence of doll's eyes.

2. Altered breathing, abnormal pulse, dropping BP.

3. Yawning.

4. Decerebrate posture.

B. Intermediate concerns include:

1. Infection.

2. Edema.

3. Other organ failure from brain derangements not sustaining their function.

C. Long-term include physiologic, psychologic, social, and educational adaptations if there are long-term sequelae.

X. Education

A. Safety becomes hallmark of focus in accidental head injury. Education and support of parenting families on safety issues and behavioral norms.

B. Prevention via use and promotion of proper head protection via safety equipment and implementation of guidelines for reentry into sports after head injury.

C. Avoidance of trauma via delivery method for high-risk delivery.

D. Implementation of appropriate discharge planning, which post-hospitalization may include multidisciplinary team and rehab or home care.

E. Promotion and proper use of child restraint systems.

MENINGITIS

Altered consciousness, 780.09	Meninges, 854.0
Brain dysfunction, 314.9	Meningitis, 322.9
Bulging fontanelle, 756.0	Papilledema, 377.00
Fever, 780.6	Seizure, 780.39
Headache, 784.0	Stiff neck, 723.5
Intracranial pressure, 781.99	Vomiting, 787.03
Irritability, 799.2	

I. Etiology

A. Infection and inflammation of meninges, a covering of brain.

B. Portal of pathogen entry can occur anywhere in body.

C. Recent advances in immunizations have led to less disease, especially those associated with *Haemophilus influenzae* and pneumococcal disease.

D. Majority are viral illnesses with most common identified etiology caused by enteroviruses (85–95%), next most prevalent are bacterial and fungal, but can be associated with drug response, disorders of immune system, or cancer.

E. Viral meningitis also is called aseptic meningitis, especially when presumed, but not proven viral.

F. Meningitis usually follows sepsis and disruption in blood–brain barrier.

II. Incidence

A. Worldwide, but increased with crowding and prolonged exposure such as day care, military, college dorms and via susceptibility factors in populations that vary by age and underlying immunologic factors.

B. Susceptibility factors in varying populations that vary by age and underlying immunologic factor.

   1. Age factors for bacterial meningitis:
      a. Neonates: in areas with high coverage via vaccine for *H. influenzae* and pneumococcal disease, about 50% of cases are Group B streptococcus, secondarily *Escherichia coli* and other gram-negative enteric bacilli, *Listeria monocytogenes,* gram-positive organisms (descending order).
      b. Other ages: strep pneumoniae and *Neisseria meningitidis,* which together account for 95% of cases.

C. Race: higher incidence in African Americans than Caucasians.

D. Sex: viral meningitis is three times more likely in males than in females.

III. Clinical manifestations

A. Signs of brain dysfunction such as fever, altered consciousness, headache, abnormal cry, seizures, sleepiness, extreme irritability, functional alterations.

B. Signs of irritation of meninges (Brudzinski's sign, Kernig's sign, stiff neck).

C. Signs of increased ICP (bulging fontanelle, sunset eyes, CN abnormalities, papilledema, vomiting, seizures).

IV. Physical findings

A. Classic triad for suspicion: fever, headache, stiff neck, but findings are age dependent to some extent (e.g., bulging fontanelle in infant versus complaint of headache in older child).

B. Following may be present in addition to those listed under clinical manifestations.

   1. Altered mental status from mild to deep coma.

   2. Tone changes, especially ominous is decorticate or decerebrate postures.

   3. Increased reflexes, clonus, positive Babinski.

   4. Incoordination.

   5. Focal neurologic signs may occur, but are less likely.

V. Diagnostic tests

A. LP in absence of increased ICP or signs of impending herniation (abnormal pupil size or reaction, abnormal tone, posturing, respiratory abnormalities, papilledema, or absent doll's eyes).

B. Collection is done for initial pressure measurement, WBC count, glucose, protein, gram stain, culture and antigen assay.

C. Head CT initially helpful due to ease of obtainment and speed to look for complications, but does not necessarily establish diagnosis. Consider MRI for later imaging of sequelae.

D. Blood cultures, CBC with differential, erythrocyte sedimentation rate (ESR).

E. Gram stain of skin lesions if present.

F. Urinalysis (UA).

G. Chemistries

H. Cultures of orifices or fluids/tissues for identification of etiologic agent.

I. Immediate serum for titers and delayed serum for convalescent titers.

VI. Differential diagnosis

Brain abscess, 324.0	Head injury, 959.01
Brain lesion, 348.8	Subdural empyema, 324.9
Encephalitis, 323.9	

A. Encephalitis (overlap possible with both coexisting at the same time).

B. Febrile manifestation of underlying illness (generally meningeal irritation signs differentiate the two from each other).

C. Brain abscess, brain tumors/lesions.

D. Subdural empyema.

E. Head injury.

F. Intoxications.

VII. Treatment

A. For suspected viral meningitis: supportive care may be done outpatient, but generally provided in hospital and consists of intravenous fluid therapy, analgesia.

B. For suspected herpes meningitis: antiviral therapy, close supervision in hospital setting.

C. For suspected/confirmed bacterial meningitis: earlier the intervention, the less the morbidity and mortality.

    1. Treatment directed to most commonly known pathogens based on child's age and setting; changes are made as indicated from test results.

    2. Most children need to be admitted, often to intensive care for appropriate management of ICP, complications, and to administer pharmacologic agents appropriate to eradicate the causative organism.

    3. For initial treatment of unspecified bacterial meningitis (before causative organism is identified

        a. Birth to 6 weeks of age: ampicillin plus a third generation cephalosporin

        b. >6 Weeks of age: vancomycin, third generation cephalosporin cefotaxime or ceftriaxone

        c. Prophylaxis for exposed contacts (e.g., meningococcal meningitis).

VIII. Follow-up

A. For viral or aseptic meningitis, frequent clinic visits for child cared for at home and in 2–4 weeks initially to ascertain if complications or sequelae to address.

B. For bacterial meningitis, may need to be transition to rehab setting and/or home care.

C. Shortly after hospitalization to ascertain understanding and transition to rehab or home is made smoothly.

D. Several months later: reassess plan and sequelae and whether plan is adequate.

E. 6 Months: assess further mental, social, functional alterations that may still be present and ensure comprehensive care. Follow up with multidisciplinary team if needed.

IX. Complications

Bacterial meningitis, 320.9	Seizures, 780.39
Emotional lability, 301.3	Viral meningitis, 047.9
Hearing loss, 389.9	

A. Up to 50% sustain sequelae from bacterial meningitis, whereas most children with nonherpetic viral meningitis recover completely.

B. Intellectual, may be global or selective.

C. Seizures.

D. Hearing loss.

E. Functional disabilities, both fine motor and gross motor.

F. Emotional consequences: emotional lability may be short term or long term (esp. common post-herpes).

G. Societal, especially for those in endemic area/scenario (e.g., college, day care).

X. Education
A. Importance of prevention via immunizations.
B. Importance of hand washing, surface cleaning in crowded locations such as day cares, barracks, dorms.
C. Importance of prophylaxis if exposure to virulent modes are noted.
D. Support and coordination of comprehensive services as needed.

SEIZURES

- Prevalence of seizures is 4–6 cases per 1000 children.
- About one third of 2 million persons in US with epilepsy are children.
- Vary with higher incidence of certain types on inherited basis.

GENERALIZED SEIZURES

Juvenile myoclonic epilepsy, 345.1	Seizures, 780.39
Lennox-Gastaut syndrome, 345.0	Tonic-clonic seizure, 345.1
Petit mal seizure, 345.0	West syndrome, 345.6

Tonic-clonic and absence seizures arise from electrical aberration of entire brain at once and are the most common type in children. Magnitude leads to loss of consciousness (LOC). There are also some less common syndromes listed below that are important to identify because they may require special treatment and/or referral.

I. Etiology
A. Those associated with inborn aberrations of brain structure, genetic/presumed metabolic aberrations. Serious: those associated with metabolic errors incompatible with normal life (e.g., amino acidurias) to presumed mild autosomal-dominant inherited types with favorable prognosis (e.g., neonatal seizures).
B. These represent minority at present, but as genetics advances, more frequent idiopathic generalized seizures are being associated with particular inheritance patterns or gene site.

II. Occurrence
A. Sporadic except for higher incidence of certain types on an inherited basis.

III. Clinical manifestations
A. LOC for generalized tonic-clonic seizure (GTCS), then alternating tonic stiffening with clonic jerking/myoclonic jerking, loss of body tone.
B. LOC for absence seizures (petit mal) may include staring, blinking, automatisms for seconds and often occur in clusters.
   1. Untreated will become 100s per day.
   2. Age: typically late preschool to teen, with predominance in school age.
C. Juvenile myoclonic epilepsy (JME): occurs in teens and usually is nocturnal or early AM. Myoclonic jerks usually involve upper extremities, may include GTCS.
D. Infantile spasms (West syndrome): syndrome of myoclonus in infancy that occurs in clusters during fatigue and often resembles Moro reflex. May progress to more exaggerated loss of tone, myoclonic jerking also in clusters.

Diagnosis includes developmental delay, characteristic EEG abnormality called hypsarrhythmia, classic myoclonic seizure description.
E. Lennox-Gastaut syndrome often develops in child who had Infantile Spasms and consists of multiple seizure types (atonic, GTCS, atypical absence) typically accompanied by mental deficiency and difficult-to-control seizures.

IV. Physical findings
A. Between seizures there may be none.
B. Fever after seizure as high as 101°F.
C. Altered consciousness and postictal confusion or fatigue.
D. Abnormal neuro exam may or may not be evident depending on causation.

V. Diagnostic tests
A. Chemistries, glucose, UA.
B. CBC with diff and platelets.
C. EEG. Initially standard awake and asleep. If problematic, consider video or prolonged.
D. CT, MRI to be considered if EEG is focally abnormal or there are residual abnormalities.
E. EKG if suspicious of cardiac or vagal disorder.

VI. Differential diagnosis

Apnea, 786.03	Hyperventilation, 786.01
Arrhythmia, 427.9	Migraine, 346.9
Behavior disorder, 312.9	Pseudoseizures, 780.39
Breath holding, 786.9	Sleep disorder, 780.50
Daydreaming, 300.13	Syncope, 780.2
Gastrointestinal disorder, 536.9	Vertigo, 780.4

A. Pseudoseizures, infantile self-stimulation, migraine.
B. Syncope, vertigo, narcolepsy, ADHD, daydreaming.
C. Apnea, breath holding, and hyperventilation.
D. Behavior disorders, sleep disorders.
E. Gastrointestinal disorders.
F. Substance exposure.
G. Cardiac episodes such as arrhythmia, abnormal perfusion states.

VII. Treatment
A. Treatment of underlying associated metabolic aberrations if found.
B. For West syndrome/infantile spasms, steroids are necessary.
C. Anticonvulsants appropriate for each seizure type, patient age (Table 31-4).
D. Ketogenic diet.
E. Behavioral interventions such as biofeedback, relaxation techniques.
F. Prevention strategies of adequate rest, nutrition, exercise, hydration.
G. Surgery such as corpus callosotomy for refractory, potentially dangerous seizure types such as those with Lennox-Gastaut. Vagal nerve stimulator for refractive cases; FDH approved for ages 12 and older, but may be considered for younger with expert input.

TABLE 31-4 • Antiseizure medications (anticonvulsants) more commonly used with children

Referral for consultation and input from neurology or child neurology resources would be best before initiation of second-line medications. Any can have allergic reaction and response may be delayed as it is related to half-life buildup of drug in system leading to systemic rash typically. Toxicity/overdose ("drunklike") behavior, such as drowsiness, ataxia, dysarthria, vomiting) for most antiseizure medications warrants reevaluation of dose.

Name	Type of seizure treated	Dosage and levels	Common side effects/adverse reactions/precautions
Carbatrol (carbamazepine, extended-release)	■ Generalized tonic–clonic ("grand mal") ■ Focal, both simple and complex partial ■ Mixed	May convert when regular carbamazepine dose reached 400 mg/d on mg/mg basis divided bid. levels: 4–12, generally toxic >15.	■ Side effects: dizziness, abdominal complaints ■ Adverse: blood dyscrasias, especially neutropenia ■ Monitor CBC before and during therapy and LFTs ■ CYP3A4 interaction precautions ■ May interfere with hormonal BC efficacy ■ Pregnancy Category D
Depakene/ Depakote (valproates)	■ Absence generalized seizures ("petit mal") ■ Tonic–clonic ■ Primary and secondary generalized ■ Mixed ■ Akinetic/myoclonic ■ Lennox–Gastaut ■ Juvenile myoclonic epilepsy	10–30 mg/kg/d divided bid–tid with max of 40 mg/kg/d. Levels 40–100, occasionally to 125 if tolerated without side effects, generally toxic above this.	■ Side effects: Fairly frequent GI complaints, may have appetite increase (more common)/decrease; alopecia ■ Adverse effects on liver function or platelets ■ Pregnancy Category D
Dilantin (phenytoin)	■ Generalized tonic–clonic ■ Partial (complex or simple) ■ Primary and secondary generalized ■ Mixed	4–7 mg/kg/day, generally given bid. Levels 10–20. Toxicity >25.	■ Side effects: gum hyperplasia, hirsutism, ataxia, nystagmus, peripheral neuropathy, osteomalacia, folate deficiency (for those not sun exposed) ■ Adverse effects: allergy; rare dyscrasias

Continued

TABLE 31-4 • Antiseizure medications (anticonvulsants) more commonly used with children—cont'd

Name	Type of seizure treated	Dosage and levels	Common side effects/adverse reactions/precautions
Mysoline (primidone)	■ Generalized tonic-clonic ■ Partial (complex and simple)	8–20 mg/kg/d generally given at bedtime or bid	■ Side effects: drowsiness, behavioral change, sleep disturbances, cognitive dulling ■ Adverse effects: allergy ■ Monitor LFTs, CBC
Phenobarbital (Phenobarbital)	■ Generalized tonic-clonic ■ Mixed	2–5 mg/kg/d. Levels 10–30; generally toxic 35	See Mysoline
Tegretol (carbamazepine)	■ Generalized tonic-clonic ■ Partial (complex and simple) ■ Mixed	8–20 mg/kg/d. Levels 4–12; generally toxic >15	Similar to Carbatrol
Trileptal (oxcarbazepine)	■ Partial (complex and simple) age 4 and up	8–10 mg/kg/d with usual increase of 5 mg/kg per day every 3rd day with targets in range up to 1.8 g/day, but dependent on weight. See literature for max doses for specific weight ranges and whether or not this is initial therapy or converting from other dibenzapines	Similar to Carbatrol except Pregnancy Category C
Zarontin (ethosuximide)	■ Exclusive use only for absence	20–40 mg/kg/d. Levels 40–100	■ Common side effects: dizziness, GI distress. ■ Adverse effects: leukopenia or kidney dysfunction. ■ Monitor CBC, chemistry profile

VIII. Follow-up

A. Single seizure may not require follow-up; encourage recontact if recurs.

B. Recurrent seizures: regular rechecks necessary, especially for some medications (to obtain therapeutic levels, assess control, reevaluate EEG, obtain other lab monitoring for side effects of medications). Reevaluate if not controlled on current regime.

IX. Complications

Behavior disturbance, 312.9
Intellectual underachievement, 313.83

A. Side effects of medications/seizures: possible intellectual, behavior effects.

B. Long-term psychologic effects (psychosocial).

X. Education

A. Initial, regarding etiology and prognosis.

B. Safety.

C. School and social advice.

D. Medication and follow-up monitoring.

E. Reevaluation parameters.

F. Encouragement of psychosocial interventions.

G. Driving restrictions pertinent to home country or state.

PARTIAL SEIZURES

Autonomic phenomena, 337.9
Partial seizure, 345.5
Seizures, 780.39

Electrical aberration leading to a manifested seizure arises from one location in brain. If consciousness is preserved, called simple; if lost, called complex (PCS). Presentation related to part of brain that is misfiring. Several are more common in children such as partial complex (movement of one site of body or alteration in ability, but with preserved consciousness), simple complex (recurrent mannerisms with altered consciousness), Jacksonian (march down one side of the body). There are also common syndromes, such as benign rolandic epilepsy, necessitating certain intervention.

I. Etiology

A. Focal disruption from injury (depressed skull fracture or parenchymal derangement), scarring (postmeningitis), innate formational (gray/white matter switch known as heterotopia), or chemical alone for unknown reasons (unknown etiology or idiopathic).

B. Idiopathic more common in children.

II. Occurrence

A. Sporadic when idiopathic, but more highly predicted risk if brain parenchyma gray matter disruption secondary to change in tissue.

III. Clinical manifestations

A. Depends on site or origin of electrical activity.

    B. Simple partial seizures may manifest as alterations in motor, sensory autonomic, or psychic phenomena.

    C. Complex partial seizures are also known as "psychomotor" and may include aforementioned elements with impaired consciousness.

    D. Remember either of the above may advance to generalized seizures.

IV. Physical findings

    A. During seizure, may or may not have alteration.

    B. May be none or may have alterations in neuro exam either postictally and transiently or permanently depending on the cause.

V. Diagnostic tests

    A. Initial workup as above in generalized seizures section but with a lower threshold to obtain a CT or MRI secondary to focal nature of disorder.

VI. Differential diagnosis

Dystonias, 333.89	Pseudoseizures, 780.39
Myoclonus, 345.1	Rage, 312.0
Obsessive compulsive disorder, 300.3	Restless leg syndrome, 333.99
Pseudohypoparathyroidism, 275.49	Tic's, 307.20

    A. Other paroxysmal movement disorders such as tics, benign myoclonus, pseudoseizures, dystonias.

    B. Behavior disorders such as rage, obsessive-compulsive disorder.

    C. Pseudohypoparathyroidism (may present with dystonia).

    D. Restless leg syndrome.

VII. Treatment

    A. Observation.

    B. Anticonvulsants.

    C. Surgical intervention, such as temporal lobectomy or hemispherectomy depending on location, severity, response to anticonvulsants. Consider immediately to avoid long-term parenchymal and personality changes.

    D. Vagal nerve stimulator for those refractory to medication.

VIII. Follow-up

    A. Dependent on therapy and seizure consequences, but often needs episodic and frequent outpatient visits for:

        1. Medication management and levels.

        2. Monitoring for side effects and favorable effects.

        3. EEG.

IX. Complications

Personality change, 310.1
Physiologic deficiency, 301.6

    A. Permanent physiologic sequelae depending on etiology and residual effects of either seizures or dysfunctional area of brain leading to seizures.

    B. Interpersonal/personality/adaptation sequelae from seizures or seizure therapy.

X. Education
   A. Medication and side effects.
   B. Follow-up.
   C. Safety.
   D. School and social interaction advice.

FEBRILE SEIZURES

Febrile seizures, 780.31
Seizures, 780.39

Seizure activity defined by brief, generalized, clonic-tonic movements. Occurs within context of febrile illness in children 6 months to 5 years of age. Simple febrile seizures are brief, generalized, not recurrent in 24-hour period. Complex febrile seizure is prolonged, may have focality, recurs in 24-hour period.

I. Etiology
   A. Likely autosomal dominant with variable penetrance.

II. Occurrence
   A. Overall population incidence of 4%.
   B. Degree of fever seems significant (105°F fever has 3 times greater risk of febrile seizure) as does risk when >2 first-degree relatives have had febrile seizures.
   C. Complex seizures comprise 20% of those with febrile seizures.

III. Clinical manifestations
   A. Simple febrile seizure:
      1. Generalized.
      2. Of short duration (<15 minutes).
      3. Single event with given illness.
      4. Fever.
   B. Complex febrile seizure:
      1. May occur >1 in given illness.
      2. May be prolonged.
      3. Recurs within 24 hours.
      4. May have focal presentation.
      5. 20% of those with febrile seizures.

IV. Physical findings
   A. Generally tonic-clonic movements or limpness associated with LOC and postictal deep lethargy or sleep.

V. Diagnostic tests
   A. Because of high suspicion with first episode of underlying brain illness, workup for meningitis or sepsis with CSF, blood cultures, UA and urine C/S, chemistries, CBC, sedimentation rate (ESR), etc.
   B. Consider an EEG to assist with prognostic factors.

VI. Differential diagnosis

Encephalitis, 323.9   Metabolic disorder, 277.9
Meningitis, 322.9   Sepsis, 995.91

     A. Meningitis.

     B. Encephalitis.

     C. Sepsis.

     D. Metabolic illness.

VII. Treatment

     A. Anticonvulsants if still seizing on presentation; otherwise reassure, review predictions for future episodes.

     B. For single first episode, perform workup for sepsis or brain illness if warranted. If nothing worrisome is found, no treatment is necessary if acceptable to parents.

     C. Immediate treatment of fever-reducing measures (pharmacologic/nonpharmacologic), but may not decrease recurrence of seizures in given illness.

     D. May prescribe rectal Valium (Diastat) during acute episode.

     E. For recurrent, worrisome complex febrile seizures, consider prophylaxis with appropriate anticonvulsant. Do not use in child <2 years.

VIII. Follow-up

     A. As needed based on exam and associated illness leading to fever.

IX. Complications

Partial seizures, 345.5

     A. Few if not complicated.

     B. Complicated may be any of above for generalized or partial seizures.

X. Education

     A. Safety and how to access EMS services.

     B. Education and support.

     C. If anticonvulsant drugs used ongoing, same as above for generalized or partial seizures.

BIBLIOGRAPHY

Aligne CA: Headaches, recurrent: migraine & others. In Garfunkel LC, Kaczorowski J, Christy C, editors: *Mosby's pediatric clinical advisor: instant diagnosis and treatment,* St. Louis, 2002, Mosby.

American Academy of Pediatrics: Adenoviruses. In Pickering LK, editor: *Red book: 2003 report of the Committee on Infectious Diseases,* ed 26, Elk Grove Village, IL, 2003, American Academy of Pediatrics.

Austin JK, et al: A feasibility study of a family seizure management program: "Be seizure smart," *J Neurosci Nursing* 34:30-37, 2002.

Barnes N, Millman G, James E: Migraine headaches in children. In *Clinical evidence concise,* issue 10, London, 2003, BMJ Publishing Group.

Brodie MJ, Kwan P: Staged approach to epilepsy management, *Neurology* 58(Suppl 5):S2-S8, 2002.

Brunquell P, et al: Prediction of outcome based on clinical seizure type in newborn infants, *J Pediatr* 140:707-712, 2002.

Buckingham SC: Rocky Mountain spotted fever: A review for the pediatrician, *Pediatr Ann* 31:163-168, 2002.

Capill B, Weinberg AR: Acupuncture: essential information for nurse practitioners, *Adv Nurse Practitioners* 81-85, February 2003.

Diamond ML: The role of concomitant headache types and non-headache co-morbidities in the underdiagnosis of migraine, *Neurology* 58(Suppl 6):S3-S8, 2002.

Edwards L: Meditation as medicine, *Adv Nurse Practitioners* 11(5):49-52, May 2003.

Fenichel GM: Infectious disorders. In *Clinical pediatric neurology: a signs and symptoms approach,* ed 4, Philadelphia, 2001, WB Saunders.

Harrison T: West Nile encephalitis, *J Pediatr Health Care* 16:278-281, 2002.

Lin J: Overview of migraine, *J Neurosci Nursing* 33:6-13, 2001.

Loman DG: The use of complementary and alternative health care practices among children, *J Pediatr Health Care* 17:58-63, 2003.

McAlhany A: Efficacy of sumatriptan in the treatment of migraine: A review of the literature, *J Neurosci Nursing* 33:270-277, 2001.

Mears D: Headache worksheet for nurse practitioners, *Am J Nurse Practitioners,* 11(2):22-28, February 2003.

Olness KN: Managing headaches without drugs, *Contemp Pediatr* 20:101-112, 2003.

Patient information: OTC pain relievers: Which one is right?, *Adv Nurse Practitioners* 11(12):30, December 2003.

Perriello VA, Jr, Barth JT: Sports concussions: coming to the right conclusions, *Contemp Pediatr* 17:132-140, 2000.

Pettit JL: Alternative medicine: ginger, *Clin Rev* 11:72-74, 2001.

Polin RA, Ditmar MF, editors: Encephalitis. In *Pediatric secrets,* ed 3, Philadelphia, 2001, Hanley & Belfus.

Reimschisel T: Breaking the cycle of medication overuse headache, *Contemp Pediatr* 20:101-114, 2003.

Rothner AD, et al: Chronic nonprogressive headaches in children and adolescents, *Semin Pediatr Neurol* 8:34-39, 2001.

Scharff L, Kemper KJ: For chronic pain, complementary and alternative medical approaches, *Contemp Pediatr* 20:117-141, 2003.

Shulman DL, et al: Neurocysticercosis: nursing perspectives, *J Neurosci Nursing* 34:237-241, 2002.

Spiro C, Spiro DM: Acute meningitis: focus on bacterial infection, *Clin Rev* 14(3):54-59, 2004.

Tan TQ: Pneumococcal infections in children, *Pediatr Ann* 31:241-247, 2002.

Tenembaum S, Chamoles N, Fejerman N: Acute disseminated encephalomyelitis: A long-term follow-up study of 84 pediatric patients, *Neurology* 59:1224-1231, 2002.

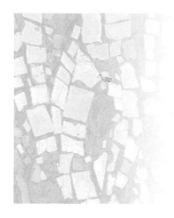

CHAPTER 32

Hematologic Disorders

BETSY ATKINSON JOYCE

IRON-DEFICIENCY ANEMIA

Anemia, 280.9	Palmar pallor, 782.61
Anemia, mild, 285.9	Poor weight gain, 263.9
Fatigue, 780.79	Splenomegaly, 789.2
GI bleeding, 578.9	Systolic flow murmurs, 785.2
Headaches, 784.0	Tachycardia, 785.0
Irritability, 799.2	

Most common anemia of childhood. Anemia is defined as reduction in red blood cell (RBC) mass or in hemoglobin concentration to level that is >2 standard deviations below mean in healthy children. Can be determined in primary care setting by physical examination, important aspects of history, and hemoglobin concentration. Screening should occur routinely around 9 months to 1 year. High-risk infants: screen earlier, more often.

I. Etiology

A. Microcytic anemia reflecting defect in production of hemoglobin during erythrocyte maturation, resulting from defect in heme synthesis due to inadequate quantities of iron:

1. Inadequate supply of iron at birth, inadequate dietary iron.
2. High demand for iron associated with growth.
3. Blood loss without replacement.

II. Occurrence

A. Common between 1 and 3 years of age because of inadequate dietary iron due to cow's milk being major staple in most children's diets.

B. Lack of adequate iron stores to meet needs for growth.

1. Affects 9% of children <2 years of age.
2. Affects 9–11% of adolescent females.

    C. Lack of adequate iron to meet needs for RBC production.

       1. Affects 3% of children <2 years of age.

       2. Affects up to 3% of adolescent females and <1% of adolescent males.

III. Clinical manifestations

    A. Mild anemia (hemoglobin of 9.5–11): may be asymptomatic; sometimes only minimal symptoms when severe anemia (hemoglobin of 8–9.5 or lower) is present. May only be detected on routine screening or discovered when blood count ordered for another reason.

    B. History of fatigue, irritability, excessive milk intake, headaches.

IV. Physical findings

    A. Mild anemia (normal physical exam).

    B. More severe anemia.

       1. Poor weight gain.

       2. Sclera or palmar pallor.

       3. Splenomegaly: 15% of affected children.

       4. Tachycardia.

       5. Systolic flow murmurs: with progression of the iron deficit.

V. Diagnostic tests

    A. Hemoglobin concentration (Table 32-1).

    B. CBC.

       1. RBC hypochromic, microcytic.

       2. Mean cell volume (MCV) decreased.

       3. Ratio of MCV/RBC > 13.

TABLE 32-1 • Maximum hemoglobin concentration and hematocrit values for iron-deficiency anemia

Sex/age, years	Hemoglobin (g/dL)	Hematocrit (%)
Both Genders		
1 to <2 years	11.0	32.9
2 to <5 years	11.1	33.0
5 to <8 years	11.5	34.5
8 to <12 years	11.9	35.4
Females		
12 to <15 years	11.8	35.7
15 to 18 years	12.0	35.9
≥18 years	12.0	35.7
Males		
12 to <15 years	12.5	37.3
15 to 18 years	13.3	39.7
≥18 years	13.5	39.9

Adapted from Centers for Disease Control and Prevention: Recommendations to prevent and control iron deficiency in the United States. *MMWR* 47(No. RR-3), April 3, 1998.

   C. Iron studies if need further information.

     1. Serum iron: decreased.

     2. Total iron-binding capacity: increased.

     3. Ferritin: decreased.

     4. % iron saturation: decreased.

VI. Differential diagnosis

Lead poisoning, **984.9**
Sideroblastic anemia, **285.0**
Thalassemia, **282.49**

   A. Thalassemia trait.

   B. Lead poisoning.

   C. Chronic infection.

   D. Sideroblastic anemia.

VII. Treatment

   A. Nutritional strategies.

   B. Reduce milk to no more than 16–24 oz/day.

     1. Increase intake of high-iron foods (i.e., beans, whole cereals, dried fruit, pork, beef).

     2. Iron therapy for infants and children:

       a. Ferrous sulfate.

        • Mild to moderate iron deficiency: 3 mg elemental iron/kg/day in 1–2 divided doses.

        • Severe iron deficiency: 4–6 mg elemental iron/kg/day in 3 divided doses.

VIII. Follow-up

   A. Recheck hemoglobin in 1 month.

   B. Treat until hemoglobin and hematocrit reach normal ranges. Then give at least 1 month additional treatment to replenish iron stores.

   C. If response not adequate within 1–2 months, consider further diagnostic testing for GI bleeding or other microcytic hypochromic anemias.

IX. Complications

Anemia, **280.9**   Developmental delays, **783.40**
Behavioral delays, **312.9**   Poor growth, **253.2**

   A. Result from long-standing iron-deficiency anemia.

     1. Increased susceptibility to infection.

     2. Poor growth.

     3. Developmental delays (lower mental and motor test scores).

     4. Behavioral delays.

X. Education

   A. Need for balanced diets and foods containing iron.

     1. Cereal, egg yolks, green/yellow vegetables, yellow fruits, red meat, potatoes, tomatoes, raisins.

   B. Amount of milk necessary/day (age dependent).

C. Information about iron medications:
1. Give after meals with orange juice to enhance absorption.
2. Do not give with milk (inhibits absorption of iron).
3. Give with straw or brush teeth after giving (may stain teeth).
4. May cause abdominal discomfort, constipation, stools to be black.
5. Extremely poisonous if taken in excessive amounts.
6. Keep out of reach of small children.

LEAD POISONING

Headache, 784.0	Poor attention span, 314.00
Irritability, 799.0	Seizures, 780.39
Lead poisoning, 984.9	Sleep disorders, 780.50
Loss of visual motor coordination, 781.3	Stomachache, 789.00
Muscular weakness, 728.87	Tiredness, 780.79
Poor appetite, 783.0	Weight loss, 783.2

Most common, widespread environmental health concern especially for children <6 years of age. Can cause decrease in gestational weight and age; may increase possibility of stillbirths and miscarriages.

I. Etiology
A. Increased lead levels in children occur by exposure to deteriorating paint, household dust, bare soil, air, drinking water, food, ceramics, home remedies, hair dyes, other cosmetics. Usually exposure is in child's own home.
B. Manufacture, use, disposal of modern products containing lead results in fine lead particles that release into environment. Lead particles enter air, water, food; also contaminate soil, dust.

II. Occurrence
A. Estimated at least 400,000 children <6 years of age have too much lead in bodies.
B. Questions for assessing risk of lead poisoning:
1. Live in, regularly visit, or have lived in a place with peeling or chipping paint built before 1960?
   a. Includes day care, preschools, homes of babysitters, relatives.
   b. Houses with recent, ongoing, planned renovation or remodeling.
2. Brother or sister, housemate, playmate being followed or treated for lead poisoning (blood level > 15 mcg/dL)?
3. Live with adult whose job or hobby involves exposure to lead?
   a. Ceramics, furniture refinishing; stained glass work; construction workers.
4. Taking home remedies such as azarcon and greta?
5. Live near active smelter, battery recycling plant, other industry likely to release lead into air?

III. Clinical manifestations
A. Many symptoms resemble common childhood complaints: headache, stomachache, irritability, tiredness, poor appetite.

  B. Other subtle symptoms: poor attention span and memory, sleep disorders.

  C. All of these can lead to coma and death because not noticed until brain damage has already occurred. Once organ systems are damaged, damage often irreversible.

IV. Physical findings

  A. Weight loss, decreased growth.

  B. Muscular weakness(diminished reflexes).

  C. Seizures (signs of anemia).

  D. Loss of visual motor coordination.

V. Diagnostic tests

  A. Lead blood levels: <10 mcg/dL. Screening tests as recommended by CDC (Table 32-2).

  B. Free erythrocyte protoporphyrin (FEP): elevated.

TABLE 32-2 • CDC recommendations for follow-up lead blood level measurements

Class	Blood lead level	Comment
I	≤9 mcg/dL	Not lead poisoned
		Low risk: 6–35 months of age, retest at 24 months
		High risk: 6–35 months of age, retest every 6 months
		>36 months of age: retest yearly until 6 years of age
IIA	10–14 mcg/dL	Rescreen frequently and consider prevention activities
		6–35 months of age, retest every 3–4 months
		>36 months of age, retest yearly
IIB	15–19 mcg/dL	Institute nutritional and educational interventions
		Retest every 3–4 months
III	20–44 mcg/dL	Evaluate environment and consider chelation therapy
		Retest every 3–4 months
IV	45–69 mcg/dL	Institute environmental intervention and chelation therapy within 48 hours
V	>70 mcg/dL	Medical emergency; requires immediate treatment

Data from Centers for Disease Control and Prevention: Recommendations for follow-up lead blood level measurements; retrieved March 2004 from www.cdc.gov/nceh/lead/about/about.htm; Cohen S: Lead poisoning: a summary of treatment and prevention, *Pediatr Nursing* 27:125, 2001.

VI. Differential diagnosis

Abdominal pain, unspecified, **789.00**	Iron-deficiency anemia, **280.9**
Behavioral disorders, **312.9**	Unexplained seizures, **780.39**

A. Neurologic problems (unexplained seizures, behavioral disorders).
B. Iron-deficiency anemia.
C. Unexplained abdominal pain.

VII. Treatment

A. Lead blood level determines treatment (Table 32-2).
B. Alteration in environment; stop unusual exposure to lead.
C. Good nutrition.
D. Chelation therapy.
    1. British antilewisite (BAL).
    2. Edetate calcium disodium (CaNa2EDTA).
    3. Dimercaptosuccinic acid (DMSA) or Succimer.
    4. D-Penicillamine.

VIII. Follow-up

A. Follow recommendations in Table 32-2 for rescreening. Treatment time is lengthy: there will be rebound levels as stored lead releases from bones and teeth.
B. After chelation therapy: obtain another blood lead level in 10–14 days.
C. Blood lead level determines subsequent treatment.

IX. Complications

Coma, **780.01**	Learning disabilities, **315.2**
Diminished fertility, **628.9**	Lower sperm counts, **792.2**
Elevated BUN, **790.6**	Mental retardation, **319.**
Headache, **784.0**	Persistent vomiting, **536.2**
Hearing loss, **389.9**	Seizures, **780.39**
Hypertension, **401.9**	Sterility, female, **628.9**
Impaired growth, **253.2**	Sterility, male, **606.9**
Kidney diseases, **593.9**	Toxicity, **323.7**
Lead encephalopathy, **984.7**	

A. Lead encephalopathy and toxicity:
    1. Headache, persistent vomiting.
    2. Seizures, coma, death.
    3. Mental retardation, learning disabilities.
    4. Impaired growth.
    5. Hearing loss.
B. Renal disorders: hypertension, kidney diseases (later in life), elevated blood urea nitrogen (BUN).
C. Reproductive system:
    1. Diminished fertility, abnormal sperm and lower counts, sterility male and female.
    2. Increased chance of miscarriage.

X. Education
A. Prevention.
B. Advice for families:
1. If suspect exposure, test child.
2. Use caution when purchasing older home.
3. Maintenance to keep old lead-based paint intact.
4. Watch for lead dust when doing home improvement projects: protect furniture from lead dust, wet mop work area after projects using detergent.
5. Wash work clothes separately from family's clothing.
6. Encourage children to play in sand, grass rather than dirt.
7. Wash hands, pacifiers before naps, bedtime.
8. Avoid folk remedies or cosmetics containing lead.
9. Test water supply for lead.
10. Wash fruits, vegetables before eating.
11. Eat healthy diet rich in iron: helps body to absorb less lead.
12. Use only cold water from tap for drinking, cooking, making baby formula. Hot water more likely to contain higher levels of lead.

SICKLE CELL DISEASE

Abdominal pain, unspecified, **789.00**	Hepatitis B, **070.30**
Angina, **413.9**	Hepatitis C, **070.51**
Aplastic crisis, **284.9**	Hepatitis D, **070.52**
Cardiomyopathy, **425.4**	Hepatitis E, **070.53**
Cerebral vascular accident, **436.**	Increased lethargy, **780.79**
Chest syndrome, acute, **517.3**	Irritability, **799.2**
Chronic hemolytic anemia, **282.9**	Leg ulcerations, **707.10**
Circulatory system disorder, unspecified, **459.9**	Maxillary hyperplasia, **524.01**
	Meningitis, **322.9**
Cytomegalovirus, **078.5**	Ocular retinopathy, **362.10**
Dehydration, **276.5**	Orthopnea, **786.02**
Delayed puberty, **259.0**	Pallor, **782.61**
Dental malocclusion, **534.9**	Pallor/jaundiced skin, **782.61**
Dyspnea, **786.09**	Persistent headaches, **784.0**
Emesis, recurrent, **787.03**	Pneumonia, **486.**
Emotional stress, **308.0**	Priapism, **607.3**
Exercise intolerance, **V47.2**	Pulmonary fibrosis, **515.**
Fatigue, **780.79**	Sickle cell disease, **282.60**
Fever, **780.6**	Splenomegaly, **789.2**
Gallbladder disease, **575.9**	Tachycardia, **785.0**
Hemolytic anemia, **282.9**	Tightness in chest, **786.59**
Hemolytic crisis, **283.9**	Urinary tract infection, **599.0**
Hemoptysis, **786.3**	Visual/speech changes, **784.49**
Hepatitis A, **070.1**	Weakness/numbness in extremities, **780.79**

Group of inherited heme disorders characterized by sickle hemoglobin (HbS); several variants within sickle cell disease. This section aimed at variant that results when one is homozygous for HbS, sometimes referred to as sickle cell anemia (HbSS).

I. Etiology
 A. Due to single defective hemoglobin module inherited as gene from both parents (autosomal-recessive disorder).
 B. Abnormal HbS is produced instead of HbA, normal hemoglobin.
 C. The abnormal hemoglobin S, when deoxygenated, deforms red cells into sickle shapes that occlude small vessels, slowing blood flow, creating vaso-occlusive crises in blood vessels and in organs such as spleen.

II. Occurrence
 A. Predominantly in black Americans with about 1 in 400 African Americans affected.
 B. Mediterranean or Arabic descendants also found to have sickle cell anemia, but in fewer numbers.

III. Clinical manifestations
 A. Chronic hemolytic anemia (aplastic crisis, hemolytic crisis, sequestration crisis).
 B. Vaso-occlusion resulting in ischemia to tissues.
   1. Painful crisis: from infarcts of muscle, bone, bone marrow, lung, intestines.
   2. Cerebrovascular accident.
   3. Acute chest syndrome.
   4. Chronic lung disease such as pulmonary fibrosis.
   5. Priapism.
   6. Ocular retinopathy.
   7. Gallbladder disease.
   8. Renal.
   9. Cardiomyopathy.
   10. Leg ulcerations.
 C. Susceptibility to infection.
 D. Growth failure, delayed puberty.
 E. Psychologic problems (narcotic addiction, chronic illness, unusual dependence).

IV. Physical findings
 A. Depends on which clinical manifestation is presenting.
 B. Chronic hemolytic anemia: pallor/jaundiced skin, tachycardia, fatigue.
 C. Susceptibility to infection: fever, other symptoms related to causative organism or system infected: e.g., meningitis; urinary tract infection (UTI); cytomegalovirus (CMV); hepatitis A, B, C, D, E; pneumonia.
 D. Vaso-occlusive crisis: again depends on location of occlusion.
 E. Splenomegaly.
 F. Maxillary hyperplasia and dental malocclusion result from compensatory bone marrow expansion.

V. Diagnostic tests
A. Newborn screening for hemoglobinopathies. Electrophoresis on cellulose acetate indicates type of hemoglobin: fetal (F), normal adult (A), sickle (S), hemoglobin C (C).
B. Repeat testing with abnormal hemoglobin (FS) pattern on newborn screen.
C. CBC with hemoglobin MCV.

VI. Differential diagnosis

Beta thalassemia anemia, 282.49
Sickle cell disease, 282.60

A. Sickle cell trait (benign), beta-thalassemia anemia.

VII. Treatment
A. Preventive care.
   1. Education of the family.
      a. Adequate fluid intake.
      b. Immediate medical help for fevers.
      c. Importance of prophylactic treatment.
   2. Immunizations per the schedule plus 23-valent pneumococcal vaccine at 2 and 5 years.
B. Pharmaceutical therapies.
   1. Penicillin prophylaxis:
      a. 2 mo–3 yrs: PenVK 125 mg PO bid.
      b. 3 yrs–5+ yrs: PenVK 250 mg PO bid.
   2. Alternative to penicillin: erythromycin (EES) 20 mg/kg/d ÷ bid.
   3. Folic acid: 1 mg/day.
   4. Multivitamin 1 daily.
   5. Hydroxyurea drug therapy.
      a. Unsickling effect of hydroxyurea can decrease frequency of vaso-occlusive crises.
      b. Starting dose: 15 mg/kg/day, increase gradually by 5 mg/kg/day while monitoring for toxicity.
      c. Toxicity manifested by falls in neutrophil count to $<2500/mm^3$ or platelet count $<80,000/mm^3$
   6. Pain medications: acetaminophen or nonsteroidal anti-inflammatory drugs (NSAIDs) (mild pain), acetaminophen with codeine (moderate pain), morphine (severe pain).

VIII. Follow-up
A. Routine well-child checks:
   1. Birth to 6 months: every 2 months, CBC every visit.
   2. 6 Months to 2 years: every 3 months.
      a. CBC every 3–6 months.
      b. Urinalysis (UA) annually.
      c. Ferritin or serum iron and total iron-binding capacity (TIBC) once at 1–2 years of age.
      d. BUN, creatinine, liver function tests (LFTs) once at 1–2 years of age.

    e. Influenza vaccine annually.
    f. Start folic acid daily at 1 year of age.
   3. 2–5 Years: visits every 6 months.
    a. CBC and UA at least yearly.
    b. BUN, creatinine, LFTs every 1–2 years.
    c. 23-Valent pneumococcal vaccine at 2 years of age, with booster at 5 years.
    d. Hearing, vision, purified protein derivative (PPD) per standard practice.
   4. >5 Years: visits every 6–12 months.
    a. CBC and UA at least annually.
    b. BUN, creatinine, LFTs every 2–3 years.
    c. Influenza vaccine yearly.
    d. Continue folic acid.
    e. May opt to stop penicillin V.
   5. Adolescent: yearly visits.
    a. CBC and UA yearly.
    b. BUN, creatinine, LFTs every 2–3 years.
    c. Ferritin or serum iron and TIBC at least once.
     • Hearing, vision, PPD as per standard practice.
     • Influenza vaccine yearly.
  B. Close monitoring by family for complications.

IX. Complications

Acute chest syndrome, 517.3	Priapism, 607.3
Anemia, 285.9	Renal dysfunction, 593.9
Aplastic crisis, 284.9	Renal failure, 586.
Avascular necrosis of hips, 733.42	Retinal detachment, 361.9
Chronic lung disease, 518.89	Retinopathy, 362.10
Febrile events, 780.6	Splenic sequestration, 289.52
Gallstones, 574.2	Stroke, 436.
Hemolysis, 283.9	Vaso-occlusive events, 459.9
Leg ulcers, 707.10	

  A. Acute and chronic complications (hemolysis, anemia, gallstones) need early recognition, prompt treatment to reduce morbidity and mortality.
  B. Acute events:
   1. Painful vaso-occlusive events.
   2. Febrile events.
   3. Acute chest syndrome.
   4. Splenic sequestration.
   5. Stroke.
   6. Aplastic crisis.
  C. Chronic events:
   1. Avascular necrosis of hips/shoulders.
   2. Priapism.

3. Chronic lung disease.
4. Leg ulcers.
5. Renal dysfunction or renal failure.
6. Retinopathy and retinal detachment.

X. Education

A. When family/patient should seek immediate medical care:
1. Fevers or persistent low-grade fever.
2. Pain unrelieved by prescribed oral medications.
3. Persistent abdominal pain, recurrent emesis.
4. Dyspnea, pain with breathing, hemoptysis, or feelings of tightness in chest.
5. Angina, exercise intolerance, or orthopnea.
6. Visual/speech changes, weakness/numbness in extremities, persistent headaches.
7. Sustained penile erections unrelieved by prescribed medications.
8. Increased lethargy, irritability, or pallor.

B. Factors that may precipitate painful vaso-occlusive crises:
1. Inadequate rest, emotional stress, fatigue.
2. Vasoconstrictive drugs, smoking, constrictive clothing.
3. Dehydration, strenuous physical exercise.
4. Extreme hot/cold temperatures, high altitudes, unpressurized aircraft.

BIBLIOGRAPHY

AAP Committee on Drugs: Treatment guidelines for lead exposure in children, *Pediatrics* 96:155, 1995.

Abshire T: Sense and sensibility: Approaching anemia in Children, *Contemp Pediatr* 9:04, 2001.

Alliance to end childhood lead poisoning, March 2004; retrieved from *www.aeclp.org/2lead101.html.*

Carley A: Anemia: When is it iron deficiency? *Pediatr Nursing* 29:127, 2003.

Centers for Disease Control and Prevention: Recommendations for follow-up lead blood level measurements, March 2004; retrieved from *www.cdc.gov/nceh/lead/about/about.htm.*

Centers for Disease Control and Prevention: Recommendations to prevent and control iron deficiency in the United States, *MMWR* 47(No. RR-3):1-36, April 3, 1998.

Cohen S: Lead poisoning: A summary of treatment and prevention, *Pediatr Nursing* 27:125, 2001.

Krause A, Sanders III W: Lead in the environment, US Environmental Protection Agency, February 2004; retrieved from *www.epa.gov/seahome/leadenv.html.*

National Safety Council: Lead poisoning, National Safety Council Fact Sheet Library, February 2004; retrieved from *www.nsc.org/library/facts/lead.htm.*

Segel GB, Hirsh MG, Feig SA: Managing anemia in pediatric office practice: Part 1, *Pediatr Rev* 23:75, 2002.

Story M, Holt K, Sofka D, editors: Iron deficiency anemia. In *Bright futures in practice: nutrition,* Arlington VA, 2000, National Center for Education in Maternal and Child Health, pp 171-177.

Tender J, Cheng TL: Iron deficiency anemia. In Burg FD, et al, editors: *Gellis & Kagan's current pediatric therapy,* Philadelphia, 2002, WB Saunders.

Zimmerman SA, Ware RE, Kinney TR: Gaining ground in the fight against sickle cell disease, *Contemp Pediatr* 14(10):154-177, October 1997.

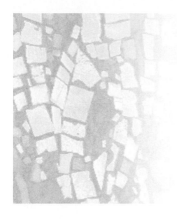

CHAPTER 33

Behavioral Disorders

DONNA HALLAS

BEHAVIORAL ASSESSMENT INSTRUMENTS

Various instruments are available for assessment of children with behavioral and emotional disorders. Refer child and parent to psychiatrist, psychologist, or social worker for completion of 1 or more of these assessment tools. Data from these evaluations will assist in understanding dynamics of family functioning and behavioral management plan (Boxes 33-1, 33-2, 33-3).

ATTENTION DEFICIT HYPERACTIVITY DISORDER (ADHD)

Arithmetical disorder, 315.1	Emotional disorder, V40.9
Attention deficit hyperactivity disorder, 314.01	Impulsivity, 314.01
	Inattentive behavior, 314.0
Behavioral disorders, 312.9	Language disorder, 315.31
Combined hyperactive/inattentive, 314.01	Learning disability, 315.2
Dyspraxia, 315.4	Reading disorder, 315.0

ADHD is characterized by levels of hyperactivity, impulsive behaviors, and/or inattentive behaviors outside the normal parameters of the psychosocial development for child's age. Symptoms are displayed by the child before 7 years of age even though diagnosis may not be established until child enters the school setting. Three subtypes of ADHD are now recognized: (1) hyperactive/impulsive (ADHD-HI), (2) inattentive (ADHD-IA), and (3) combined (ADHD-CT).

I. Etiology
    A. Specific etiology unknown. Believed that abnormal dopamine transport and uptake at nerve synapse may account for symptoms displayed.

II. Occurrence
    A. 3–5% of all children have some form of ADHD with/without hyperactivity.
    B. More prevalent in males than females, approximate ratio of 4:1 C. Prevalence of comorbid conditions ranges from 9% to 50% depending on specific comorbid condition. Refer to Table 33-1.

BOX 33-1 • Behavioral Assessment Rating Scales

Achenbach Child Behavior Checklist System
- Parent Form (CBCL)
- Teacher Report Form (TRF)

Attention Deficit Disorders Evaluation Scales (ADDES)
- Home Version
- School Version

Behavior Assessment System for Children (BASC)
- Parent Rating Scale (PRS)
- Teacher Rating Scale (TRS)

Connor's Parent/Teacher Rating Scale
Personality Inventory for Children–Revised (PIC-R)
Social Skills Rating Scale (SSRS)
Walker Problem Behavior Identification Checklist (WPBIC)

BOX 33-2 • Behavioral Assessment: Self-Report Rating Scales

Achenbach Child Behavior Checklist System (CBCL)
- Youth Self-Report

Behavior Assessment System for Children (BASC)
- Self-Report of Personality

Child Anxiety Scale
Children's Personality Questionnaire (CPQ)
Early School Personality Questionnaire (ESPQ)
High School Personality Questionnaire (HSPQ)
Revised Children's Manifest Anxiety Scale (RCMAS)
Social Skills Rating System (SSRS)–Student Form

BOX 33-3 • Behavioral Assessment: Protective Measures

Draw a Person: Screening Procedure for Emotional Disturbance (DAP: SPED)
Minnesota Multiphasic Personality Inventory–A (MMPI-A)
Tell Me a Story (TEMAS)

TABLE 33-1 • Prevalence of comorbid conditions in children with ADHD

Comorbid condition	Prevalence rate (%)
Conduct disorder, 312.9	25
Oppositional defiant disorder, 313.81	33
Depressive disorder, 311.	9–38
Anxiety disorder, 300.00	25
Learning disorder, 315.2	12–30

Adapted from Agency for Health Care Policy and Research, US Department of Health & Human Services.

III. Clinical manifestations

A. Child displays and/or parents and teachers report inappropriate degrees of:

    1. Hyperactivity.

    2. Impulsivity.

    3. Inattentive behaviors.

B. DSM-IV diagnostic criteria delineate clinical manifestations of ADHD and clarify criteria utilized to make definitive diagnosis (Box 33-4).

BOX 33-4 • DSM-IV Diagnostic Criteria for ADHD

A. Either 1 or 2

    1. Six or more of the following symptoms of inattention have persisted for at least 6 months to degree that is maladaptive and inconsistent with developmental level:

    Inattention

      a. Often fails to give close attention to details or makes careless mistakes in schoolwork, work, or other activities

      b. Often has difficulty sustaining attention in tasks or play activities

      c. Often does not seem to listen when spoken to directly

      d. Often does not follow through on instructions and fails to finish schoolwork, chores, or duties in workplace (not due to oppositional behavior or failure to understand instructions)

      e. Often has difficulty organizing tasks and activities

      f. Often avoids, dislikes, or is reluctant to engage in tasks requiring sustained mental effort (such as schoolwork or homework)

      g. Often loses things necessary for tasks or activities (e.g., toys, school assignments, pencils, books, or tools)

      h. Is often easily distracted by extraneous stimuli

      i. Is often forgetful in daily activities

    2. Six or more of the following symptoms of hyperactivity-impulsivity have persisted for at least 6 months to degree that is maladaptive and inconsistent with developmental level:

    Hyperactivity

      a. Often fidgets with hands/feet or squirms in seat

      b. Often leaves seat in classroom or in other situations in which remaining seated is expected

      c. Often runs about or climbs excessively in situations in which it is inappropriate (in adolescents or adults, may be limited to subjective feelings of restlessness)

      d. Often has difficulty playing or engaging in leisure activities quietly. Is often "on the go" or often acts as if "driven by a motor"

      e. Often talks excessively

    Impulsivity

      a. Often blurts out answers before questions have been completed

      b. Often has difficulty awaiting turn

      c. Often interrupts or intrudes on others (e.g., butts into conversations or games)

Continued

BOX 33-4 • DSM-IV Diagnostic Criteria for ADHD—cont'd

B. Some hyperactive-impulsive or inattentive symptoms that caused impairment were present before 7 years of age.

C. Some impairment from the symptoms is present in 2 or more settings (e.g., at school [or work] or at home).

D. There must be clear evidence of clinically significant impairment in social, academic, or occupational functioning.

E. Symptoms do not occur exclusively during course of pervasive developmental disorder, schizophrenia, or other psychotic disorder and are not better accounted for by another mental disorder (e.g., mood disorder, anxiety disorder, dissociative disorder, or personality disorder).

Code based on type:

314.01 attention-deficit/hyperactivity disorder, combined type: if both criteria A1 and A2 are met for past 6 months

314.00 attention-deficit/hyperactivity disorder, predominantly inattentive type: if criterion A1 is met but criterion A2 is not met for the past 6 months

314.01 attention-deficit/hyperactivity disorder, predominantly hyperactive, impulsive type: if criterion A2 is met but criterion A1 is not met for past 6 months

314.9 attention-deficit/hyperactivity disorder not otherwise specified

---

Reprinted with permission from the *Diagnostic and statistical manual of mental disorders,* text revision, 4th ed (DSM-IV). Copyright 2000, American Psychiatric Association.

C. Identifying at-risk child.
 1. Nurse practitioner plays integral role in identifying children at risk for ADHD by evaluating comprehensive medical history.
 2. Positive family history of 1 or more of hyperactivity, conduct disorders, learning disorders, substance abuse, psychiatric disorders.
 3. Intrauterine exposure to smoking and drug/alcohol use, especially during first trimester.
 4. Parent, schoolteacher report that child displays impulsive and inattentive behaviors.
 a. School-age children tend to steal, tell lies, deliberately destroy property.
 b. Adolescents display behaviors associated with anger and mood lability: alcohol/substance abuse, smoking, sexually transmitted infections, early pregnancy, low self-esteem, involvement in motor vehicle accidents.
D. Comprehensive medical history: include questions that elicit details concerning each of following parameters:
 1. Parental concerns.
 a. Onset and duration of symptoms.
 b. Parental approaches to displayed symptoms.
 2. Behavioral history.
 a. Hyperactivity as described by parents, caregivers, teachers.
 b. Behaviors that display impulsivity, inattentiveness to details.

    c. Ability to focus on interactive video games.

    d. Sleep patterns.

    e. General behavior at home and in school settings.

    f. Previous results of Denver Developmental Screening Tests and any formal psychologic testing.

    g. School performance.

    h. Identification of any learning disabilities.

    i. Behaviors displayed while playing with other children.

3. Significant past medical history.

    a. Prenatal, birth, neonatal history.

    b. Evaluation of growth charts.

    c. Evaluation of previous diagnostic testing including CBC results, lead levels, visual and hearing test results.

    d. Seizures/seizure-like behaviors including staring episodes, tics, head trauma.

    e. Medication history (prescribed, OTC, illicit).

4. Developmental history.

    a. Achievement of developmental milestones.

    b. Speech and language development.

    c. Gross motor and fine motor development.

    d. Coordination.

5. Educational history.

    a. Type of educational program.

    b. Early intervention.

    c. Special education program.

    d. Participation in mainstream programs.

    e. One-to-one programs.

    f. Success/failure in each educational program.

6. Behaviors at school.

    a. Reports from teachers, counselors.

    b. Relationships with children at school.

7. Family history.

    a. Parents or siblings diagnosed with ADHD.

    b. Substance abuse.

    c. Mental illness.

    d. Learning disabilities.

8. Psychosocial history.

    a. Family structure, function.

    b. Head of family.

    c. Parents occupation, employment, level of education.

    d. Substance abuse by parents/child.

    e. Evaluations family–child interactions.

E. Manifestations consistent with comorbid conditions:

1. Lack of motor control; clumsiness (developmental coordination disorder [dyspraxia]).

2. Preschooler with speech, language delay (learning disability).
3. Writes number in reverse order after age 7 (learning disability).
4. Poor school performance: unable to learn to read, write, or do mathematics (learning disability).
5. Insomnia.
6. Enuresis, encopresis.
7. Negative, hostile, defiant behaviors lasting at least 6 months (oppositional defiant disorder, ODD).
8. Violation of home/school rules (conduct disorder).
9. Symptoms of depression.
10. Inappropriate levels of anxiety.
11. Low self-esteem.

IV. Physical findings
A. For diagnosis without comorbid conditions, physical examination is usually unremarkable.
B. Behavior during physical examination is often inappropriate for age.
C. Dysmorphic features may be consistent with comorbid conditions.
D. Neurocutaneous lesions may be consistent with comorbid conditions.

V. Diagnostic tests
A. No specific diagnostic tests for definitive diagnosis.
B. Some laboratory tests may assist in ruling out or verifying comorbid conditions. Following laboratory tests may be helpful:
   1. CBC with differential.
   2. Basic metabolic panel.
   3. Liver function panel.
   4. Thyroid studies including thyroid-stimulating hormone (TSH).
   5. ECG: to evaluate heart rate and QT interval.
   6. EEG: recommended for all children who may be placed on medication therapy and have a past medical history of seizures and/or a family history of a seizure disorder.
C. Diagnosis of ADHD.
   1. For definitive diagnosis, must use DSM-IV diagnostic criteria for ADHD (Box 33-4).
   2. American Academy of Pediatrics (AAP) published evidenced-based guidelines for primary care diagnosis and clinical evaluation of children suspected of having ADHD. AAP guidelines based on DSM-IV diagnostic criteria as well as number of scientific studies that evaluated treatment of children with diagnosis of ADHD.

VI. Differential diagnosis
A. Because diagnosis has several significant comorbid conditions, comprehensive history and physical examination essential to establish definitive diagnosis and formulate treatment plan.
B. Differential diagnosis included in Table 33-2.

VII. Treatment (Box 33-5)
A. Aimed at alleviating major symptoms child displays and improving child's ability to function within family unit, social and educational environments.

TABLE 33-2 • Differential diagnosis of ADHD

Differential diagnosis	Characteristic symptoms or presentation
Learning disability, 315.2	Language delay especially in preschool years
	Persistent reversal of numbers after 7 years of age
	Unsuccessful in achieving reading, writing, math skills
	Difficulty understanding concept of left and right
Sleep disorders, 780.50	Insomnia leading to attention deficit in school activities
	Sleeping during class
	Extended daytime naps at home or in school (preschool or kindergarten)
	Frequent episodes of night terrors or nightmares
Mild mental retardation, 317.	Children who present with learning difficulties in elementary grades
Tourette syndrome, 307.23	Usually symptoms are evident after 7 years of age
	Reports by parents/caregivers that child has had 2+ motor tics and 1 vocal tic during 1-year interval
Oppositional defiant disorder, 313.81	Negativistic
	Hostile
	Defiant behaviors
	Uncontrolled temper
	Angry
	Refuses to comply with social rules at home, school
	Behaviors are associated with poor school performance
Conduct disorder, 312.9	Violates rights of others
	Violates societal norms
	Violates rules at home, school
	Participates in at-risk behaviors: smoking, substance abuse
	Often suspended from school
Anxiety disorder, 300.00	Feels threatened without apparent reason, cannot identity source of threat
	Feelings of uneasiness
	Apprehension
	History of breathlessness, palpitations, restlessness, chest tightness, trembling
Depression, 311.	Low self-esteem, low self-image
	Reports feeling depressed
	Poor social relationships, does not participate in school activities
Bipolar disorder, 296.7	Mood lability, irritability
	Evidence of depression
Pervasive developmental disorders, 299.8: autism, Asperger's syndrome, 299.8; childhood disintegrative disorder, 299.1; Rett syndrome, 330.8	Language delay
	Abnormal social behaviors
	Ritualistic movements
	Impaired intellectual functioning

BOX 33-5 • Role of Nurse Practitioner in Managing Children with ADHD

1. Establish rapport with psychiatrist or psychologist to identify treatment plan.
2. Include parents, child, school personnel in the treatment plan.
3. Monitor effects of stimulant medication to ensure desired treatment plan outcomes.
4. Follow-up should include biannual physical examinations and appropriate laboratory studies.

    B. In addition, if child also displays symptoms of 1 or more comorbid conditions, treatment is highly recommended to reduce or alleviate these symptoms.

    C. Mental health referrals for all children suspected of having comorbid psychiatric conditions.

    D. Characteristics of treatment plan.

      1. Parent education.

        a. Provide education about ADHD and appropriate comorbid condition.

        b. Identify available resources and support groups for parents.

      2. School-based strategies.

        a. Structured classroom setting.

        b. Consistent instruction and application of rules of conduct.

        c. Meets educational needs of child as identified through in-school testing.

      3. Behavior modification.

        a. Strategies are consistent and followed at home and at school.

        b. Inform child of rules of acceptable behavior.

        c. Appropriate behaviors are consistently rewarded.

      4. Medication therapy.

        a. Basic principles.

          • Begin with lowest dosage and increase dosage every 5–7 days based on parent and teacher assessment of child's response (changes in behavior) to medication.

          • Once positive response to medication therapy is reported, increase dose at least 1 more time.

          • Medication administered every 12 hours has been shown to be most effective in controlling symptoms of ADHD.

        b. Drugs of choice.

          • May use immediate-release tablets: methylphenidate (Ritalin), dextroamphetamine levoamphetamine (Adderall), dextroamphetamine (Dexedrine).

          • May use sustained-release tablets: methylphenidate (Ritalin SR; Concerta; Metadate ER; Metadate CD), dextroamphetamine levoamphetamine (Adderall XR), dextroamphetamine (Dexedrine spansule).

        c. Potential side effects:

          • Decreased appetite, weight loss.

          • Sleep problems.

- Increased heart rate, blood pressure, dizziness.
- Growth suppression.
- Exacerbations of tics and Tourette's syndrome.
  d. Management of side effects:
  - Administer dose after meals to improve appetite; frequent high-calorie snacks.
  - Avoid caffeine intake.
  - Modify time of administration if sleep problems.
  5. New drug therapy for ADHD.
  a. Atomoxetime (Strattera), a nonstimulant medication.
  b. Maximum dose may not be achieved for at least 4 weeks after drug therapy is initiated. Therefore, if changing from psychostimulant medication to atomoxetime, administer psychostimulant with atomoxetime for first 4 weeks of therapy, then taper and discontinue.

VIII. Follow-up
  A. Monitor height, weight, heart rate, blood pressure every 3 months in children <12 years of age. School nurse can play integral role in monitoring these measurements in child every 3 months and report these findings to primary care provider.
  B. In children >12 years of age, monitor height, weight, heart rate, blood pressure every 6 months.
  C. Monitor CBC every 6 months. Children are at increased risk for anemia while on psychostimulant drug therapy.
  D. Perform interval history, physical assessment every 6 months to evaluate child's response to treatment program.
  E. Consult with teacher and school psychologist prior to each 6-month health care evaluation for continuity of care.
  F. Follow up with psychiatric referrals, as appropriate.

IX. Complications

High blood pressure, 401.9	Tourette's syndrome, 307.23
Increased heart rate, 785.0	Weight loss, 783.21
Tic's, 307.20	

  A. Complications from medication therapy include weight loss, increased heart rate and blood pressure, growth suppression, exacerbations of tics and Tourette's syndrome.
  B. Once medication is discontinued, symptoms related to complications of medication therapy resolve; however, symptoms of ADHD may return even with continuous behavior modification therapy.

X. Education
  A. Parent education is key to successful management.
  1. Parents should receive initial and updated education related to behavior modification strategies for successful treatment as child reaches each new developmental stage.

2. Parents need to understand medication management.
3. Know possible side effects of medication therapy.
4. Support groups.
5. Internet resources.

AUTISTIC SPECTRUM DISORDER

Asperger's syndrome, 299.8	Echolalia, 784.69
Autistic disorder, 299.	Language disorder, 315.31
Autistic spectrum disorder, 299.	Rett syndrome, 330.8
Childhood disintegrative disorder, 299.1	Social disorder, 313.22

Also called pervasive developmental disorders. Includes autistic disorder, Asperger's syndrome, childhood disintegrative disorder, Rett syndrome. Characterized by impairment in verbal and nonverbal communication as well as impaired social interactions.

I. Etiology
  A. Cause unknown.
  B. Multiple theories include genetics, association with fragile X, abnormal neurochemical findings.

II. Occurrence
  A. More common in males than in females.
  B. Occurs in 3–4 of every 10,000 children.

III. Clinical manifestations
  A. Symptoms develop before 30 months of age.
    1. Lack of (or poorly developed) verbal and nonverbal communication skills.
      a. Abnormal speech patterns; echolalia, nonsense rhyming.
    2. Abnormal social play, solitary play, no friendships.
    3. Repetitive body movements.
      a. Ritualistic behaviors; need for sameness.
      b. Tantrums when ritual is disrupted.
      c. Rocking behaviors.
    4. Impaired intellectual functioning.
      a. May have mental retardation.
      b. Occasionally child has particular talent, i.e., art; music.

IV. Physical findings
  A. Physical examination is normal.
  B. Lack of communication skills and psychosocial skills lead examiner to suspect autism.

V. Diagnostic tests
  A. Refer to psychologist for cognitive and psychologic testing.
  B. Refer to neurologist for full neurologic diagnostic workup including blood work, MRI with contrast, CT scan, EEG.
  C. Refer for early intervention services.
  D. Autistic measures (Box 33-6).

BOX 33-6 • Autistic Measures

Autistic Diagnostic Observation Schedule (ADOS)
Childhood Autism Rating Scale (CARS)

VI. Differential Diagnosis

Asperger's syndrome, 299.8	Mental retardation, 319.
Childhood disintegrative disorder, 299.1	Obsessive-compulsive disorder, 300.3
Conduct disorder, 312.9	Pervasive disorder, 299.8
Fragile X syndrome, 759.83	Rett syndrome, 330.8
Hearing disorder, 389.9	Schizophrenia, 299.9
Lead poisoning, 984.9	Tourette's syndrome, 307.23

   A. Obsessive-compulsive disorder, Tourette's syndrome.
   B. Conduct disorder, mental retardation, hearing disorder.
   C. Schizophrenia of childhood.
   D. Lead poisoning.
   E. Fragile X syndrome.
   F. Additional pervasive disorders.
   G. Asperger's syndrome.
      1. Impairment is primarily in social interactions, which includes repetitive and obsessive behaviors.
      2. Children usually do not have language impairments characteristic of autism.
      3. Rare disorder characterized by normal development until 2–4 years old at which time, there is severe mental and social deterioration.
   H. Childhood disintegrative disorder.
   I. Rett syndrome.
      1. Development normal until 1 year of age at which time language and motor development regress.
      2. Microcephaly is usually evident by 1 year of age.

VII. Treatment
   A. Implement all early intervention services in home and school: speech therapy; occupational and physical therapy; behavior modification strategies.
   B. Diagnosis.
      1. Denver Developmental II screening test: valuable tool used to assist in early recognition.
      2. Refer to developmental neurologist as soon as symptoms are suspected.

VIII. Follow-up
   A. Recognize early signs and symptoms of autism, Asperger's syndrome, childhood disintegrative disorder, Rett syndrome and make appropriate referrals.

B. Support for parents, other primary caregivers is essential. Families may benefit from connecting with the Autism Society of America (*www.autism-society.org*).

C. Encourage parents to find respite care for child.

IX. Complications

Autism, **299.**

A. Autism is a chronic disease with no cure.

X. Education

A. Families need education about the disorder, what treatments have been proven to be successful; multidisciplinary interventions.

B. Families need to be careful when investigating treatment programs and determine proven benefits from these programs. Families must consider own safety and that of their child.

BREATH HOLDING

Apnea, **786.03**
Bradycardia, **427.89**
Breath holding spells, **786.9**
Breath holding, **312.81**
Cerebral anoxia, **348.1**
Clonic jerks, **333.2**

Cyanosis, **782.5**
Cyanotic spells, **782.5**
Loss of consciousness, **780.09**
Pallid spells, **782.61**
Tonic seizure activity, **345.1**

Characterized by episodes in which infant/young child holds breath, which leads to cerebral anoxia resulting in limp body and extremities, unresponsiveness. Two types: cyanotic spells and pallid spells.

I. Etiology

A. Unknown.

II. Occurrence

A. Usually begins after 6 months old.

B. Highest incidence is at 2 years old.

C. Usually resolves by 5 years old.

III. Clinical manifestations

A. Cyanotic spells.

 1. Brief shrill cry followed by forced expiration and apnea.

 2. Onset of cyanosis.

 3. Loss of consciousness.

 4. Generalized clonic jerks.

 5. Bradycardia.

B. Pallid spells.

 1. Usually follows fall in which child strikes head, causing pain.

 2. Cessation of normal breathing pattern; prolonged apneic episode.

 3. Loses consciousness.

 4. Pallor.

 5. Tonic seizure activity (occasional).

IV. Physical findings
A. Normal physical exam findings.
V. Diagnostic tests
A. EEG. Referral to neurologist is recommended.
VI. Differential diagnosis

Seizure disorder, 780.39

A. Seizure disorder.
VII. Treatment
A. Parental support and reassurance.
VIII. Follow-up
A. Call within a few days to assess how family is dealing and answer questions.
B. Parents' level of comfort with breath-holding spells determines further follow-up.
IX. Complications
A. None.
X. Education
A. Discussion of management plan that parents can follow consistently. Parents must feel comfortable with plan.
B. Provide safe environment for child during and at conclusion of episode.
C. Avoid reinforcement of these behaviors.

NIGHTMARES AND NIGHT TERRORS

Dilated pupil, 379.43   Nightmares, 307.47
Hyperventilation, 300.11   Tachycardia, 785.0
Night terrors, 307.46

I. Etiology
A. Actual cause unknown.
B. Dysfunctional family relationships should be suspected.
II. Occurrence
A. Occurs in 1–3% of children, mostly in boys between 5 and 7 years old.
III. Clinical manifestations
A. Sudden unexpected screams during sleep usually between 12 midnight and 2 AM.
B. Appears frightened; pupils dilated.
C. Tachycardia, hyperventilation.
D. Thrashing of extremities.
E. Inconsolable, not aware of parents presence.
F. Returns to sleep.
G. No recall of night terror in morning.
IV. Physical findings
A. None.
V. Diagnostic tests
A. None necessary.

VI. Differential diagnosis

Anxiety, **300.00**	Emotional disorder, **V40.9**
Depression, **311.**	Seizure, **780.39**

    A. Rule out emotional disorder; anxiety; depression.

    B. Seizures.

VII. Treatment

    A. Child should be encouraged to lie down and helped back to sleep (e.g., talking quietly, rubbing back).

    B. Encourage family to wake child before episode for 1–2 weeks to attempt to break cycle.

    C. Protect child from injury.

    D. Provide comfort, reassurance to child.

    E. Counseling may be necessary for children who have severe nighttime fears.

    F. May use diazepam or imipramine for short time period depending on family functional pattern.

VIII. Follow-up

    A. Refer to psychologist or psychiatrist if night terrors persist.

    B. Complete family evaluation may be necessary.

IX. Complications

Night terrors, **307.46**

    A. Injury.

    B. Continued nighttime fears.

X. Education

    A. Often night terrors are self-limiting.

    B. Family support may necessary to reduce parental anxiety.

BIBLIOGRAPHY

Adesman A: A diagnosis of ADHD? Don't overlook the probability of comorbidity! *Contemp Pediatr* 20:91-106, 2003.

Agency for Health Care Policy and Research: *Diagnosis of attention deficit/hyperactivity disorder* [Technical Review No. 3], Rockville, MD, 1999, US Department of Health and Human Services.

American Psychiatric Association: *Diagnostic and statistical manual of mental disorders,* ed 4, Washington, DC, 1994, American Psychiatric Association.

Behrman RE, Liegman RM, Jenson HB: *Nelson textbook of pediatrics,* ed 16, Philadelphia, 2000, WB Saunders.

Conners CK: ADHD therapy: Optimizing functional outcomes, *Contemp Pediatr* 20(Suppl): 4-6, 2003.

Liu YH, Leslie LK: Diagnosing ADHD: Putting AAP guidelines to the test—and into practice. *Contemp Pediatr* 20:51-73, 2003.

Wolraich ML: ADHD therapy: Optimizing functional outcomes, *Contemp Pediatr* 20(Suppl):7-10, 2003.

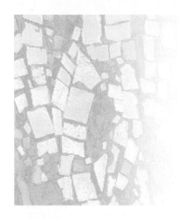

CHAPTER 34

Mental Health Disorders

KIM WALTON

ANXIETY DISORDERS

Anxiety disorders, 300.00	Overanxious disorder in children, 313.0
Compulsions, 307.9	Panic disorder, 300.01
Dermatitis, 692.9	Post-traumatic stress disorder (PTSD), 309.81
Diarrhea, 787.91	Restlessness, 799.2
Dizziness, 780.4	School problems, 312.9
Fatigue, 780.79	Separation anxiety, 309.21
Headaches, 784.0	Shortness of breath, 786.05
Irritability, 799.2	Sleep disturbance, 780.50
Muscle tension, 729.82	Sweating, 780.8
Nausea, 787.02	Temper tantrums, 312.1
Obsessive compulsive disorder (OCD), 300.3	Tiredness, 780.89

Presentation of anxiety disorder; includes both physical and emotional characteristics.

I. Etiology
  A. Biochemical changes in brain.
   1. Possible genetic vulnerability.
   2. Post-traumatic stress disorder (PTSD), present in children who survive severe or terrifying physical or emotional event.
   3. Separation anxiety, note relative frequency in children of mothers with panic disorder.

II. Occurrence
  A. Most common mental illness group occurring in children and adolescents.
  B. Estimated prevalence of any anxiety disorder among children and adolescents is 13% in 6-month period.

III. Clinical manifestations
  A. Generalized anxiety disorder (also known as overanxious disorder in children).

435

1. Characterized by at least 6 months of persistent, excessive anxiety/worry over everyday events; difficult to control the worry.
2. Anxiety and worry are associated with at least 1 of following:
   a. Restlessness.
   b. Being easily fatigued.
   c. Difficulty concentrating.
   d. Irritability.
   e. Muscle tension.
   f. Sleep disturbance.
3. Symptoms must cause significant distress or impairment in functioning.
B. Obsessive compulsive disorder (OCD).
   1. Obsessions: recurring thoughts or images that are disturbing, intrusive, cannot be controlled through rational reasoning.
      a. Common obsessions:
         • Contamination.
         • Fear of harm to self/family member.
         • Worry about acting on aggressive impulses.
         • Concern about order and symmetry.
      b. Thoughts or images are not simply excessive worries about real-life problems.
      c. Attempts to ignore or suppress such thoughts or images with some other thought/action.
   2. Compulsions: repetitive behaviors that one feels obliged to complete. Performance of compulsive behavior, at least temporarily, decreases anxiety, thereby reinforcing behavior.
      a. Common compulsions:
         • Hand washing.
         • Cleaning rituals.
         • Requesting reassurance.
         • Ordering and arranging.
         • Complex touching habits.
         • Checking, counting, and repetition of routine activities.
      b. Behaviors are aimed at preventing or reducing distress.
   3. Obsessions or compulsions must be time consuming (take >1 hour a day), cause marked distress, interfere with daily activities.
   4. Often seen with comorbidities.
   5. Strong familial component.
   6. Immune response to streptococcal infections.
C. PTSD.
   1. Must have exposure to traumatic event with *both* of following:
      a. Actual or threatened death/serious injury or threat to physical integrity of self/others **AND**
      b. Response involving intense fear, helplessness, horror. May be expressed as disorganized/agitated behavior in children.

2. Traumatic event is persistently reexperienced in 1 or more of following ways:
   a. Recurrent, intrusive, distressing thoughts of event. In young children, may include repetitive play.
   b. Recurrent distressing dreams. In children, may be frightening dreams without recognizable content.
   c. Acting or feeling as if trauma were reoccurring. In young children, may include trauma specific reenactment, often through play.
   d. Intense psychologic distress on exposure to internal/external cues reminiscent of traumatic event.
   e. Physiologic reactivity on exposure to internal/external cues reminiscent of traumatic event.
3. Persistent *avoidance* of stimuli, numbing of general responsiveness with 3 or more of following:
   a. Efforts to avoid thoughts, feelings, or talking about trauma.
   b. Efforts to avoid activities, places, people that arouse memories.
   c. Inability to recall important aspect of event.
   d. Diminished interest/participation in activities.
   e. Feelings of detachment/estrangement.
   f. Restricted range of affect.
   g. Sense of foreshortened future.
4. Persistent symptoms of *arousal* with 2 or more of following:
   a. Difficulty falling asleep/staying asleep.
   b. Irritability or outbursts of anger.
   c. Difficulty concentrating.
   d. Hypervigilance.
   e. Exaggerated startle response.
5. Duration of symptoms for >1 month.
6. Disturbance causes significant distress or impairment in functioning.
7. Diagnosis may be acute (symptoms <3 months), chronic (symptoms ≥3 months), or delayed (onset of symptoms at least 6 months after stressor).

D. Separation anxiety.
1. Onset of excessive anxiety on separation from home/major attachment figure *beyond what is expected* for developmental level as evidenced by 3 or more of following:
   a. Recurrent excessive distress on separation from home or major attachment figure.
   b. Persistent/excessive worry about losing or harm coming to major attachment figure.
   c. Worry that untoward event will lead to separation (e.g., getting lost or kidnapped).
   d. Reluctance or refusal to go to school.
   e. Fearful or reluctant to be alone.
   f. Reluctance or refusal to go to sleep without being near attachment figure or to sleep away from home.

    g. Repeated nightmares with themes of separation.

    h. Repeated physical complaints when separation occurs or is anticipated.

  2. Symptoms must be present for at least 4 weeks and must begin before age 18.

  3. Symptoms must cause significant distress/impairment at home, school, with friends.

IV. Physical findings

  A. May present with symptoms of sleep disturbance, tiredness, school problems, restlessness, irritability, somatic complaints (sweating, nausea, diarrhea, shortness of breath, dizziness, headaches).

  B. For OCD, parents generally bring children in due to increase in temper tantrums, decline in school performance, food restriction, dermatitis. Children rarely request help, may be secretive about thoughts, behaviors.

V. Diagnostic tests

  A. None. Requires interview with child and parent/caregiver.

  B. Consider collateral contact with school personnel, especially with separation anxiety.

  C. Assess recent life stressors (family move, death, divorce, new school setting, etc.).

VI. Differential diagnosis

Anxiety disorder, **300.00**	Post-traumatic stress disorder (PTSD), **309.81**
Attention deficit hyperactive disorder (ADHD), **314.00**	Separation anxiety, **309.21**
Obsessive-compulsive disorder (OCD), **300.3**	Stress reaction, acute, **308.9**

  A. Attention deficit hyperactivity disorder (ADHD).

  B. Differentiate among anxiety disorders such as PTSD, separation anxiety, generalized anxiety disorder, OCD.

  C. Consider acute stress reaction if exposed to traumatic event, symptoms present <1 month.

VII. Treatment

  A. May require use of medications to reduce anxiety symptoms. Consider use of selective serotonin reuptake inhibitors (SSRIs). These may include:

    1. Clomipramine (Anafranil): starting dose of 10 mg/day; increase to 75–100 mg/day for children; 100–200 mg/day for teens.

    2. Fluoxetine (Prozac): starting dose of 5 mg/day; increase to 15–30 mg/day for children; 10–40 mg/day for teens.

    3. Fluvoxamine (Luvox): starting dose of 25 mg/day; increase to 50–200 mg/day for children; 150–300 mg/day for teens.

    4. Sertraline (Zoloft): starting dose of 25 mg/day; increase to 50–100 mg/day for children; 50–200 mg/day for teens.

    B. Cognitive behavioral therapy to help identify anxiety triggers, awareness of physiologic responses to anxiety. Develop plan for coping, evaluation of success of strategies.

    C. Family therapy to address ways family can support the child.

VIII. Follow-up

    A. Follow-up appointment to monitor effectiveness of medications, address side effects of medications, compliance issues.

    B. Collaboration with family, mental health treatment provider, school personnel to assess success of treatment approaches and medications.

IX. Complications

    A. Poor school performance.

    B. Poor self-esteem, social skills, avoidance of peers.

    C. Potential for family stress and conflict.

    D. Development of comorbid diagnosis of substance abuse or major depression.

X. Education

    A. Parent/caregiver and child need education about nature of anxiety, ways to identify, evaluate, change anxious thoughts.

    B. Child needs to learn to recognize physiologic symptoms of anxiety, use of positive "self-talk."

    C. Relaxation training may be beneficial.

EATING DISORDERS

Abdominal pain, 789.00	Hair loss, 704.00
Anorexia nervosa, 307.1	Hypotension, 458.9
Arrhythmias, 427.9	Hypothermia, 996.1
Brittle nails, 703.8	Insomnia, 780.52
Bulimia nervosa, 783.6	Lethargy, 780.79
Cold intolerance, 788.90	Leukopenia, 288.0
Constipation, 564.00	Metabolic acidosis, 276.2
Dehydration, 276.5	Metabolic alkalosis, 276.3
Dental caries, 525.09	Mild anemia, 285.9
Dental enamel erosion, 521.3	Nausea, 787.02
Dry skin, 701.1	Scars, 709.2
Eating disorders, 307.50	Sinus bradycardia, 427.89
Enlarged parotid glands, 240.9	Vomiting, 787.03
Expected weight gains, 783.41	Weakness, 780.79
Fatigue, 780.79	Weight loss, 783.21
Fluid and electrolyte imbalances, 276.9	

Serious, sometimes life threatening; tend to be chronic, usually arise in adolescence.

    I. Etiology

        A. Combination of genetic, neurochemical, psychodevelopmental, sociocultural factors.

1. Increased risk among first-degree biological relatives of individuals with disorder. Often co-occurs with other mental health problems such as depression, anxiety, substance abuse, personality disorders.

II. Occurrence

A. >90% of all eating disorders occur in females.

B. Estimated 0.5% of adolescent females have anorexia nervosa; 1–5% meet criteria for bulimia nervosa.

C. Rarely begins before puberty, most common in ages 14–18 years.

D. Onset may be associated with stressful life event.

III. Clinical manifestations

A. Anorexia nervosa.

1. Most severe consequence with mortality rate from starvation, suicide, electrolyte imbalance.

2. Characterized by refusal to maintain minimally normal body weight for age and height (<85% of expected weight).

3. Intense fear of gaining weight or becoming fat.

4. Significant disturbance in perception of shape or size of body; sees self as overweight even when dangerously thin.

5. In postmenarchal females, presence of amenorrhea.

B. Bulimia nervosa.

1. Repeated episodes of binge eating characterized by:

a. Eating in discrete period of time (e.g., within 2 hours) amount of food larger than most people would eat during same period of time and under similar circumstances.

b. Sense of lack of control over eating during episode.

2. Recurrent inappropriate compensatory behaviors to prevent weight gain such as self-induced vomiting, misuse of laxatives, diuretics, enemas, other medications, fasting, excessive exercise.

3. Occurrence of *both* of above behaviors, on average at least twice a week for 3 months. Individuals place excessive emphasis on body shape, weight in self-evaluation.

IV. Physical findings

A. Anorexia nervosa.

1. Reported by family members, individual presents with weight loss or failure to make expected weight gains.

2. Leukopenia, mild anemia are common.

3. May present with signs/symptoms of dehydration, sinus bradycardia, arrhythmias.

4. May present with constipation, abdominal pain, cold intolerance, lethargy, hypotension, hypothermia, dry skin, dental enamel erosion.

B. Bulimia nervosa.

1. Typically presents within normal weight range to slightly overweight.

2. May present with complaints of abdominal pain, nausea, hair loss, brittle nails, fatigue, insomnia, or weakness.

3. Fluid and electrolyte imbalances: metabolic alkalosis from vomiting or metabolic acidosis from laxative abuse.
4. Loss of dental enamel, increased frequency of dental caries.
5. Enlarged parotid glands.
6. Possible calluses/scars on dorsal surface of hand from repeated self-induced vomiting.

V. Diagnostic tests
A. Ask all preteens, adolescents screening questions about eating patterns, satisfaction with body appearance.
B. Monitor height, weight, body mass index on all visits.
C. Laboratory studies: CBC, electrolyte measurement, liver function tests, urinalysis, thyroid-stimulating hormone (TSH) test.
D. Electrocardiogram.

VI. Differential diagnosis

AIDS, 042.	Major depression, 311.
Anxiety disorder, **300.00**	Substance abuse, **995.50**
Brain tumors, 348.8	Weight gain, **783.1**
GI disease, 569.9	Weight loss, **783.21**

A. Rule out other possible medical causes for significant weight loss/failure to gain weight (GI disease, brain tumors, malignancies, AIDS, etc.), although these do not present with distorted body image.
B. Comorbid diagnosis of substance abuse, major depression, anxiety disorder.

VII. Treatment
A. Anorexia nervosa.
   1. Requires comprehensive treatment plan including medical care, monitoring, psychotherapy, nutritional counseling, medication (when appropriate). Involves 3 phases:
      a. Restoring weight loss due to severe dieting, purging.
      b. Treating psychologic disturbances such as distorted body image, low self-esteem, interpersonal conflicts.
      c. Achieving long-term remission, rehabilitation.
   2. Treatment with medication, such as SSRIs; consider *only* after weight gain established.
   3. Acute inpatient hospitalization may be required to restore weight, address fluid and electrolyte imbalance or cardiac disturbances. May require nutrition via nasogastric tube/IV therapy.
   4. Intensive treatment may be needed in specialized day treatment program or intensive outpatient program.
   5. Refer for cognitive behavioral therapy and family therapy.
B. Bulimia nervosa.
   1. Requires comprehensive treatment plan including medical care, monitoring, psychotherapy, nutritional counseling, medication (when appropriate).

   2. Primary goal: reduce/eliminate binge eating, purging behavior.
      a. Establish pattern of regular, nonbinging eating.
      b. Improve attitudes related to eating disorder.
      c. Encourage healthy, not excessive exercise.
      d. Resolution of co-occurring disorders such as depression, anxiety.
   3. Treatment approaches may include individual, group/family therapy.
   4. Cognitive behavioral therapy: useful to address cognitive distortions related to body image and to develop adaptive coping skills.
   5. Antidepressant medications, especially SSRIs, have been found to be effective.

VIII. Follow-up

   A. May need weekly visits to monitor weight, lab work.
   B. To achieve long-term remission and rehabilitation, treatment must include ongoing behavioral therapy, continued assessment of weight and physical health status.
   C. Ongoing assessment of anxiety/depressive symptoms.
   D. Collaboration between family and mental health provider to assess effectiveness of treatment approaches.
   E. Pharmacologic support has found conflicting evidence as benefit.

IX. Complications

Anorexia nervosa, 307.1	Fluid and electrolyte imbalances, 276.9
Bulimia nervosa, 783.6	Gastric rupture, 537.89
Cardiac arrhythmias, 427.9	Loss of dental enamel, 521.3
Cardiac complications, 429.9	Potential for development of depression, 311.
Dehydration, 276.5	Potential for suicide, 300.9
Dental caries, 525.09	Renal failure, 584.9
Depression, 300.4	Starvation, 994.2
Esophagitis, 530.10	Ulceration of esophagus, 530.20
Family stress and conflict, 308.9	Vomiting, 787.03

   A. Anorexia nervosa.
      1. Starvation, fluid and electrolyte imbalances, dehydration.
      2. Cardiac complications.
      3. Renal failure.
      4. Potential for suicide.
      5. Development of anxiety/depression.
      6. Potential for family stress and conflict.
   B. Bulimia nervosa.
      1. Dental caries, loss of dental enamel.
      2. Potential for development of depression, substance abuse.
      3. Gastric rupture from acute gastric dilatation secondary to vomiting.
      4. Esophagitis and ulceration of esophagus.
      5. Potential for cardiac arrhythmias.

X. Education
A. Educate family on potential complications of disorder, as well as how to best support adolescent in treatment.
B. Adolescent and family may benefit from nutritional counseling.

MOOD DISORDERS

Appetite changes, 783.0	Mania, 296.90
Attention deficit hyperactive disorder (ADHD), 314.01	Mood disorders, 296.90
	Oppositional behavior, 313.81
Bipolar disorder, 296.7	Self harm, 300.9
Depression, 311.	Sleep, 307.40
Fatigue, 780.79	Stomachache, 789.00
Headache, 784.0	

I. Etiology
A. Close family member with depression or bipolar disorder may be single largest contributor to likelihood of disorder in child.

II. Occurrence
A. For depression, prevalence is 2% in children, 6% in adolescents with lifetime prevalence in adolescents estimated to be 20%.
B. 1% of adolescents 14–18 years of age meet criteria for bipolar.

III. Clinical manifestations
A. Major depression.
   1. Characterized by 5 or more of these symptoms present daily for at least 2 weeks:
      a. Persistent sadness or irritable mood.
      b. Loss of interest in activities once enjoyed.
      c. Significant change in appetite or body weight.
      d. Difficulty sleeping or oversleeping.
      e. Psychomotor agitation or slowing.
      f. Loss of energy.
      g. Feelings of worthlessness or inappropriate guilt.
      h. Difficulty concentrating.
      i. Recurrent thoughts of death or suicide.
   2. Other signs associated with depression include:
      a. Frequent, vague, nonspecific physical complaints such as stomachaches, headaches, muscle aches, tiredness.
      b. Frequent absences from school or poor school performance.
      c. Talk of/efforts to run away from home.
      d. Outbursts of shouting, complaining, unexplained irritability or crying.
      e. Being bored or lack of interest in playing with friends.
      f. Alcohol or substance abuse.
      g. Social isolation, poor communication, difficulty with relationships.
      h. Fear of death.

      i. Extreme sensitivity to rejection/failure.

      j. Increased irritability, anger, hostility.

      k. Reckless behavior.

B. Bipolar disorder.

  1. Bipolar I: experiences alternating episodes of intense mania and depression.

  2. Bipolar II: experiences episodes of hypomania (markedly elevated or irritable mood with increased physical and mental energy) between recurrent periods of depression.

  3. *Manic symptoms* include:

    a. Severe or rapid changes in mood: extremely irritable or overly silly, elated mood.

    b. Overly inflated self-esteem, grandiosity.

    c. Exaggerated beliefs about personal talents/abilities.

    d. Increased energy, decreased need for sleep; able to go with very little/ no sleep for days without tiring.

    e. Talks too much, too fast, changes subjects too quickly.

    f. Distractibility, hyperactivity: attention shifts from one thing to another quickly.

    g. Increased sexual thoughts, feelings, behaviors or use of explicit sexual language.

    h. Increased goal-directed activity or physical agitation.

    i. Excessive involvement in risky, daredevil behaviors/activities.

  4. *Depressive symptoms* include:

    a. Pervasive/overwhelming sadness, crying spells.

    b. Sleeping too much or inability to sleep.

    c. Agitation, irritability.

    d. Withdrawal from activities formerly enjoyed.

    e. Drop in grades, inability to concentrate.

    f. Thoughts of death and suicide.

    g. Low energy.

    h. Significant loss of appetite.

  5. May also present: explosive/destructive rages, separation anxiety, defiance of authority, bedwetting, night terrors, strong and frequent cravings, impaired judgment, impulsivity.

  6. Presents with depressive symptoms and also exhibits ADHD-like symptoms that are very severe: refer to mental health professional for further evaluation, particularly if family history of bipolar disorder.

IV. Physical findings

A. Specifically ask about thoughts of suicide or self-harm: suicide is third leading cause of death among 10- to 24-year-olds.

B. Major depression may present with multiple, vague somatic complaints (i.e., headache, stomachache, fatigue, sleep, appetite changes).

C. Bipolar disorder may present with symptoms of ADHD, depression, mania, oppositional behavior.

V. Diagnostic tests

A. Several screening tools useful for children/adolescents include Children's Depression Inventory for ages 7–17 and Beck Depression Inventory for adolescents. Positive screens indicate need for comprehensive diagnostic evaluation by mental health professional.

B. Requires intensive interview with child/adolescent and family as well as detailed family history.

VI. Differential diagnosis

Adjustment disorder, **309.9**	Intermittent explosive disorder, **312.34**
Attention deficit hyperactivity disorder (ADHD), **314.01**	Oppositional defiant disorder, **313.81**

A. Adjustment disorder.

B. ADHD.

C. Intermittent explosive disorder.

D. Oppositional defiant disorder.

VII. Treatment

A. Major depression.

   1. Antidepressant medication may be indicated.

   a. Consider SSRI medications:

   - Fluoxetine (Prozac): starting dose of 5 mg/day; increase to 15–40 mg/day for children, 10–60 mg/day for teens.
   - Fluvoxamine (Luvox): starting dose of 25 mg/day; increase to 50–200 mg/day for children, 100–300 mg/day for teens.
   - Sertraline (Zoloft): starting dose of 25 mg/day; increase to 50–150 mg/day for children, 50–200 mg/day for teens.

   b. Following remission of symptoms, continue medications *with* therapy for at least several months given high rate of relapse, recurrence of depression. Gradually discontinue medications over 6 weeks or longer.

   2. Short-term psychotherapy such as cognitive behavioral therapy (CBT).

   a. CBT based on premise that young people with depression have distorted view of themselves, world, future. CBT focuses on changing distortions through time-limited therapy.

   b. Continued therapy for several months after remission of symptoms may help consolidate skills learned, cope with after effects of depression, address environmental stressors, understand how young person's thoughts, behaviors could contribute to relapse.

B. Bipolar disorder.

   1. Use of mood-stabilizing medications such as lithium (Eskalith, Lithobid, lithium carbonate), valproic acid (Depakote), carbamazepine (Tegretol), gabapentin (Neurontin), tiagabine (Gabitril).

   a. Start lithium at 25 mg/kg/day, gradually increase until serum level reaches therapeutic range of 0.9–1.1 mEq/L.

    b. Valproic acid (Depakote): start at 15 mg/kg/day, gradually increase until serum level reaches therapeutic range of 80–120 mg/ml.

    c. Carbamazepine (Tegretol): starting dose of 100 mg/day with increase to 300–800 mg/day in children, 800–1000 mg/day in teens; monitor for serum level to reach therapeutic range of 8–12 mcg/mL.

    d. Gabapentin (Neurontin): starting dose of 10–15 mg/kg per day in 3 divided doses.

2. Consider polypharmacy with addition of antipsychotic medications, calcium channel blockers, antianxiety agents.

3. Do not use antidepressant medication alone; may lead to mania or rapid cycling.

4. Psychostimulant medications frequently used to treat ADHD may worsen manic symptoms.

5. CBT, interpersonal therapy, multifamily support groups essential part of overall treatment plan.

VIII. Follow-up

A. Monitor effectiveness of medications; address side effects, compliance issues.

B. Monitor closely for suicidal thoughts and/or behaviors. NOTE: FDA Black Box warning on use of SSRI antidepressants in children and teens.

C. Monitor blood levels to assess appropriate medication dosing.

D. Collaborate with family, mental health treatment provider, school personnel to assess success of treatment approaches.

IX. Complications

Conduct disorder, 312.9	Risk for suicide, 300.9
Poor psychosocial functioning, V71.02	Substance abuse, 995.50

A. Increased risk for suicidal behavior: attempts may rise, particularly among adolescent males, if depression accompanied by conduct disorder or substance abuse.

B. Increased risk for poor psychosocial functioning.

C. School truancy or poor academic performance.

D. Substance use.

X. Education

A. Monitor effectiveness of medications.

B. Educate families on signs/symptoms of both depression and mania and signs/symptoms of suicidal ideation.

BIBLIOGRAPHY

American Psychiatric Association: *Diagnostic and statistical manual of mental disorders,* ed 4, text revision, Washington, DC, 2000, American Psychiatric Association.

Kaplan DW, et al: Identifying and treating eating disorders, *Pediatrics* 111:1, 2003.

National Institute of Mental Health: Brief notes on the mental health of children and adolescents, Bethesda, MD, 2002, National Institute of Mental Health.

National Institute of Mental Health: NIH Publication No. 01-4901, Bethesda, MD, 2002, National Institute of Mental Health.

National Institute of Mental Health: NIH Publication No. 00-4744, Bethesda, MD, 2002, National Institute of Mental Health.

National Institute of Mental Health: NIH Publication No. 00-4778, Bethesda, MD, 2002, National Institute of Mental Health.

Scahill L: Child and adolescent psychiatric nursing. In Keltner NL, Schwecke LH, Bostrom CE, editors: *Psychiatric nursing,* ed 3, St. Louis, 2001, Mosby.

Recommended Immunization Schedule

Recommended Childhood and Adolescent Immunization Schedule UNITED STATES • 2005

Vaccine ▼ / Age ▶	Birth	1 month	2 months	4 months	6 months	12 months	15 months	18 months	24 months	4–6 years	11–12 years	13–18 years
Hepatitis B[1]	HepB #1	HepB #2			HepB #3					HepB Series		
Diphtheria, Tetanus, Pertussis[2]			DTaP	DTaP	DTaP		DTaP			DTaP	Td	Td
Haemophilus influenzae type b[3]			Hib	Hib	Hib	Hib						
Inactivated Poliovirus			IPV	IPV		IPV				IPV		
Measles, Mumps, Rubella[4]						MMR #1				MMR #2	MMR #2	
Varicella[5]						Varicella				Varicella		
Pneumococcal[6]			PCV	PCV	PCV	PCV				PCV	PPV	
Influenza[7]						Influenza (Yearly)				Influenza (Yearly)		
Hepatitis A[8]										Hepatitis A Series		

Vaccines below red line are for selected populations

This schedule indicates the recommended ages for routine administration of currently licensed childhood vaccines, as of December 1, 2004, for children through age 18 years. Any dose not administered at the recommended age should be administered at any subsequent visit when indicated and feasible.

░ Indicates age groups that warrant special effort to administer those vaccines not previously administered. Additional vaccines may be licensed and recommended during the year. Licensed combination vaccines may be used whenever any components of the combination are indicated and other components of the vaccine are not contraindicated. Providers should consult the manufacturers' package inserts for detailed recommendations. Clinically significant adverse events that follow immunization should be reported to the Vaccine Adverse Event Reporting System (VAERS). Guidance about how to obtain and complete a VAERS form are available at **www.vaers.org** or by telephone, **800-822-7967**.

▓ Range of recommended ages	▨ Only if mother HBsAg(−)
▒ Preadolescent assessment	▓ Catch-up immunization

DEPARTMENT OF HEALTH AND HUMAN SERVICES
CENTERS FOR DISEASE CONTROL AND PREVENTION

The Childhood and Adolescent Immunization Schedule is approved by:
Advisory Committee on Immunization Practices www.cdc.gov/nip/acip
American Academy of Pediatrics www.aap.org
American Academy of Family Physicians www.aafp.org

Recommended Immunization Schedule
for Children and Adolescents Who Start Late or Who Are More Than 1 Month Behind
UNITED STATES • 2005

The tables below give catch-up schedules and minimum intervals between doses for children who have delayed immunizations.
There is no need to restart a vaccine series regardless of the time that has elapsed between doses. Use the chart appropriate for the child's age.

CATCH-UP SCHEDULE FOR CHILDREN AGED 4 MONTHS THROUGH 6 YEARS

Vaccine	Minimum Age for Dose 1	Minimum Interval Between Doses			
		Dose 1 to Dose 2	**Dose 2 to Dose 3**	**Dose 3 to Dose 4**	**Dose 4 to Dose 5**
Diphtheria, Tetanus, Pertussis	6 wks	**4 weeks**	**4 weeks**	**6 months**	**6 months**[1]
Inactivated Poliovirus	6 wks	**4 weeks**	**4 weeks**	**4 weeks**[2]	
Hepatitis B[3]	Birth	**4 weeks**	**8 weeks** (and 16 weeks after first dose)		
Measles, Mumps, Rubella	12 mo	**4 weeks**[4]			
Varicella	12 mo				
Haemophilus influenzae type b[5]	6 wks	**4 weeks** if first dose given at age <12 months **8 weeks (as final dose)** if first dose given at age 12-14 months **No further doses needed** if first dose given at age ≥15 months	**4 weeks**[6] if current age <12 months **8 weeks (as final dose)**[6] if current age ≥12 months and second dose given at age <15 months **No further doses needed** if previous dose given at age ≥15 mo	**8 weeks (as final dose)** This dose only necessary for children aged 12 months–5 years who received 3 doses before age 12 months	
Pneumococcal[7]	6 wks	**4 weeks** if first dose given at age <12 months and current age <24 months **8 weeks (as final dose)** if first dose given at age ≥12 months or current age 24–59 months **No further doses needed** for healthy children if first dose given at age ≥24 months	**4 weeks** if current age <12 months **8 weeks (as final dose)** if current age ≥12 months **No further doses needed** for healthy children if previous dose given at age ≥24 months	**8 weeks (as final dose)** This dose only necessary for children aged 12 months–5 years who received 3 doses before age 12 months	

CATCH-UP SCHEDULE FOR CHILDREN AGED 7 YEARS THROUGH 18 YEARS

Vaccine	Minimum Interval Between Doses		
	Dose 1 to Dose 2	**Dose 2 to Dose 3**	**Dose 3 to Booster Dose**
Tetanus, Diphtheria	**4 weeks**	**6 months**	**6 months**[8] if first dose given at age <12 months and current age <11 years **5 years**[8] if first dose given at age ≥12 months and third dose given at age <7 years and current age ≥11 years **10 years**[8] if third dose given at age ≥7 years
Inactivated Poliovirus[8]	**4 weeks**	**4 weeks**	IPV[2,9]
Hepatitis B	**4 weeks**	**8 weeks** (and 16 weeks after first dose)	
Measles, Mumps, Rubella	**4 weeks**		
Varicella[10]	**4 weeks**		

DEPARTMENT OF HEALTH AND HUMAN SERVICES
CENTERS FOR DISEASE CONTROL AND PREVENTION

The Childhood and Adolescent Immunization Schedule is approved by:
Advisory Committee on Immunization Practices www.cdc.gov/nip/acip
American Academy of Pediatrics www.aap.org
American Academy of Family Physicians www.aafp.org

Recommended Dietary Fluoride Supplement Schedule

Recommended Dietary Fluoride Supplement* Schedule

Age	Fluoride concentration in community drinking water†		
	<0.3 ppm	0.3–0.6 ppm	>0.6 ppm
0–6 months	None	None	None
6 months–3 years	0.25 mg/day	None	None
3–6 years	0.50 mg/day	0.25 mg/day	None
6–16 years	1.0 mg/day	0.50 mg/day	None

*Sodium fluoride (2.2 mg sodium fluoride contains 1 mg fluoride ion).
†1.0 parts per million (ppm) = 1 mg/L.

Approved by the American Dental Association, American Academy of Pediatrics, and American Academy of Pediatric Dentistry.

Sources:
American Academy of Pediatric Dentistry. Special issue: reference manual 1994–95. *Pediatr Dent* 16(Special issue):1-96, 1995.
American Academy of Pediatrics Committee on Nutrition: Fluoride supplementation for children: interim policy recommendations. *Pediatrics* 95:777, 1995.
Meskin LH, editor: Caries diagnosis and risk assessment: a review of preventive strategies and management. *J Am Dent Assoc* 126(Suppl):1S-24S, 1995.

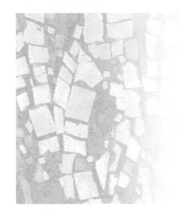

Children's Growth Charts

Birth to 36 months: Boys
Length-for-age and Weight-for-age percentiles

NAME _____

RECORD# _____

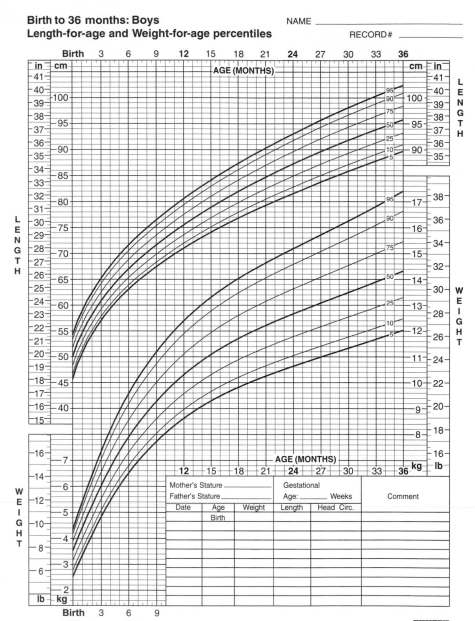

Published May 30, 2000 (modified 4/20/01).
SOURCE: Developed by the National Center for Health Statistics in collaboration with
the National Center for Chronic Disease Prevention and Health Promotion (2000).
http://www.cdc.gov/growthcharts

SAFER · HEALTHIER · PEOPLE™

Birth to 36 months: Boys
Head circumference-for-age and
Weight-for-length percentiles

NAME _____

RECORD# _____

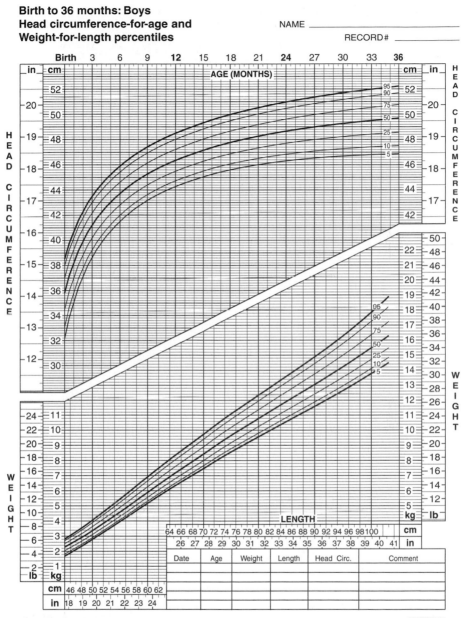

Published May 30, 2000 (modified 10/16/00).
SOURCE: Developed by the National Center for Health Statistics in collaboration with
the National Center for Chronic Disease Prevention and Health Promotion (2000).
http://www.cdc.gov/growthcharts

SAFER·HEALTHIER·PEOPLE™

Birth to 36 months: Girls
Length-for-age and Weight-for-age percentiles

NAME _____

RECORD # _____

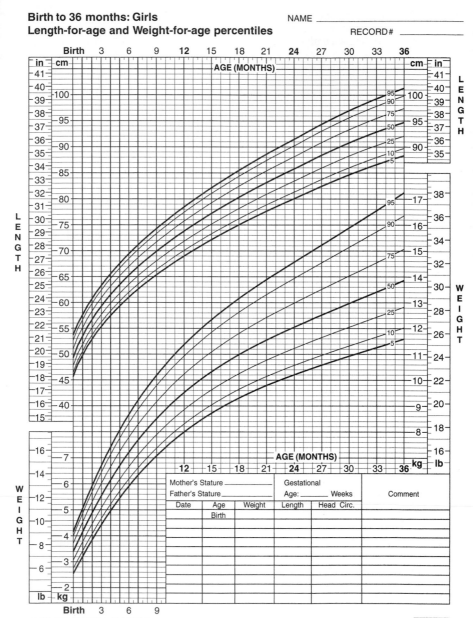

Published May 30, 2000 (modified 4/20/01).
SOURCE: Developed by the National Center for Health Statistics in collaboration with
   the National Center for Chronic Disease Prevention and Health Promotion (2000).
   http://www.cdc.gov/growthcharts

SAFER · HEALTHIER · PEOPLE™

Birth to 36 months: Girls
Head circumference-for-age and
Weight-for-length percentiles

NAME _____

RECORD# _____

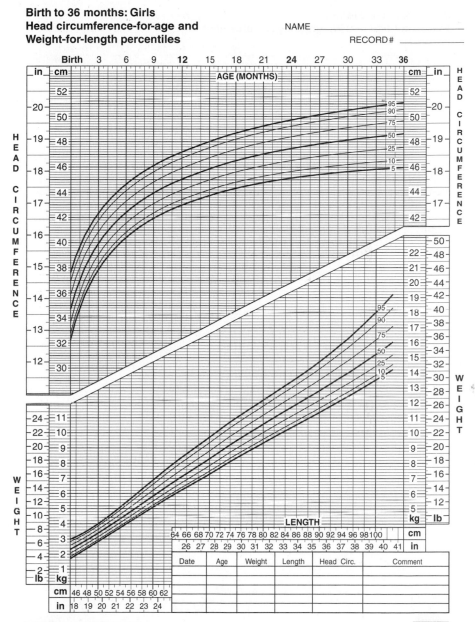

Date	Age	Weight	Length	Head Circ.	Comment

Published May 30, 2000 (modified 10/16/00).
SOURCE: Developed by the National Center for Health Statistics in collaboration with
the National Center for Chronic Disease Prevention and Health Promotion (2000).
http://www.cdc.gov/growthcharts

SAFER · HEALTHIER · PEOPLE™

2 to 20 years: Boys
Stature-for-age and Weight-for-age percentiles

NAME _____

RECORD# _____

Mother's Stature		Father's Stature			AGE (YEARS)
Date	Age	Weight	Stature	BMI*	

*To Calculate BMI: Weight (kg) ÷ Stature (cm) ÷ Stature (cm) x 10,000
or Weight (lb) ÷ Stature (in) ÷ Stature (in) x 703

Published May 30, 2000 (modified 11/21/00).
SOURCE: Developed by the National Center for Health Statistics in collaboration with
the National Center for Chronic Disease Prevention and Health Promotion (2000).
http://www.cdc.gov/growthcharts

SAFER · HEALTHIER · PEOPLE™

2 to 20 years: Boys
Body mass index-for-age percentiles

NAME _____

RECORD # _____

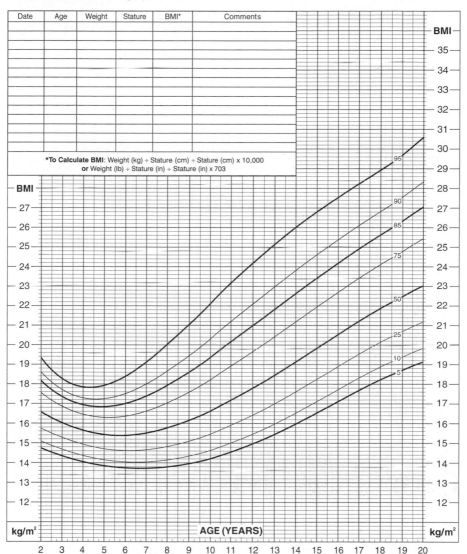

Date	Age	Weight	Stature	BMI*	Comments

*To Calculate BMI: Weight (kg) ÷ Stature (cm) ÷ Stature (cm) x 10,000
or Weight (lb) ÷ Stature (in) ÷ Stature (in) x 703

AGE (YEARS)

Published May 30, 2000 (modified 10/16/00).
SOURCE: Developed by the National Center for Health Statistics in collaboration with
the National Center for Chronic Disease Prevention and Health Promotion (2000).
http://www.cdc.gov/growthcharts

SAFER · HEALTHIER · PEOPLE

2 to 20 years: Girls
Stature-for-age and Weight-for-age percentiles

NAME _____

RECORD# _____

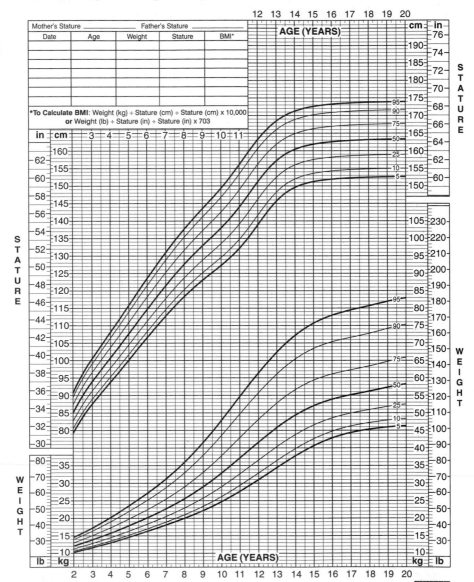

Published May 30, 2000 (modified 11/21/00).
SOURCE: Developed by the National Center for Health Statistics in collaboration with
the National Center for Chronic Disease Prevention and Health Promotion (2000).
http://www.cdc.gov/growthcharts

CDC

SAFER·HEALTHIER·PEOPLE™

2 to 20 years: Girls
Body mass index-for-age percentiles

NAME _____
RECORD # _____

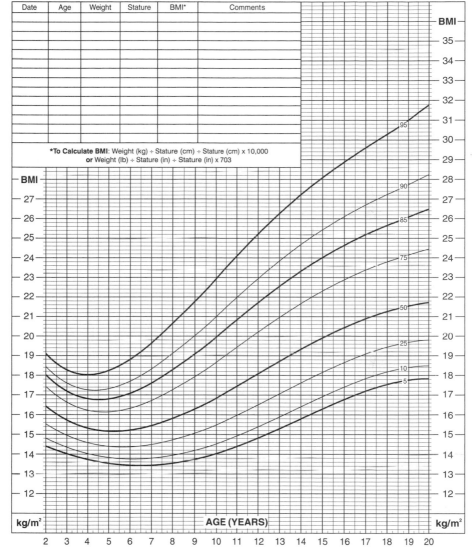

*To Calculate BMI: Weight (kg) ÷ Stature (cm) ÷ Stature (cm) x 10,000
or Weight (lb) ÷ Stature (in) ÷ Stature (in) x 703

Published May 30, 2000 (modified 10/16/00).
SOURCE: Developed by the National Center for Health Statistics in collaboration with
the National Center for Chronic Disease Prevention and Health Promotion (2000).
http://www.cdc.gov/growthcharts

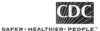

SAFER · HEALTHIER · PEOPLE™

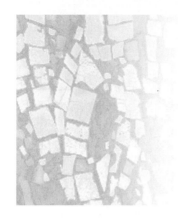

Children's Body Mass Index (BMI) Tables

Children's BMI Tables[*]

BMI	13	14	15	16	17	18	19	20	21	22	23	24	25	26	27	28	29	30	31	32	33	34	35	36
Height (inches)																								
33	20	21	23	24	26	27	29	30	32	34	35	37	38	40	41	43	44	46	48	49	51	52	54	55
34	21	23	24	26	27	29	31	32	34	36	37	39	41	42	44	46	47	49	50	52	54	55	57	59
35	22	24	26	27	29	31	33	34	36	38	40	41	43	45	47	48	50	52	54	55	57	59	60	62
36	23	25	27	29	31	33	35	36	38	40	42	44	46	47	49	51	53	55	57	58	60	62	64	66
37	25	27	29	31	33	35	37	38	40	42	44	46	48	50	52	54	56	58	60	62	64	66	68	70
38	26	28	30	32	34	36	39	41	43	45	47	49	51	53	55	57	59	61	63	65	67	69	71	73
39	28	30	32	34	36	38	41	43	45	47	49	51	54	56	58	60	62	64	67	69	71	73	75	77
40	29	31	34	36	38	40	43	45	47	50	52	54	56	59	61	63	66	68	70	72	75	77	79	81
41	31	33	35	38	40	43	45	47	50	52	54	57	59	62	64	66	69	71	74	76	78	81	83	86
42	32	35	37	40	42	45	47	50	52	55	57	60	62	65	67	70	72	75	77	80	82	85	87	90
43	34	36	39	42	44	47	49	52	55	57	60	63	65	68	71	73	76	78	81	84	86	89	92	94
44	35	38	41	44	46	49	52	55	57	60	63	66	68	71	74	77	79	82	85	88	90	93	96	99
45	37	40	43	46	48	51	54	57	60	63	66	69	72	74	77	80	83	86	89	92	95	97	100	103
46	39	42	45	48	51	54	57	60	63	66	69	72	75	78	81	84	87	90	93	96	99	102	105	108
47	40	43	47	50	53	56	59	62	65	69	72	75	78	81	84	87	91	94	97	100	103	106	109	113
48	42	45	49	52	55	58	62	65	68	72	75	78	81	85	88	91	95	98	101	104	108	111	114	117
49	44	47	51	54	58	61	64	68	71	75	78	81	85	88	92	95	99	102	105	109	112	116	119	122
50	46	49	53	56	60	64	67	71	74	78	81	85	88	92	96	99	103	106	110	113	117	120	124	128
51	48	51	55	59	62	66	70	73	77	81	85	88	92	96	99	103	107	110	114	118	122	125	129	133
52	50	53	57	61	65	69	73	76	80	84	88	92	96	100	103	107	111	115	119	123	126	130	134	138
53	51	55	59	63	67	71	75	79	83	87	91	95	99	103	107	111	115	119	123	127	131	135	139	143
54	53	58	62	66	70	74	78	82	87	91	95	99	103	107	111	116	120	124	128	132	136	141	145	149
55	55	60	64	68	73	77	81	86	90	94	98	103	107	111	116	120	124	129	133	137	141	146	150	154
56	57	62	66	71	75	80	84	89	93	98	102	107	111	115	120	124	129	133	138	142	147	151	156	160
57	60	64	69	73	78	83	87	92	97	101	106	110	115	120	124	129	134	138	143	147	152	157	161	166
58	62	66	71	76	81	86	90	95	100	105	110	114	119	124	129	133	138	143	148	153	157	162	167	172
59	64	69	74	79	84	89	94	99	103	108	113	118	123	128	133	138	143	148	153	158	163	168	173	178
60	66	71	76	81	87	92	97	102	107	112	117	122	128	133	138	143	148	153	158	163	168	174	179	184
61	68	74	79	84	89	95	100	105	111	116	121	127	132	137	142	148	153	158	164	169	174	179	185	190
62	71	76	82	87	92	98	103	109	114	120	125	131	136	142	147	153	158	164	169	174	180	185	191	196
63	73	79	84	90	95	101	107	112	118	124	129	135	141	146	152	158	163	169	175	180	186	191	197	203
64	75	81	87	93	99	104	110	116	122	128	134	139	145	151	157	163	168	174	180	186	192	198	203	209
65	78	84	90	96	102	108	114	120	126	132	138	144	150	156	162	168	174	180	186	192	198	204	210	216
66	80	86	92	99	105	111	117	123	130	136	142	148	154	161	167	173	179	185	192	198	204	210	216	223
67	83	89	95	102	108	114	121	127	134	140	146	153	159	166	172	178	185	191	197	204	210	217	223	229
68	85	92	98	105	111	118	124	131	138	144	151	157	164	171	177	184	190	197	203	210	217	223	230	236
69	88	94	101	108	115	121	128	135	142	148	155	162	169	176	182	189	196	203	209	216	223	230	237	243
70	90	97	104	111	118	125	132	139	146	153	160	167	174	181	188	195	202	209	216	223	230	236	243	250
71	93	100	107	114	121	129	136	143	150	157	164	172	179	186	193	200	207	215	222	229	236	243	250	258
72	95	103	110	117	125	132	140	147	154	162	169	176	184	191	199	206	213	221	228	235	243	250	258	265
73	98	106	113	121	128	136	144	151	159	166	174	181	189	197	204	212	219	227	234	242	250	257	265	272
74	101	109	116	124	132	140	148	155	163	171	179	186	194	202	210	218	225	233	241	249	257	264	272	280
75	104	112	120	128	136	144	152	160	168	176	184	192	200	208	216	224	232	240	248	256	264	272	280	288
76	106	115	123	131	139	147	156	164	172	180	188	197	205	213	221	230	238	246	254	262	271	279	287	295
77	109	118	126	134	143	151	160	168	177	185	193	202	210	219	227	236	244	253	261	269	278	286	295	303
78	112	121	129	138	147	155	164	173	181	190	199	207	216	225	233	242	250	259	268	276	285	294	302	311

Weight (pounds)

[*]To use the table, find the appropriate height in the left-hand column labeled **Height**. Move across to a given **Weight**. The number at the top of the column is the **BMI** at that height and weight. Pounds have been rounded off.

Children's Metric BMI Tables*

pediatrics.About.com

BMI	13	14	15	16	17	18	19	20	21	22	23	24	25	26	27	28	29	30	31	32	33	34	35	36
Height (cm)																								
90	10	11	12	12	13	14	15	16	17	17	18	19	20	21	21	22	23	24	25	25	26	27	28	29
93	11	12	12	13	14	15	16	17	18	19	19	20	21	22	23	24	25	25	26	27	28	29	30	31
96	11	12	13	14	15	16	17	18	19	20	21	22	23	23	24	25	26	27	28	29	30	31	32	33
99	12	13	14	15	16	17	18	19	20	21	22	23	24	25	26	27	28	29	30	31	32	33	34	35
102	13	14	15	16	17	18	19	20	21	22	23	24	26	27	28	29	30	31	32	33	34	35	36	37
105	14	15	16	17	18	19	20	22	23	24	25	26	27	28	29	30	31	33	34	35	36	37	38	39
108	15	16	17	18	19	20	22	23	24	25	26	27	29	30	31	32	33	34	36	37	38	39	40	41
111	16	17	18	19	20	22	23	24	25	27	28	29	30	32	33	34	35	36	38	39	40	41	43	44
114	16	18	19	20	22	23	24	25	27	28	29	31	32	33	35	36	37	38	40	41	42	44	45	46
117	17	19	20	21	23	24	26	27	28	30	31	32	34	35	36	38	39	41	42	43	45	46	47	49
120	18	20	21	23	24	25	27	28	30	31	33	34	36	37	38	40	41	43	44	46	47	48	50	51
123	19	21	22	24	25	27	28	30	31	33	34	36	37	39	40	42	43	45	46	48	49	51	52	54
126	20	22	23	25	26	28	30	31	33	34	36	38	39	41	42	44	46	47	49	50	52	53	55	57
129	21	23	24	26	28	29	31	33	34	36	38	39	41	43	44	46	48	49	51	53	54	56	58	59
132	22	24	26	27	29	31	33	34	36	38	40	41	43	45	47	48	50	52	54	55	57	59	60	62
135	23	25	27	29	30	32	34	36	38	40	41	43	45	47	49	51	52	54	56	58	60	61	63	65
138	24	26	28	30	32	34	36	38	39	41	43	45	47	49	51	53	55	57	59	60	62	64	66	68
141	25	27	29	31	33	35	37	39	41	43	45	47	49	51	53	55	57	59	61	63	65	67	69	71
144	26	29	31	33	35	37	39	41	43	45	47	49	51	53	55	58	60	62	64	66	68	70	72	74
147	28	30	32	34	36	38	41	43	45	47	49	51	54	56	58	60	62	64	66	69	71	73	75	77
150	29	31	33	36	38	40	42	45	47	49	51	54	56	58	60	63	65	67	69	72	74	76	78	81
153	30	32	35	37	39	42	44	46	49	51	53	56	58	60	63	65	67	70	72	74	77	79	81	84
156	31	34	36	38	41	43	46	48	51	53	55	58	60	63	65	68	70	73	75	77	80	82	85	87
159	32	35	37	40	42	45	48	50	53	55	58	60	63	65	68	70	73	75	78	80	83	85	88	91
162	34	36	39	41	44	47	49	52	55	57	60	62	65	68	70	73	76	78	81	83	86	89	91	94
165	35	38	40	43	46	49	51	54	57	59	62	65	68	70	73	76	78	81	84	87	89	92	95	98
168	36	39	42	45	47	50	53	56	59	62	64	67	70	73	76	79	81	84	87	90	93	95	98	101
171	38	40	43	46	49	52	55	58	61	64	67	70	73	76	78	81	84	87	90	93	96	99	102	105
174	39	42	45	48	51	54	57	60	63	66	69	72	75	78	81	84	87	90	93	96	99	102	105	108
177	40	43	46	50	53	56	59	62	65	68	72	75	78	81	84	87	90	93	97	100	103	106	109	112
180	42	45	48	51	55	58	61	64	68	71	74	77	81	84	87	90	93	97	100	103	106	110	113	116
183	43	46	50	53	56	60	63	66	70	73	77	80	83	87	90	93	97	100	103	107	110	113	117	120
186	44	48	51	55	58	62	65	69	72	76	79	83	86	89	93	96	100	103	107	110	114	117	121	124
189	46	50	53	57	60	64	67	71	75	78	82	85	89	92	96	100	103	107	110	114	117	121	125	128
192	47	51	55	58	62	66	70	73	77	81	84	88	92	95	99	103	106	110	114	117	121	125	129	132
195	49	53	57	60	64	68	72	76	79	83	87	91	95	98	102	106	110	114	117	121	125	129	133	136

Weight (kg)

*To use the table, find the appropriate height in the left-hand column labeled **Height**. Move across to a given **Weight**. The number at the top of the column is the **BMI** at that height and weight. Pounds have been rounded off.

Food Guide Pyramids

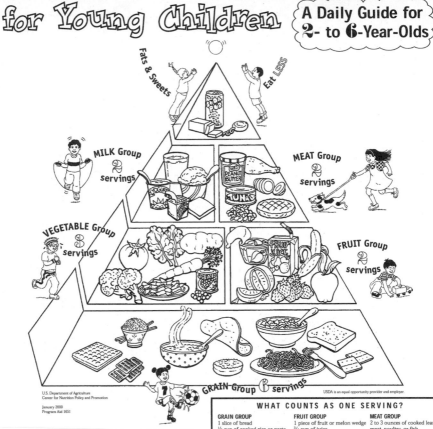

FOOD Guide PYRAMID

for Young Children

A Daily Guide for 2- to 6-Year-Olds

Fats & Sweets — Eat LESS

MILK Group — 2 servings

MEAT Group — 2 servings

VEGETABLE Group — 3 servings

FRUIT Group — 2 servings

GRAIN Group — 6 servings

U.S. Department of Agriculture
Center for Nutrition Policy and Promotion

January 2000
Program Aid 1651

USDA is an equal opportunity provider and employer.

FOOD IS FUN and learning about food is fun, too. Eating foods from the Food Guide Pyramid and being physically active will help you grow healthy and strong.

WHAT COUNTS AS ONE SERVING?

GRAIN GROUP
1 slice of bread
½ cup of cooked rice or pasta
½ cup of cooked cereal
1 ounce of ready-to-eat cereal

VEGETABLE GROUP
½ cup of chopped raw or cooked vegetables
1 cup of raw leafy vegetables

FRUIT GROUP
1 piece of fruit or melon wedge
¾ cup of juice
½ cup of canned fruit
¼ cup of dried fruit

MILK GROUP
1 cup of milk or yogurt
2 ounces of cheese

MEAT GROUP
2 to 3 ounces of cooked lean meat, poultry, or fish.
½ cup of cooked dry beans, or 1 egg counts as 1 ounce of lean meat. 2 tablespoons of peanut butter count as 1 ounce of meat.

FATS AND SWEETS
Limit calories from these.

Four- to 6-year-olds can eat these serving sizes. Offer 2- to 3-year-olds less, except for milk.
Two- to 6-year-old children need a total of 2 servings from the milk group each day.

EAT a variety of FOODS AND ENJOY!

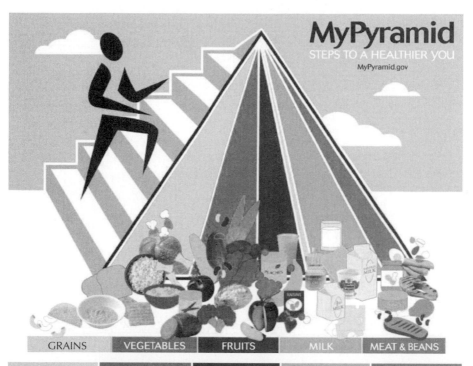

MyPyramid
STEPS TO A HEALTHIER YOU
MyPyramid.gov

GRAINS	VEGETABLES	FRUITS	MILK	MEAT & BEANS
GRAINS Make half your grains whole	**VEGETABLES** Vary your veggies	**FRUITS** Focus on fruits	**MILK** Get your calcium-rich foods	**MEAT & BEANS** Go lean with protein
Eat at least 3 oz. of whole-grain cereals, breads, crackers, rice, or pasta every day 1 oz. is about 1 slice of bread, about 1 cup of breakfast cereal, or ½ cup of cooked rice, cereal, or pasta	Eat more dark-green veggies like broccoli, spinach, and other dark leafy greens Eat more orange vegetables like carrots and sweetpotatoes Eat more dry beans and peas like pinto beans, kidney beans, and lentils	Eat a variety of fruit Choose fresh, frozen, canned, or dried fruit Go easy on fruit juices	Go low-fat or fat-free when you choose milk, yogurt, and other milk products If you don't or can't consume milk, choose lactose-free products or other calcium sources such as fortified foods and beverages	Choose low-fat or lean meats and poultry Bake it, broil it, or grill it Vary your protein routine — choose more fish, beans, peas, nuts, and seeds

For a 2,000-calorie diet, you need the amounts below from each food group. To find the amounts that are right for you, go to MyPyramid.gov.

Eat 6 oz. every day	Eat 2½ cups every day	Eat 2 cups every day	Get 3 cups every day; for kids aged 2 to 8, it's 2	Eat 5½ oz. every day

Find your balance between food and physical activity
- Be sure to stay within your daily calorie needs.
- Be physically active for at least 30 minutes most days of the week.
- About 60 minutes a day of physical activity may be needed to prevent weight gain.
- For sustaining weight loss, at least 60 to 90 minutes a day of physical activity may be required.
- Children and teenagers should be physically active for 60 minutes every day, or most days.

Know the limits on fats, sugars, and salt (sodium)
- Make most of your fat sources from fish, nuts, and vegetable oils.
- Limit solid fats like butter, margarine, shortening, and lard, as well as foods that contain these.
- Check the Nutrition Facts label to keep saturated fats, trans fats, and sodium low.
- Choose food and beverages low in added sugars. Added sugars contribute calories with few, if any, nutrients.

MyPyramid.gov
STEPS TO A HEALTHIER YOU

U.S. Department of Agriculture
Center for Nutrition Policy and Promotion
April 2005
CNPP-15

USDA

USDA is an equal opportunity provider and employer

Predicted Peak Flow Measurements

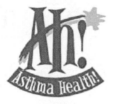

**Predicted
Peak Flow
Measurements** (liters per minute)
(based on Personal Best peak flow meter)

Normal Children & Adolescents		
Height (in)	(cm)	Males & Females
43	109	147
44	112	160
45	114	173
46	117	187
47	119	200
48	122	214
49	124	227
50	127	240
51	130	254
52	132	267
53	135	280
54	137	293
55	140	307
56	142	320
57	145	334
58	147	347
59	150	360
60	152	373
61	155	387
62	157	400
63	160	413
64	163	427
65	165	440
66	168	454

Normal Adult Males					
		Height			
Age (Years)	(in) (cm)	60" 152	65" 165	70" 178	75" 191	80" 203
20		554	575	594	611	626
25		580	603	622	640	656
30		594	617	637	655	672
35		599	622	643	661	677
40		597	620	641	659	675
45		591	613	633	651	668
50		580	602	622	640	656
55		566	588	608	625	640
60		551	572	591	607	622
65		533	554	572	588	603
70		515	535	552	568	582
75		496	515	532	547	560

Normal Adult Females					
		Height			
Age (Years)	(in) (cm)	55" 140	60" 152	65" 165	70" 178	75" 191
20		444	460	474	486	497
25		455	471	485	497	509
30		458	475	489	502	513
35		458	474	488	501	512
40		453	469	483	496	507
45		446	462	476	488	499
50		437	453	466	478	489
55		427	442	455	467	477
60		415	430	443	454	464
65		403	417	430	441	451
70		390	404	416	427	436
75		377	391	402	413	422

Ah! Asthma Health is a program of Maine Health, a non profit
health system based in Portland, Maine (*www.maine health.org*).

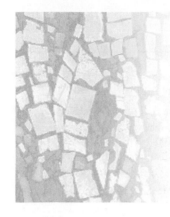

Asthma Management Plan

Date: _____   Personal Best PEFR _____

ASTHMA MANAGEMENT PLAN FOR _____

Green Zone = Good control

Green Zone: _____ to _____ Peak Flow Rate (80–100% of personal best; no symptoms)

To keep your asthma under control: Stay away from things that make your asthma worse (such as animals, smoke, etc.; talk to your doctor about these things). **Take your medicine(s).**

Name of Medicine	How Much To Take	How Often/ When To Take It

Yellow Zone = Caution

Yellow Zone: _____ to _____ Peak Flow Rate (50–79% of personal best)

Take medicine listed below to get your asthma back under control.

Symptoms: Coughing, wheezing, shortness of breath, tightness in the chest, or other symptoms of an asthma episode. Symptoms may be mild.

Early signs your asthma is getting worse: _____

Take your Yellow Zone medicine when these early signs occur.

Name of Medicine	How Much To Take	How Often/ When To Take It

- Peak flow rate or symptoms not better in _____ minutes after taking the medicine listed above? Call the doctor.

- Keep taking your Green Zone medicine(s). Keep staying away from things that make your asthma worse.

Red Zone = Danger!

Red Zone: Below _____ Peak Flow Rate (below 50% of personal best)

Take the medicine listed below. Then call your doctor.

Symptoms: Coughing, very short of breath, trouble walking and talking, tightness in the chest, other symptoms.

Name of Medicine	How Much To Take	How Often/ When To Take It

- Call your doctor or emergency room NOW, say this is an emergency, and ask what you should do next.

- Go to the doctor or hospital **right away** or call an ambulance without delay if:

  - You are struggling to breathe or your lips or fingernails turn a little blue or grey.

  - Your peak flow remains in the Red Zone level 20 minutes after taking your medicine.

- Keep taking your Green Zone medicine(s).

Doctor: _____

Office Phone: _____

Phone Number After Office Hours: _____

Emergency Room: _____

Notes

_____
_____
_____
_____
_____
_____
_____

Nurses: Partners in Asthma Care, National Asthma Education and Prevention Program, National Heart, Lung, and Blood Institute, NIH Publication No. 95-3308, 1995.

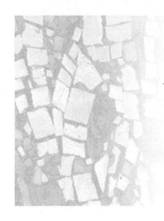

Pediatric
Dosage Schedules

IBUPROFEN SUSPENSION (ADVIL, MOTRIN) every 6 hours

Age	Weight (lb)	Fever 102.5°F (39.2°C) or below 5 mg/kg		Fever 102.5°F (39.2°C) or below 10 mg/kg	
		mg	tsp	mg	tsp
6-11 mo	13-17	25	¼	50	½
12-23 mo	18-23	50	½	100	1
2-3 yr	24-35	75	¾	150	1 ½
4-5 yr	36-47	100	1	200	2
6-8 yr	48-59	125	1 ¼	250	2 ½
9-10 yr	60-71	150	1 ½	300	3
11-12 yr	72-95	200	2	400	4

ACETAMINOPHEN (TYLENOL) every 4–6 hours

Age	Weight (lb)	Drops	Susp	Chewables 80 mg	Chewables 160 mL
6 wk–4 mo	Under 12	½ dropper (.4 mL)	¼ tsp	-	-
5-11 mo	12-17	1 dropper (.8 mL)	½ tsp	-	-
12-23 mo	18-23	1 ½ dropper (1.2 mL)	¾ tsp	-	-
2-3 yr	24-35	2 droppers (1.6 mL)	1 tsp	2	-
4-5 yr	36-47	3 droppers (2.4 mL)	1 ½ tsp	3	-
6-8 yr	48-59	-	2 tsp	4	2
9-10 yr	60-71	-	2 ½ tsp	5	2 ½
11 yr	72-95	-	3 tsp	6	3
12 yr	96 or over	-	4 tsp	8	4

TRIAMINIC / TRIAMINIC-DM / TRIAMENIC EXPECTORANT

Age	Weight (lb)	Dosage–tid
6 mo to under 1 yr	12-17	¼ tsp (1.25 mL)
1 yr to under 2 yr	18-23	½ tsp (2.5 mL)
2 yr to under 6 yr	24-47	1 tsp (5 mL)
6 yr to under 12 yr	49-95	2 tsp (10 mL)

DIMETAPP AND ROBITUSSIN / ROBITUSSIN–DM

Age	Dosage–tid
6 mo to under 1 yr	¼ tsp
1 yr to under 3 yr	½ tsp
3 yr to under 5 yr	¾ tsp
5 yr or older	1 tsp

RONDEC / RONDEC-DM DROPS AND SYRUP

Age	Dosage–tid, qid, or q6h
1-3 mo	¼ dropper (¼ mL)
3-6 mo	½ dropper (½ mL)
6-9 mo	¾ dropper (¾ mL)
9-18 mo	1 dropper (1mL)
18 mo-6yr	½ tsp (2.5 mL) syrup
6yr or older	1 tsp (5 mL) syrup

DELSYM COUGH FORMULA (DEXTROMETHORPHAN)

Age	Dosage–q12h
1-2 yr	¼ tsp
2-6 yr	½ tsp
6-12 yr	1 tsp
12 yr or older	2 tsp

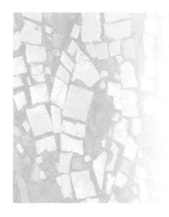

Pediatric Medications

ACYCLOVIR—ANTIVIRAL

BRAND NAME:
Zovirax, Avirax

USES:
Antiviral, used to treat initial and recurrent episodes of mucocutaneous herpes simplex virus (HSV-1 and HSV-2) infections in immunocompromised patients; varicella (chickenpox) infections in immunocompromised patients; acute herpes zoster infection in immunocompetent patients; herpes simplex encephalitis.

AVAILABILITY:
Suspension: 200 mg/5 mL. **Tablets:** 400 mg, 800 mg. **Capsules:** 200 mg. **Injection:** 500 mg/vial, 1 g/vial

INDICATIONS/ROUTES/DOSAGE:
Varicella infection in immunocompromised patients: **Children ≥ 12 yrs:** 800 mg PO q4h (5 times/day while awake) for 5 days. **Children ≥ 2 yrs and weighing < 40 kg:** 20 mg/kg (max: 800 mg/dose) PO qid for 5 days.

Acute herpes zoster: **Children ≥ 12 yrs:** 800 mg PO q4h (5 times/day) for 7–10 days.

Genital herpes (initial episode): **Adults:** 200 mg q4h (5 times/day) for 10 days.

Genital herpes (recurrent episode): **Adults:** 200 mg q4h (5 times/day) for 5 days.

Usual topical dosage: **Adults:** 3–6 times/day for 7 days.

Data from *Saunders Nursing Drug Handbook 2004* and *Mosby's Nursing Drug Reference 2004.*
Note: all patients weighing >100 lbs should be dosed according to adult dosage guidelines.

ADVERSE REACTIONS:

Malaise, headache, encephalopathic changes, nausea, vomiting, diarrhea hematuria, acute renal failure, thrombocytopenia, leukopenia, rash, itching, urticaria, inflammation or phlebitis at injection site

IMPLICATIONS:

- May increase BUN and creatinine levels. May decrease WBC, and increase or decrease platelet count.
- Use cautiously in patients with neurologic problems, renal disease, or dehydration. Monitor renal function.
- Drink adequate fluids, do not touch lesions with fingers to prevent spreading infection to new site, use finger cot or rubber glove to apply topical ointment.
- Avoid sexual intercourse while lesions present to prevent spread to partner.

ALBUTEROL—BRONCHODILATOR

BRAND NAME:

Ventolin, Proventil

USES:

Relaxes bronchial, uterine, and vascular smooth muscle, to prevent or treat bronchospasm.

AVAILABILITY:

Aerosol inhaler: 90 mcg/metered spray, 100 mcg/metered spray. *Albuterol sulfate:* **Capsules for inhalation:** 200 mcg. **Solution for inhalation:** 0.083% mg/mL, 0.5% mg/mL, 0.63 mg/mL, 1.25 mg/3 mL. **Syrup:** 2 mg/5 mL. **Tablets:** 2 mg, 4 mg. **Tablets, extended-release:** 4 mg, 8 mg

INDICATIONS/ROUTES/DOSAGE:

Prevention/treatment of bronchospasm in patients with reversible obstructive airway disease: *Aerosol inhalation:* **Children ≥ 4 yrs:** 1 or 2 inhalations q4–6h. *Capsules for inhalation:* **Children ≥ 4 yrs:** 200 mcg inhaled q4–6h. *Solution for inhalation:* **Children ≥ 12 yrs:** 2.5 mg tid or qid by nebulizer. **Children 2–12 yrs:** initially, 0.1–0.15 mg/kg by nebulizer, with subsequent dosing titrated to response, not to exceed 2.5 mg tid or qid by nebulization.

Syrup or oral tablets: **Children 2–6 yrs:** initially, 0.1 mg/kg PO tid. Starting dose should not exceed 2 mg (1 tsp) tid. Do not exceed 4 mg tid. **Children 6–14 yrs:** 2 mg PO tid or qid. Do not exceed 24 mg daily. **Adults, children ≥ 14 yrs:** 2–4 mg PO tid or qid. Do not exceed 8 mg qid.

Extended-release tablets: **Children 6–12 yrs:** 4 mg PO q12h. **Adults, children > 12 yrs:** 4–8 mg PO q12h.

To prevent exercise-induced bronchospasm: 2 aerosol inhalations 15–30 min before exercise.

ADVERSE REACTIONS:
Nervousness, dizziness, headache, weakness, insomnia, nasal congestion, hoarseness, tachycardia, hypertension, nausea, vomiting, heartburn, increased appetite, hypokalemia, muscle cramps, bronchospasm, cough, increased sputum

IMPLICATIONS:
- Use caution in patients with diabetes mellitus, hypertension, or hyperthyroidism.
- Teach family how to use inhaler properly.
- Increase fluid intake.
- Do not take more than 2 inhalations at any one time to prevent paradoxical bronchoconstriction.
- Rinse mouth after inhalation.

AMOXICILLIN—ANTIBIOTIC

BRAND NAME:
Amoxil (generic also available)

USES:
Treat otitis media, upper and lower respiratory tract, soft tissue, skin, GI, GU, and gonorrhea infections. Used to treat: **Gram-positive cocci:** *Staphylococcus aureus, Streptococcus pyogenes, Streptococcus faecalis, Streptococcus pneumoniae.* **Gram-negative cocci:** *Neisseria gonorrhoeae, Neisseria meningitides.* **Gram-positive bacillus:** *Corynebacterium diphtheriae, Listeria monocytogenes.* **Gram-negative bacillus:** *Haemophilus influenzae, Escherichia coli, Proteus mirabilis, Salmonella;* also used in bacterial endocarditis prophylaxis.

AVAILABILITY:
Suspension: 125/5 mL, 200/5 mL, 250/5 mL, 400/5 mL. **Tablets:** 500 mg, 875 mg. **Pediatric drops:** 50 mg/mL. **Tablets, chewable:** 125 mg, 200 mg, 250 mg, 400 mg. **Capsules:** 250 mg, 500 mg.

INDICATIONS/ROUTES/DOSAGE:
Ear, nose, throat, GU, skin/structure infections: **Children < 20 kg:** 20–40 mg/kg/day divided q8–12h. **Children, adults > 20 kg:** 250–500 mg/q8h or 500–875 mg 2 times/day

Lower respiratory tract infections: **Children < 20 kg:** 40 mg/kg/day divided q8–12h. **Children, adults > 20 kg:** 500 mg/q8h or 875 mg tablets 2 times/day

Acute uncomplicated gonorrhea, epididymitis-orchitis: **Adults:** 3 g once with 1 g probenecid PO follow with tetracycline or erythromycin

Acute otitis media: **Children:** 80–90 mg/kg/day divided bid for those at high risk

ADVERSE REACTIONS:
Mild diarrhea, rash, oral/vaginal candidiasis; superinfection, colitis, allergic reaction–anaphylaxis

IMPLICATIONS:
- Take all of medication.
- Report rash or severe diarrhea.
- Discard suspension after 14 days.

AMOXICILLIN AND CLAVULANATE POTASSIUM—ANTIBIOTIC

BRAND NAME:
Augmentin

USES:
Treat lower respiratory infection, otitis media, sinusitis, skin infections, urinary tract infections caused by susceptible strains of gram-positive and gram-negative organisms.

AVAILABILITY:
Oral suspension: 125 mg/5 mL, 200 mg/5 mL, 250 mg/5 mL, 400 mg/5mL. **Tablets:** 250 mg, 500 mg, 875 mg. **Tablets, chewable:** 125 mg, 200 mg, 250 mg, 400 mg

INDICATIONS/ROUTES/DOSAGE:
Recurrent or persistent otitis media caused by **Streptococcus pneumoniae, Haemophilus influenzae,** *or* **Moraxella catarrhalis:** Augmentin ES-600. **Children > 3 mos:** 90 mg/kg/day, based on amoxicillin component, PO q12h for 10 days.

Lower respiratory infections, otitis media, sinusitis, skin infections, urinary tract infections caused by susceptible strains of gram-positive and gram-negative organisms: **Adults, children weighing >40 kg:** 250 mg (based on amoxicillin component) PO q8h or 500 mg q12h. May use 500 mg PO q8h **OR** 875 mg PO q12h for more severe infections. **Children weighing <40 kg:** 20 to 45 mg/kg, based on amoxicillin component and severity of infection, PO daily in divided doses q8–12h.

Children ≤ 3 months: 30 mg/kg/day PO in divided doses q12h.

ADVERSE REACTIONS:
Nausea, vomiting, diarrhea, agitation, confusion, dizziness, insomnia, enterocolitis, pseudomembranous colitis, abdominal pain, vaginitis, anemia, thrombocytopenia, hypersensitivity reactions

IMPLICATIONS:
- May decrease effectiveness of hormonal contraceptives.
- *Note:* oral suspensions have varying clavulanic acid content.
- Continue antibiotic for full length of treatment, take with meals.

AZITHROMYCIN—MACROLIDE ANTIBIOTIC

BRAND NAME:
Zithromax

USES:
Treat otitis media, pharyngitis, tonsillitis, dental prophylaxis in patients allergic to penicillin, uncomplicated gonococcal infections, chlamydial infections.

AVAILABILITY:
Powder for oral suspension: 100 mg/5 mL, 200 mg/5 mL, 1000 mg/packet. **Tablets:** 250 mg, 500 mg, 600 mg. **Injection:** 500 mg

INDICATIONS/ROUTES/DOSAGE:
Otitis media: **Children ≥ 6 mos:** 10 mg/kg PO daily for 3 days **OR** 10 mg/kg PO on day 1 then 5 mg/kg once daily on days 2–5.

Pharyngitis, tonsillitis: **Children ≥ 2 yrs:** 12 mg/kg (max. of 500 mg) PO daily for 5 days.

Dental prophylaxis: **Adults:** 500 mg PO 1 h before procedure. **Children:** 15 mg/kg PO 1 h before procedure.

Chlamydial infections: **Adults, adolescents ≥ 16 yrs:** 1 g PO as a single dose.

ADVERSE REACTIONS:
Dizziness, headache, fatigue, palpitations, chest pain, nausea, vomiting, diarrhea, abdominal pain, cholestatic jaundice, pseudomembranous colitis, candidiasis, vaginitis, rash, photosensitivity, angioedema

IMPLICATIONS:
■ Use cautiously with liver impairment.
■ Give oral suspension 1 hour before or 2 hours after meals.
■ Do not give with antacids.

BENZOCAINE—TOPICAL OTIC ANALGESIC

BRAND NAME:
Auralgan Otic Solution

USES:
Topical analgesic to reduce pain associated with acute otitis media.

AVAILABILITY:
10-mL bottle

INDICATIONS/ROUTES/DOSAGE:
Instill drops until ear canal is full, put wick into ear canal. May repeat every 1–2 hours as needed.

ADVERSE REACTIONS:
Irritation of ear canal

IMPLICATIONS:
- Do not let dropper touch ear canal, do not rinse ear dropper after use, keep out of the reach of children.
- Have child lay on side and tilt the affected ear upward, pull ear lobe up and instill medication, have child lay on side for 5 minutes then insert wick.
- Do not use on perforated ear drum.

BUDESONIDE—INHALATION CORTICOSTEROID ANTIINFLAMMATORY

BRAND NAME:
Entocort EC, Pulmicort, Rhinocort

USES:
Manage symptoms of seasonal or perennial allergic rhinitis.

AVAILABILITY:
Nasal inhaler: 32 mcg/metered spray (Rhinocort AQ). **Nasal spray:** 50 mcg/dose (Pulmicort). **Powder for inhalation:** 200 mcg/inhalation (Pulmicort Turbuhaler). **Suspension for oral inhalation:** 0.25 mg/2 mL, 0.5 mg/2 mL (Pulmicort Respules)

INDICATIONS/ROUTES/DOSAGE:
Intranasal: **Children > 6 yrs, adults: Rhinocort:** 2 sprays each nostril 2 times/day or 4 sprays to each nostril in morning. **Rhinocort Aqua:** 1 spray to each nostril once daily. **Children < 12 yrs:** 4 sprays/day. **Children > 12 yrs:** 8 sprays/day.

Nebulization: **Children 1–8 yrs:** 0.25–1 mg/day titrated to lowest effective dosage.

Inhalation: **Children > 6 yrs, adults:** initially 200–400 mcg 2 times/day to max 400 mcg 2 times/day.

Rhinitis: Nasal inhalation: **Children > 6 yrs:** initial, 2 sprays/nostril twice daily. **Adult:** initial 2 sprays/nostril bid or 4 sprays/nostril in the morning. Max. 4 sprays/nostril per day. *Nasal spray:* **Children > 6 yrs:** initial, 1 spray/nostril once a day. Max dose 4 sprays/nostril/day. **Children < 12 yrs:** 2 sprays/nostril once a day. Not recommended for children < 6 yrs. **Children > 12 yrs:** 4 sprays/nostril, once a day. **Nasal spray:** initial, 1 spray/nostril once daily, max. 4 sprays/nostril once a day.

ADVERSE REACTIONS:
Mild nasopharyngeal irritation, burning stinging, headache, throat irritation, epistaxis, Cushing's syndrome, cataract; adrenal suppression; glaucoma

IMPLICATIONS:
- Use caution in patients with cataracts, diabetes mellitus, exposure to viral infections, glaucoma, liver cirrhosis, peptic ulcer.
- Do not consume grapefruit juice during oral treatment.
- Reduce dose for hepatic insufficiency.
- May take 3–7 days for full effect.

CEFDINIR—3RD-GENERATION CEPHALOSPORIN ANTIBIOTIC

BRAND NAME:
Omnicef

USES:
Treat susceptible infections due to *Streptococcus pyogenes, S. pneumoniae, Haemophilus influenzae, H. parainfluenzae, Moraxella catarrhalis,* acute maxillary sinusitis, chronic bronchitis; community-acquired pneumonia, otitis media, pharyngitis/tonsillitis, skin infections.

AVAILABILITY:
Suspension: 125 mg/5 mL. **Capsule:** 300 mg

INDICATIONS/ROUTES/DOSAGE:
Children > 6 mos: 7 mg/kg PO q12h for 10 days or 14 mg/kg PO once a day for 10 days; max. 600 mg/day.

Children: <20 kg: 2.5 mL (½ tsp) q12h or 5 mL (1 tsp) q24h. **20–40 lbs:** 5 mL (1 tsp) q12h or 10 mL (2 tsp) q24h. **41–60 lbs:** 7.5 mL (1½ tsp) q12h or 15 mL (3 tsp) q24h. **61–80 lbs:** 10 mL (2 tsp) q12h or 20 mL (4 tsp) q24h. **81–85 lbs:** 12 mL (2½ tsp) q12h or 24 mL (5 tsp) q24h.

Adults: 300 mg PO q12h or 600 mg PO once a day for 10 days.

ADVERSE REACTIONS:
Diarrhea, nausea, oral and vaginal candidiasis, headache

IMPLICATIONS:
- May take with or without food.
- Take antacids 2 hours before or after taking medication.
- Take for full length of treatment.

- Suspension can be stored at room temperature, discard after 10 days.
- Adjust dose in renal impairment.

CEFPROZIL—2ND-GENERATION CEPHALOSPORIN ANTIBIOTIC

BRAND NAME:
Cefzil

USES:
Treat susceptible infections due to *Streptococcus pneumoniae, S. pyogenes, Staphylococcus aureus, Haemophilus influenzae, Moraxella catarrhalis,* acute or chronic bronchitis, secondary bacterial infection, acute sinusitis; otitis media, pharyngitis/tonsillitis, skin infections.

AVAILABILITY:
Oral suspension: 125 mg/5 mL, 250 mg/5 mL. **Tablets:** 250 mg, 500 mg

INDICATIONS/ROUTES/DOSAGE:
Acute sinusitis: **Children 6 mos–12 yrs:** 7.5–15 mg/kg PO q12h for 10 days. **Adults:** 250–500 mg PO q12h for 10 days.

Otitis media: **Children 6 mos–12 yrs:** 15 mg/kg PO q12h for 10 days (max 1 g/day).

Bronchitis: **Adult:** 500 mg PO q12h for 10 days.

Pharyngitis/tonsillitis: **Children 2–12 yrs:** 7.5 mg/kg PO q12h for 10 days. **Adults:** 500 mg PO q24h for 10 days.

Skin infections: **Children 2–12 yrs:** 20 mg/kg PO q24h for 10 days. **Adults:** 250 mg–500 mg PO q12–24h for 10 days.

ADVERSE REACTIONS:
Diarrhea, nausea, vomiting; diaper rash, oral and vaginal candidiasis, dizziness, elevation of liver enzymes, severe hypersensitivity reactions

IMPLICATIONS:
- Refrigerate suspension, discard after 14 days.
- May take with or without food.
- Adjust dose for renal impairment.

CEFTRIAXONE—3RD-GENERATION CEPHALOSPORIN ANTIBIOTIC

BRAND NAME:
Rocephin

USES:

Treat susceptible infections due to gram-negative bacilli, *Haemophilus influenzae, Escherichia coli, Proteus mirabilis, Klebsiella, Enterobacter, Salmonella, Shigella, Neisseria, Serratia;* gram-positive organisms, *Streptococcus pneumoniae, S. pyrogenes, Staphylococcus aureus,* serious lower respiratory tract, urinary tract, gonorrhea, meningitis, septicemia, bone, joint infections.

AVAILABILITY:

Powder for injection: 500 mg, 1 g, 2 g, 10 g

INDICATIONS/ROUTES/DOSAGE:

Children: 50–75 mg/kg/day divided q12h; adult 1–2 g daily. Max 2 g q12h.

Uncomplicated gonorrhea: **adults:** 250 mg IM as a single dose.

Meningitis: **Children, adult:** 100 mg/kg/day IM divided q12h. Max 4 g/day.

ADVERSE REACTIONS:

Nausea, vomiting, diarrhea, anorexia, hypersensitivity, nephrotoxicity

IMPLICATIONS:

- Assess sensitivity to penicillin and other cephalosporins (10% cross over).
- Watch for adverse reactions.

CEFUROXIME SODIUM, AXETIL—2ND-GENERATION CEPHALOSPORIN ANTIBIOTICS

BRAND NAME:

Kefurox, Zinacef, Cefuroxime Axetil, Ceftin

USES:

Treat susceptible infections due to Group B streptococci, pneumococci, staphylococci, *Haemophilus influenzae, Escherichia coli, Enterobacter, Klebsiella,* bone and joint infection, gonorrhea, lower respiratory tract infections, meningitis, preoperative prophylaxis, septicemia, urinary tract infections.

AVAILABILITY:

Suspension: 125 mg/5 mL, 250 mg/5 mL. **Tablet:** 250 mg, 500 mg. **Infusion:** 1.5 g/50 mL, 750 mg/50 mL. **Injection:** 1.5 g, 7.5 g, 750 mg

INDICATIONS/ROUTES/DOSAGE:

Pharyngitis/tonsillitis: **Tablets:** 125 mg PO bid for 10 days. **Children 3 mos–12 yrs:** 30 mg/kg/day PO in 2 divided doses for 10 days. Max 500 mg/day.

Impetigo, otitis media, Sinusitis: **Children 3 mos–12 yrs:** 30 mg/kg/day PO in 2 divided doses for 10 days. Max 1 g/day. **Tablets:** 250 mg PO bid for 10 days.

Susceptible infections: **Neonates:** 20–100 mg/kg/day IV in divided doses q12h. **Children ≥ 3 mos:** 50–100 mg/kg/day IV/IM divided q6–8h.

Bone and joint infections: **Children ≥ 3 mos:** 150 mg/kg/day IV/IM divided q8h.

Meningitis: **Children ≥ 3 mos:** 200–240 mg/kg/day IV/IM divided q6–8h. Max 9 g/day.

Bronchitis: **Adults:** 250 or 500 mg PO bid for 10 days.

Gonorrhea: **Adults:** 1 g PO as a single dose; 1.5 g IM as a single dose with 1.5 g probenecid PO.

Gonococcal infections: **Adults:** 750 mg IV/IM q8h.

Pharyngitis/tonsillitis/sinusitis: **Adults:** 250 mg PO bid for 10 days.

Skin infections: **Adults:** 250–500 mg PO bid for 10 days.

Urinary tract infections: **Adults:** 125mg or 250 mg PO bid for 7–10 days.

ADVERSE REACTIONS:
Local reactions at IV/IM site; diarrhea, abdominal cramping, nausea, oral and vaginal candidiasis

IMPLICATIONS:
- Adjust dose for renal impairment.
- Take antibiotic for full length of treatment.

CEPHALEXIN HYDROCHLORIDE—1ST-GENERATION CEPHALOSPORIN ANTIBIOTIC

BRAND NAME:
Keftab, Keflex, Biocef

USES:
Treat infections of respiratory tract, GI tract, skin, soft tissue, bone, joints, and otitis media caused by *Escherichia coli* and other coliform bacteria, Group A beta-hemolytic streptococci, *Klebsiella* species, *Proteus mirabilis, Streptococcus pneumoniae,* and staphylococci.

AVAILABILITY:
Cephalexin hydrochloride: **Tablets:** 500 mg. *Cephalexin monohydrate:* **Oral suspension:** 125 mg/5 mL, 250 mg/5 mL. **Tablets:** 250 mg, 500 mg, 1 g. **Capsules:** 250 mg, 500 mg

INDICATIONS/ROUTES/DOSAGE:
Children: 25–50 mg/kg/day PO in 2 to 4 equally divided doses. **Adults:** 250 mg–1 g PO q6h or 500 mg q12h. Max 4 g daily. Dose can be doubled in severe infections.

ADVERSE REACTIONS:
Dizziness, headache, confusion, fatigue, hallucinations, nausea, vomiting, diarrhea, pseudomembranous colitis, oral candidiasis, vaginitis, genital pruritus, interstitial nephritis, neutropenia, anemia, thrombocytopenia, arthritis, joint pain, rash, urticaria, hypersensitivity reactions

IMPLICATIONS:
- Take with food or milk.
- There is a possibility of cross-sensitivity with penicillin and other beta-lactam antibiotics.
- Adjust dose for renal impairment.
- Avoid using with aminoglycosides, increases risk of nephrotoxicity.

CETIRIZINE-ANTIHISTAMINE

BRAND NAME:
Zyrtec

USES:
Rhinitis, allergic symptoms

AVAILABILITY:
Syrup: 5 mg/5 mL. **Tablets:** 5 mg, 10 mg

INDICATIONS/ROUTES/DOSAGE:
Child 2–6 yrs: 2.5 mg daily may increase to 5 mg daily or 2.5 mg bid.

Child > 6 yrs, adult: 5–10 mg daily.

ADVERSE REACTIONS:
Thickening of bronchial secretions, dry mouth, headache, drowsiness

IMPLICATIONS:
- Avoid driving if drowsiness occurs, use sunscreen when in sunlight.

CHLORPHENIRAMINE-ANTIHISTAMINE

BRAND NAME:
Pedia Care, Chlor-Trimeton

USES:
Treat rhinitis, allergy symptoms.

AVAILABILITY:
Syrup: 1 mg/5 mL, 2 mg/5 mL, 2.5 mg/5 mL. **Tablets:** 4 mg, 8 mg, 12 mg. **Tablets, chewable:** 2 mg. **Time-released:** 8 mg, 12 mg

INDICATIONS/ROUTES/DOSAGE:
Child 2–5 yrs: 1 mg q4–6h not to exceed 4 mg/day. Time-released not recommended for child < 6 yrs. **Child 6–12 yrs:** 2 mg q4–6h not to exceed 12 mg/day; time-released 8 mg at bedtime or daily. **Child > 12 yrs, adult:** 2–4 mg tid–qid not to exceed 24 mg/day. **Time-released:** 8–12 mg bid–tid not to exceed 24 mg/day.

ADVERSE REACTIONS:
Dizziness, drowsiness, fatigue, anxiety, dry mouth, nose, urinary retention, increased CNS depression with alcohol, tricyclics, hypnotics, opiates

IMPLICATIONS:
- Do not crush, chew or break sustained-release forms.
- Avoid driving if drowsiness occurs.
- No alcohol.
- Notify provider of difficulty voiding.

CIPROFLOXACIN HYDROCHLORIDE— FLUOROQUINOLONE ANTIINFECTIVE

BRAND NAME:
Cipro

USES:
Treat conjunctival keratitis, keratoconjunctivitis, corneal ulcers, blepharitis, dacryocystitis, blepharoconjunctivitis.

AVAILABILITY:
Ophthalmic: 0.03%

INDICATIONS/ROUTES/DOSAGE:
Conjunctivitis: 1–2 drops q2h for 2 days, then q4h next 5 days.

Corneal ulcer: 2 drops q15min for 6h, then 2 drops q30min remainder first day; 2 drops q1h second day; then q4h days 3–14.

ADVERSE REACTIONS:
Ophthalmic: sensitization may contraindicate later systemic use of ciprofloxacin

IMPLICATIONS:
- Tilt patient's head back, put drops in conjunctival sac.
- Do not use ophthalmic solution as injection.

CLARITHROMYCIN—MACROLIDE ANTIBIOTIC

BRAND NAME:
Biaxin, Biaxin XL

USES:
Treat bronchitis, otitis media, acute maxillary sinusitis, pharyngitis, tonsillitis, pneumonia, skin infections.

AVAILABILITY:
Suspension: 125/5 mL, 250/5 mL. **Tablets:** 250 mg, 500 mg. **Tablets, extended-release:** 500 mg

INDICATIONS/ROUTES/DOSAGES:
Acute otitis media: **Children:** 15 mg/kg/day in 2 divided doses for 10 days.

Respiratory/skin infections: **Children:** 15 mg/kg/day in 2 divided doses for 7–14 days. **Usual adult dose:** 250–500 mg q12h for 7–14 days. **Extended release:** Two 500-mg tablets daily for 7–14 days

ADVERSE REACTIONS:
Antibiotic-associated colitis (severe abdominal pain, fever, watery diarrhea), superinfection, hepatotoxicity, thrombocytopenia

IMPLICATIONS:
- Monitor bowel activity and stool consistency.
- For minor GI effects take with food.
- Doses should be evenly spaced.
- Take with 8 oz water.

CLINDAMYCIN—ANTIBIOTIC

BRAND NAME:
Cleocin

USES:
Treat infections from staphylococci, streptococci, Rickettsia, *Pneumocystis carinii* pneumonia

AVAILABILITY:
Oral solution: 75 mg/mL. **Capsules:** 75 mg, 150 mg, 300 mg

INDICATIONS/ROUTES/DOSAGE:
Children < 1 mo: 15–20 mg/kg/day divided q6–8h. **Children > 1 mo:** 8–25 mg/kg/day divided q6–8h. **Adult:** 150–450 mg q6h. Max 1.8 g/day.

ADVERSE REACTIONS:
Nausea, vomiting, diarrhea, pseudomembranous colitis (severe diarrhea), urinary frequency, vaginitis

IMPLICATIONS:
- Take with full glass of water.
- Give with food to reduce GI symptoms.
- Antiperistaltic drugs may worsen diarrhea.
- Do not break, crush, or chew capsules.
- Call provider for diarrhea.

CLOMIPRAMINE HYDROCHLORIDE—TRICYCLIC ANTIDEPRESSANT

BRAND NAME:
Anafranil

USES:
Treat obsessive-compulsive disorder manifested as repetitive tasks producing marked distress; unlabeled: mental depression, panic disorder, neurogenic pain, bulimia.

AVAILABILITY:
Capsules: 25 mg, 50 mg, 75 mg

INDICATIONS/ROUTES/DOSAGE:
Children: starting dose of 10 mg/day; increase to 75–100 mg/day **Teens:** starting dose of 10 mg/day increase to 100–200 mg/day.

ADVERSE REACTIONS:
Dry mouth, dizziness, sleepiness, tremors, decreased libido, headache, aggressiveness, high doses may produce cardiovascular effects (severe postural hypotension, dizziness, tachycardia, palpitations, arrhythmias, seizures). Abrupt withdrawal from prolonged therapy may produce headache, malaise, nausea, vomiting

IMPLICATIONS:
- Contraindicated within 14 days of MAO inhibitor ingestion.
- Caution with history of seizures, hyperthyroidism, cardiac/hepatic/renal disease, diabetes mellitus.
- May cause dry mouth, blurred vision, constipation, drowsiness.
- Ability to tolerate postural hypotension, sedative, and anticholinergic effects occurs during early therapy.
- Maximum therapeutic effect occurs in 2–4 weeks.

- Do not abruptly stop medication.
- Avoid tasks that require alertness, motor skills until drug response is established.
- Wear sunscreen to prevent photosensitivity.

CO-TRIMOXAZOLE SULFAMETHOXAZOLE—TRIMETHOPRIM ANTIINFECTIVE

BRAND NAME:
Bactrim, Septra

USES:
Treat acute/complicated and recurrent urinary tract infections, shigella, enteritis, otitis media, traveler's diarrhea, enteritis, *Pneumocystis carinii* pneumonia.

AVAILABILITY:
Oral suspension: 40 mg trimethoprim/200 mg, 400 mg sulfamethoxazole/5 mL.
Tablets: 80 mg trimethoprim/400 mg sulfamethoxazole; 160 mg/800 mg

INDICATIONS/ROUTES/DOSAGE:
Urinary tract infection caused by **Escherichia coli, Klebsiella, Proteus mirabilis, Enterobacter,** *enteritis, acute otitis media:* **Children > 2 mos:** 7.5–8 mg/kg/day divided q12h for 10 days. **Adults:** 160 mg q12h for 7–14 days.

Weight (lb) (kg)		Suspension	Tablets
22	10	1 tsp (5 mL)	$\frac{1}{2}$
44	20	2 tsp (10 mL)	1
66	30	3 tsp (15 mL)	$1\frac{1}{2}$
88	40	4 tsp (20 mL)	2 tablets or 1 DS tablet

Travelers diarrhea, bronchitis: **Adults:** 1 DS tablet q12h × 5 days.

ADVERSE REACTIONS:
Anorexia, nausea, vomiting urticaria, diarrhea, abdominal pain, rash, fever, sore throat, cough, shortness of breath

IMPLICATIONS:
- Take each dose with 1 glass water and increase fluid intake.
- Take for full treatment time as prescribed.
- Do not use in children < 2 months.
- Do not use in patients sensitive to sulfa drugs.

CROTAMITON—SCABICIDE, ANTIPRURITIC

BRAND NAME:
Eurax

USES:
Treat parasitic infestation (scabies), pruritus.

AVAILABILITY:
Topical cream: 10%. **Topical lotion:** 10%

INDICATIONS/ROUTES/DOSAGE:
For itching, apply locally, massaging affected area until medication absorbed.

ADVERSE REACTIONS:
Dermatitis, skin irritation

IMPLICATIONS:
- Patient should wash entire body with soap and water.
- Avoid application to face, eyes, mouth, or mucous membranes; avoid applying to inflamed skin or raw, oozing skin surfaces.
- Remove any crusting and apply a thin layer of cream over entire body from the chin down.
- Apply 2nd coat. Wash medication off 48 hours after second coat applied.
- Repeat treatment in 7–10 days if new lesions develop.

DESMOPRESSIN ACETATE—ENURESIS, INCONTINENCE

BRAND NAME:
DDAVP, Desmospray, Stimate

USES:
Used to treat primary nocturnal enuresis; hemophilia A and von Willebrand's disease, nonnephrogenic diabetes insipidus, temporary polyuria, and polydipsia R/T pituitary trauma.

AVAILABILITY:
Nasal solution: 0.1 mg/mL, 1.5 mg/mL. **Tablets:** 0.1 mg, 0.2 mg. **Injection:** 4 mcg/mL; 15 mcg/mL

INDICATIONS/ROUTES/DOSAGE:
Nocturnal enuresis: **Children ≥ 6 yrs:** 20 mcg intranasally at bedtime initially. May increase to a max of 40 mcg daily **OR** 0.2 mg PO at bedtime initially up to a max 0.6 mg PO.

Hemophilia A and von Willebrand's disease: **Nasal:** 300 mcg of 1.5 mcg/mL solution. **For patients weighing <50 kg:** 150 mcg may be adequate. Dose should be given 2h before surgery.

Nonnephrogenic diabetes insipidus, temporary polyuria and polydipsia R/T pituitary trauma: **Children 3 mos–12 yrs:** 0.05–0.3 mL intranasal daily in 1–2 doses. **12 yrs–adult:** 0.1–0.4 mL intranasal daily IV or 0.5–1 mL in 2 divided doses.

ADVERSE REACTIONS:
Systemic: headache, flushing, lethargy, disorientation, abdominal cramps, nausea, cough. *Intranasal:* nausea, congestion, cramps, headache. *IV/IM:* burning or swelling at injection site.

IMPLICATIONS:
- Teach correct technique for intranasal administration.
- Keep intranasal solution in refrigerator.
- Avoid OTC cough, hay fever products.
- Monitor BP and pulse during infusion.
- Monitor intake and output, weigh daily, and keep a log.
- Use cautiously in patients with coronary artery disease, hypertension, and conditions linked to fluid and electrolyte imbalances, such as cystic fibrosis. These patients are prone to hyponatremia.

DIPHENHYDRAMINE HYDROCHLORIDE— ANTIHISTAMINE, ANTIPRURITIC, ANTITUSSIVE

BRAND NAME:
Benadryl, Nytol, Allerdryl

USES:
Treat allergy symptoms, rhinitis, motion sickness, urticaria.

AVAILABILITY:
Elixir: 125 mg/5 mL. **Syrup:** 12.5 mg/5 mL. **Tablets:** 25 mg, 50 mg. **Tablets, chewable:** 25 mg. **Capsules:** 25 mg, 50 mg

INDICATIONS/ROUTES/DOSAGE:
Children 2–6 yrs: 6.25 mg q4–6h. Max 37.5 mg/day. **6–12 yrs:** 12.5–25 mg q4–6h. Max 150 mg/day. **Children > 12 yrs, adults:** 25–50 mg q4–6h. Max 300 mg/day.

Moderate to severe allergic reaction: **Children:** 5 mg/kg/day divided q6–8h. Max 300 mg/day. **Adults:** 25–50 mg q4h. Max 400 mg/day.

ADVERSE REACTIONS:
Dizziness, drowsiness, dry nose, throat

IMPLICATIONS:
- Avoid tasks that require alertness, motor skills until response to drug is established, avoid alcohol.

ERYTHROMYCIN—ANTIBIOTIC

BRAND NAME:
Erythromycin, EES

USES:
Treat upper and lower respiratory infections such as pneumonia, bronchitis, pharyngitis, otitis media, pertussis, Legionnaires' disease, prophylaxis for rheumatic fever, oral surgery, intestinal and skin infections, gonorrheal pelvic inflammatory infection (if penicillin is contraindicated), Lyme disease (<9 years).

AVAILABILITY:
Tablets: 250 mg, 333 mg, 500 mg. **Tablets, delayed-release:** 333 mg. **Capsules, delayed-release:** 250 mg

Estolate: **Oral suspension:** 125 mg/5 mL, 250 mg/5 mL. **Tablets:** 500 mg. **Capsules:** 250 mg

Ethylsuccinate: **Oral suspension:** 200 mg/5 mL, 400 mg/5 mL. **Tablets:** 400 mg. **Tablets, chewable:** 200 mg

Stearate: **Tablets:** 250 mg, 500 mg

INDICATIONS/ROUTES/DOSAGE:
Base and ethylsuccinate: **Children:** 30–50 mg/kg/day divided q6–8h up to 60–100 mg/kg/day for severe infections for 10 days, not to exceed 2 g/day. **Adults: delayed-release:** 333 mg q8h increase up to 4 g/day.

Ethylsuccinate: **Adults:** 400–800 mg q6–12h.

Estolate: 30–50 mg/kg/day divided q6–12h. Do not exceed 2 g/day. **Adults:** 250–500 mg q6–12h.

Stearate: 30–50 mg/kg/day divided q6h. Do not exceed 2 g/day. **Adults:** 250–500 mg q6–12h.

Pertussis: 40–50 mg/kg/day divided q6h for 14 days.

Prophylaxis for rheumatic fever: 250 mg bid if penicillin allergy.

Chlamydia trachomatis: 50 mg/kg/day divided q6h for 10–14 days.

ADVERSE REACTIONS:
Nausea, vomiting, abdominal pain, diarrhea, rash, anaphylaxis

IMPLICATIONS:
- Avoid milk and acidic beverages 1 hour before or after a dose.
- Take with food or snack to decrease GI upset.
- Do not break or chew tablets or capsules.
- Suspension is stable for 14 days at room temperature.

FERROUS SULFATE—IRON PREPARATION

BRAND NAME:
Feosol, Fer-In-Sol

USES:
Treat iron-deficiency anemia.

AVAILABILITY:
Feosol: **Tablets:** 200 mg (65 mg elemental iron). *Fer-In-Sol:* **Drops:** 75 mg/0.6 mL (15 mg elemental iron/0.6 mL)

INDICATIONS/ROUTES/DOSAGE:
Mild to moderate iron deficiency: 3 mg elemental iron/kg/day in 1–2 divided doses.
Severe iron deficiency: 4–6 mg elemental iron/kg/day in 3 divided doses.

ADVERSE REACTIONS:
Nausea, diarrhea, black stools, constipation, black urine, teeth staining

IMPLICATIONS:
- **Interactions:** antacids, tetracycline will reduce absorption. Vitamin C enhances absorption.
- Give between meals with orange juice; do not give with milk. Give with a straw or brush teeth after giving.
- May cause abdominal discomfort, keep out of the reach of small children.

FEXOFENADINE HYDROCHLORIDE—ANTIHISTAMINE

BRAND NAME:
Allegra

USES:
Treat seasonal allergic rhinitis.

AVAILABILITY:
Tablets: 30 mg, 60 mg, 180 mg. **Capsules:** 60 mg. **Capsules, extended-release:** 180 mg

INDICATIONS/ROUTES/DOSAGE:
Children > 12 yrs: 60 mg bid or 180 mg once daily.

Children 6–11 yrs: 30 mg bid.

ADVERSE REACTIONS:
Dry mouth, nose, headache, fatigue, nausea, vomiting

IMPLICATIONS:
- Avoid tasks that require alertness, motor skills until response to drug is known.
- Avoid alcohol, coffee or tea; may decrease drowsiness.

FLUOXETINE—SELECTIVE SEROTONIN REUPTAKE INHIBITOR, ANTIDEPRESSANT

BRAND NAME:
Prozac, Sarafem (Prozac weekly)

USES:
Treat major depression, obsessive-compulsive disorder (OCD), bulimia nervosa, premenstrual dysphonia disorder (PMDD).

AVAILABILITY:
Oral solution: 20 mg/5 mL. **Tablets:** 10 mg, 20 mg. **Capsules:** 10 mg, 20 mg, 40 mg

INDICATIONS/ROUTES/DOSAGE:
Anxiety disorders: starting dose of 5 mg/day, increase to 15–30 mg/day for children and 10–40 mg/day for teens.

Major depression: starting dose of 5 mg/day increase to 15–40 mg per day for children, 10–60 mg/day for teens.

ADVERSE REACTIONS:
Headache, nervousness, insomnia, drowsiness, anxiety, tremor, dizziness, sedation, poor concentration, abnormal dreams, decreased libido, dry mouth, diarrhea, weight loss

IMPLICATIONS:
- Take with food and milk for GI symptoms.
- Can crush tablet if patient unable to swallow.
- Take at night to decrease oversedation.
- Therapeutic effect may take 1–4 weeks.
- Use sunscreen to prevent photosensitivity.
- Avoid alcohol and other CNS depressants.

- Notify prescriber if pregnant, plan to become pregnant, or are breast-feeding.
- Change position slowly due to orthostatic hypotension.
- Educate parents about FDA concerns of suicide risk in patients on SSRI antidepressants, monitor suicidal risk closely during course of treatment especially in the first 30 days of treatment.

FLUVOXAMINE—SELECTIVE SEROTONIN REUPTAKE INHIBITOR, ANTIDEPRESSANT, ANTIANXIETY

BRAND NAME:
Luvox

USES:
Treat obsessive-compulsive disorder (OCD), major depression, anxiety disorders.

AVAILABILITY:
Tablets: 25 mg, 50 mg, 100 mg

INDICATIONS/ROUTES/DOSAGE:
Starting dose of 25 mg/day, increase to 50–200 mg/day for children and 150–300 mg/day for teens.

ADVERSE REACTIONS:
Headache, drowsiness, dizziness, convulsions, nausea, vomiting, anorexia, constipation, diarrhea, decreased libido, increased effect with St. John's wort. Fatal reactions: MAO inhibitor interactions increase action of propranolol, diazepam, lithium, warfarin, carbamazepine, theophylline

IMPLICATIONS:
- Give with food, milk for GI distress.
- Therapeutic effects may take 2–3 weeks. Use caution when driving.
- Do not use with other CNS depressants alcohol, barbiturates, benzodiazepines, St. John's wort.
- Educate parents about FDA concerns of suicide risk in patients on SSRI antidepressants; monitor suicidal risk closely during course of treatment especially in the first 30 days of treatment.

FOLIC ACID—NUTRITION SUPPLEMENT

BRAND NAME:
Folate, Folvite

USES:
Treat anemia due to folate deficiency, nutritional supplement to prevent neural tube defects.

AVAILABILITY:
Tablets: 0.4 mg, 0.8 mg, 1.0 mg

INDICATIONS/ROUTES/DOSAGE:
Recommended daily intake for children: **6 mos–3 yrs:** 50 mcg (15 mcg/kg/day). **4–6 yrs:** 75 mcg. **7–10 yrs:** 100 mcg. **11–14 yrs:** 150 mcg. **>15 yrs:** 200 mcg.

Dosage: **Infants:** 15 mcg/kg/daily. **Children:** 1 mg/day initial dosage. **Maintenance dose, 1–10 yrs:** 0.1–0.4 mg/day. **Children > 11 yrs, adults:** 1 mg/day initial dose; maintenance dose 0.5 mg/day.

ADVERSE REACTIONS:
Flushing, irritability, difficulty sleeping, malaise, rash, itching, GI upset, hypersensitivity reactions

IMPLICATIONS:
- Take everyday.
- Call provider if adverse reactions.

LACTULOSE—HYPEROSMOTIC LAXATIVE

BRAND NAME:
Constilac, Constulose, Enulose

USES:
Treat constipation.

AVAILABILITY:
Syrup: 10 mg/15 mL. **Packets:** 10 g, 20 g

INDICATIONS/ROUTES/DOSAGE:
Children: 7.5 mL/day after breakfast. **Adults:** 15–30 mL/day up to 60 mL/day.

ADVERSE REACTIONS:
Cramping, flatulence, increased thirst, abdominal discomfort, diarrhea indicates an overdose

IMPLICATIONS:
- Drink water, juice, milk with each dose.
- Evacuation occurs in 24–48 hours of initial dose.
- Patients should also be on a high-fiber diet and exercise to promote defecation.

LEVALBUTEROL—BRONCHODILATOR

BRAND NAME:
Xopenex

USES:
Prevention of bronchospasm due to reversible obstructive airway disease.

AVAILABILITY:
Solution for nebulization: 0.63 mg **OR** 1.25 mg in 3-mL vials (no dilution necessary)

INDICATIONS/ROUTES/DOSAGE:
Children >12 yrs: 0.63–1.25 mg q6–8h (tid), with max of 1.25 mg tid.

ADVERSE REACTIONS:
Tremors, nervousness, headache, throat dryness/irritation, palpitations, chest pain, extrasystole

IMPLICATIONS:
- Monitor rate, depth, rhythm, and type of respiration.
- Increase fluid intake.
- Rinse mouth with water after inhalation.
- Avoid caffeine.

LITHIUM CARBONATE—ANTIMANIC, ANTIDEPRESSANT

BRAND NAME:
Eskalith, Duralith

USES:
Prophylaxis, treatment of acute mania, manic phase of bipolar disorder.

AVAILABILITY:
Syrup: 300 mg/5 mL. **Tablets:** 300 mg. **Tablets, slow-release:** 300 mg, 450 mg. **Capsules:** 150 mg, 300 mg, 600 mg

INDICATIONS/ROUTES/DOSAGE:
Start at 25 mg/kg/day, gradually increase until serum level reaches therapeutic range of 0.9–1.1 mEq/L.

ADVERSE REACTIONS:
Headache, drowsiness, dizziness, anorexia, nausea, vomiting, diarrhea, hypotension, dry mouth. May increase effects of antithyroid medication, iodinate glycerol, potassium iodide. NSAIDS and diuretics may increase concentration, toxicity. May decrease absorption of phenothiazines

IMPLICATIONS:
- Give with meals, milk.
- Limit alcohol, caffeine.

- May cause dry mouth.
- Do not crush, chew, or break extended-release or film-coated tablets.
- Assess serum lithium levels q3–4days during initial phase of therapy, q1–2mos thereafter and weekly if no improvement.
- Monitor for signs of lithium toxicity vomiting, diarrhea, drowsiness, incoordination, hand tremor, muscle twitching, mental confusion, ataxia.

LORATADINE—ANTIHISTAMINE

BRAND NAME:
Claritin

USES:
Treat seasonal rhinitis.

AVAILABILITY:
Syrup: 5 mg/5 mL. **Tablet:** 10 mg

INDICATIONS/ROUTES/DOSAGE:
Children 2–12 yrs: 5 mg daily. **Children >12 yrs, adult:** 10 mg daily.

ADVERSE REACTIONS:
Sedation is more common with larger doses, headache

IMPLICATIONS:
- Use sunscreen (photosensitive).
- Avoid driving if drowsiness occurs.
- Additive CNS effects with alcohol and antidepressants.

MEBENDAZOLE—ANTIHELMINTIC

BRAND NAME:
Vermox

USES:
Treatment of *Enterobiasis vermicularis* (pinworms), *Ascaris lumbricoides* (roundworm), *Trichuris trichiura* (whipworm), and *Ancylostoma duodenale* (common hookworm).

AVAILABILITY:
Tablets, chewable: 100 mg

INDICATIONS/ROUTES/DOSAGE:
Enterobiasis: **Children, adults:** 100 mg PO as a single dose. *Other infestations:* **Children, adults:** 100 mg 2 bid for 3 days.

ADVERSE REACTIONS:
GI transient abdominal pain. Carbamazepine and phenytoin can increase metabolism of mebendazole

IMPLICATIONS:
- Tablets may be chewed, swallowed, or crushed and mixed with food.
- Do not administer to children < 2 years or pregnant and lactating women.
- If patient is not cured in 3 weeks following treatment, retreatment is necessary.
- All family members should be treated at the same time.
- Discuss hygiene, transmission, and reinfection.

MONTELUKAST (ANTIASTHMATIC)

BRAND NAME:
Singulair

USES:
Prophylaxis and chronic treatment of asthma.

AVAILABILITY:
Tablets: 10 mg. **Tablets, chewable:** 4 mg, 5 mg. **Oral granules:** 4 mg

INDICATIONS/ROUTES/DOSAGES:
Children 1–5 yrs: one 4-mg tablet taken in the evening. **6–14 yrs:** one 5-mg chewable tablet taken in the evening. **Children > 14, adults:** 10 mg daily taken in the evening.

ADVERSE EFFECTS:
Headache, abdominal pain, fever, restlessness, irritability

IMPLICATIONS:
- Do not use to reverse bronchospasm as in an acute asthma attack.
- Increase fluid intake.
- Continue other asthma medications while taking this one.
- Chewable table contains phenylalanine.
- Patients sensitive to aspirin should avoid aspirin and nonsteroidal anti-inflammatory drugs (NSAIDS) while on this medication.

NITROFURANTOIN—ANTIBIOTIC

BRAND NAME:
Furadantin, Macrobid, Macrodantin

USES:
Treat urinary tract infections caused by *Escherichia coli, Klebsiella, Pseudomonas, Proteus vulgaris, Staphylococcus aureus, Salmonella, Shigella.*

AVAILABILITY:
Suspension: 25 mg/5 mL. **Tablets:** 50 mg, 100 mg. **Capsules:** 25 mg, 50 mg, 100 mg

INDICATIONS/ROUTES/DOSAGE:
Active infections: **Children 1 mos–3 yrs:** 5–7 mg/kg/day divided qid; 1–3 mg/kg/day for long-term treatment. **Children > 12 yrs, adult:** 50–100 mg qid PO or 50–100 mg at bedtime for long-term treatment.

Chronic suppression: **Children:** 1 mg/kg/day every night. **Adults:** 50–100 mg every night.

ADVERSE REACTIONS:
Dizziness, headache, nausea, vomiting, abdominal pain, diarrhea.

IMPLICATIONS:
- Do not use in infants < 1 mo.
- Take with food or milk.
- Avoid alcohol.
- Drowsiness may occur, do not drive or operate machinery until response to drug is established.
- Do not crush tabs or open capsules.
- May turn urine rust-yellow to brown.

OFLOXACIN—FLUOROQUINOLONE ANTIINFECTIVE

BRAND NAME:
Floxin Optic, Floxin Otic Drops, Ocuflox

USES:
Ophthalmic: Treat bacterial conjunctivitis, corneal ulcers. *Otic:* Treat otitis externa, acute/chronic otitis media.

AVAILABILITY:
Ophthalmic solution: 3 mg/mL. **Otic solution:** 0.3%

INDICATIONS/ROUTES/DOSAGE:
Bacterial conjunctivitis: 1–2 drops q2–4h for 2 days then 4 times/day for 5 days.

Corneal ulcers: **Ophthalmic:** 1–2 drops q30min while awake for 2 days, then q60min while awake for 5–7 days, then 4 times/day. **Otic:** twice daily.

ADVERSE REACTIONS:
Allergic reaction

IMPLICATIONS:
Ophthalmic:
- Tilt patient's head back, place solution in conjunctival sac.
- Do not use ophthalmic solution for injection.

Otic
- Eardrops should be at room temperature.
- Instruct patient to lie down with head turned so affected ear is upright.
- Pull the auricle down and posterior in children, up and posterior in older adolescents and adults.
- Instill toward canal wall.

OMEPRAZOLE—GASTRIC ACID PUMP INHIBITOR

BRAND NAME:
Prilosec

USES:
Short-term treatment (4–8 wks) and maintenance of erosive esophagitis, gastro-esophageal reflux disease (GERD), poorly responsive to other treatments. Unlabeled treatment of *Helicobacter pylori*–associated duodenal ulcer.

AVAILABILITY:
Tablets: 10 mg, 20 mg, 40 mg

INDICATIONS/ROUTES/DOSAGE:
Children > 2 yrs: 20 mg/day < 20 kg 10 mg/day.

ADVERSE REACTIONS:
May increase concentration of oral anticonvulsants diazepam, phenytoin may increase serum glutamic-oxaloacetic transaminase (SGOT), serum glutamic-pyruvic transaminase (SGPT), alanine aminotransferase (ALT)

IMPLICATIONS:
- Report headache to provider.
- Take before meals.
- Swallow capsule whole, do not crush or chew.

PAROXETINE HYDROCHLORIDE—SELECTIVE SEROTONIN REUPTAKE INHIBITOR, ANTIDEPRESSANT, ANTIPANIC, ANTIANXIETY

BRAND NAME:
Paxil, Paxil CR

USES:

Treat major depressive disorder, obsessive-compulsive disorder (OCD), panic and generalized anxiety disorders.

AVAILABILITY:

Oral suspension: 10 mg/kg. **Tablets:** 10 mg, 20 mg, 30 mg, 40 mg. **Tablets, controlled-release (CR):** 12.5 mg, 25 mg, 37.5 mg

INDICATIONS/ROUTES/DOSAGE:

Children, adolescents: initial dose 5–10 mg, titrate up to 20 mg and monitor for side effects. *Paxil CR:* **Children, adolescents:** initial dose 12 mg titrate up to 25 mg.

ADVERSE REACTIONS:

Nausea, headache, nervousness, insomnia, sedation, agitation, fatigue, dry mouth, constipation, diarrhea, decreased libido/sexual dysfunction

IMPLICATIONS:

- Dose changes should occur at 1-wk intervals for both drugs.
- Do not use with MAO inhibitor.
- Use with Cimetidine may increase concentrations.
- Use with phenytoin may decrease concentrations.
- Use with risperidone may increase paroxetine concentration enough to cause extrapyramidal symptoms.
- May cause dry mouth, avoid alcohol.
- Therapeutic effect may occur in 1–4 weeks.
- Do not abruptly discontinue medication.
- Avoid tasks that require alertness or motor skills until response to drug is established.
- Give with food or milk if GI symptoms.
- Educate parents about FDA concerns of suicide risk in patients on SSRI antidepressants, monitor suicidal risk closely during course of treatment especially in the first 30 days of treatment.

PENICILLIN V POTASSIUM—ANTIBIOTIC

BRAND NAME:

Pen VK, V-cillin-K

USES:

Treatment of mild to moderate infections of respiratory tract, skin/skin structures, otitis media, prophylaxis for rheumatic fever, dental procedures.

AVAILABILITY:

Oral solution: 125 mg/5 mL, 250 mg/5 mL. **Tablets:** 125 mg, 250 mg, 500 mg

INDICATIONS/ROUTES/DOSAGE:
Children < 12 yrs: 25–50 mg/kg/day divided q6–8h. Max 3 g/day. **Children >12 yrs, adults:** 125–500 mg q6–8h.

Rheumatic fever prophylaxis: **Children, adults:** 250 mg 2–3 times/day.

ADVERSE REACTIONS:
Hypersensitivity reaction, colitis, fever, rash, pruritus

IMPLICATIONS:
- Question history of drug allergies.
- Continue antibiotic for full treatment.
- Notify provider of rash, sensitivity reaction.

PREDNISOLONE—ANTIINFLAMMATORY

BRAND NAME:
Pediapred, Prelone, Orapred

USES:
Treat reactive airway disease and asthma flare.

AVAILABILITY:
Syrup: 5 mg/5 mL, 15 mg/5 mL. **Tablets:** 5 mg

INDICATIONS/ROUTES/DOSAGE:
1–2 mg/kg/day in divided doses bid usually for 5 days, although longer may be required.

ADVERSE REACTIONS:
Insomnia, heartburn, nervousness, abdominal distention, mood swings, increased sweating and delayed healing. **Long term:** hypocalcemia, hypokalemia, muscle wasting especially the arms and legs, osteoporosis, spontaneous fractures, amenorrhea, cataracts, glaucoma, peptic ulcer disease

IMPLICATIONS:
- Notify health care provider of fever, sore throat, muscle aches, swelling, weight gain.
- Avoid alcohol, caffeine.
- Avoid exposure to chickenpox or measles.

SERTRALINE—SEROTONIN SELECTIVE REUPTAKE INHIBITOR, ANTIDEPRESSANT, ANTIPANIC AGENT

BRAND NAME:
Zoloft

USES:
Treat major depression, obsessive-compulsive disorder (OCD), post-traumatic stress disorder, panic disorder, premenstrual dysphoric disorder.

AVAILABILITY:
Oral liquid: 20 mg/mL. **Tablets:** 25 mg, 50 mg, 100 mg

INDICATIONS/ROUTES/DOSAGE:
Anxiety: **Children:** starting dose of 25 mg/day increase to 50–100 mg/day; 50–200 mg/day for teens.

Major depression: **Children:** starting dose of 25 mg/day increase to 50–150 mg/day; 50–200 mg/day for teens.

ADVERSE REACTIONS:
Headache, nausea, diarrhea, insomnia, drowsiness, fatigue, rash, dry mouth, anxiety, sexual dysfunction

IMPLICATIONS:
- Do not give within 14 days of MAO inhibitor.
- Therapeutic effect may take 2–3 weeks.
- Avoid tasks that require alertness, motor skills until response to drug is established.
- Take with food or milk, avoid alcohol.
- Weigh weekly: appetite may decrease.
- Notify provider if intending to become pregnant, are pregnant, or are breast-feeding.
- Do not use with St. John's wort, Sam-e.
- Avoid CNS depressants.
- Do not stop quickly, need to taper.
- Educate parents about FDA concerns of suicide risk in patients on SSRI anti-depressants, monitor suicidal risk closely during course of treatment especially in the first 30 days of treatment.

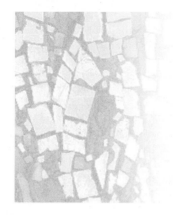

Index

H

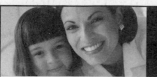
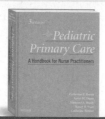
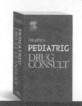
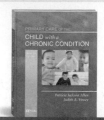

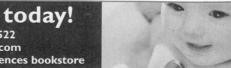